NATURAL REMEDIES

An A–Z Reference Guide to Tried-and-True Cures for Common Complaints

MIM BEIM

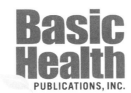

Basic Health
PUBLICATIONS, INC.

The information contained in this book is based upon the research and personal and professional experiences of the author. It is not intended as a substitute for consulting with your physician or other healthcare provider. Any attempt to diagnose and treat an illness should be done under the direction of a healthcare professional.

The publisher does not advocate the use of any particular healthcare protocol but believes the information in this book should be available to the public. The publisher and author are not responsible for any adverse effects or consequences resulting from the use of the suggestions, preparations, or procedures discussed in this book. Should the reader have any questions concerning the appropriateness of any procedures or preparation mentioned, the author and the publisher strongly suggest consulting a professional healthcare advisor.

Basic Health Publications, Inc.

28812 Top of the World Drive

Laguna Beach, CA 92651

949-715-7327 • www.basichealthpub.com

Library of Congress Cataloging-in-Publication Data

Beim, Mim

  Natural remedies : an A/Z reference guide to tried-and-true cures for common complaints / Mim Beim.

    pages cm

  Includes bibliographical references and index.

  ISBN 978-1-59120-369-8

  1. Naturopathy—Popular works. I. Title.

  RZ440.B44   2014

  615.5'35—dc23

                                                              2014009334

In-house Editor: Carol Killman Rosenberg

Typesetting/Book design: Gary A. Rosenberg & Theresa Wiscovitch

Cover design: Mike Stromberg

Printed in the United States of America

10   9   8   7   6   5   4   3   2   1

CONTENTS

Acknowledgments, vii

Introduction, 1

How to Use This Book, 2

A General Guide to Using Remedies, 3

Acne, 6

Anemia, 10

Anorexia Nervosa, 13

Anxiety, 17

Arthritis (Osteoarthritis), 22

Arthritis (Rheumatoid Arthritis), 26

Asthma, 31

Atherosclerosis, 36

Bad Breath (Halitosis), 39

Baldness (Alopecia), 42

Body Odor, 45

Boils, 48

Bronchitis, 51

Bruising, 53

Bulimia, 56

Cancer, 60

Cancer Treatments (dealing with), 67

Candida, 73

Cataracts, 76

Cellulite, 78

Chickenpox, 81

Chilblains (Perniosis), 83

Cholesterol, High, 86

Chronic Fatigue Syndrome, 90

Cold Sores, Herpes, and Shingles, 94

Colds and Flue, 97

Conjunctivitis, 102

Constipation, 104

Cough, 109

Cystitis, 112

Dandruff, 115

Depression, 118

Diabetes (Type 2), 123

Diarrhea, 127

Diverticulitis, 130

Ear Infection, 133

Eczema and Dermatitis, 137

Endometriosis, 141

Erectile Dysfunction (Impotence), 143

Fatigue, 146

Flatulence, 148

Food Sensitivity, Allergy, and Intolerance, 152

Fungal Infections, 160

Gallstones, 163

Glandular Fever (Mononucleosis), 166

Gluten Intolerance (Celiac Disease and
  Gluten Sensitivity), 168

Gout, 172

Gum Disease, 175

Hay Fever, 177

Headaches and Migraines, 181

Hemochromatosis, 187

Hemorrhoids, 189

High Blood Pressure, 192

Infertility, 196

Inflammatory Bowel Disease (IBD), 201

Insomnia, 206

Irritable Bowel Syndrome (IBS), 211

Jet Lag, 214

Kidney Stones, 218

Memory and Concentration, 221

Menopause, 225

Mouth Ulcer, 229

Multiple Sclerosis, 231

Nausea and Vomiting, 234

Osteoporosis, 240

Overweight, 243

Peptic Ulcer, 250

Pregnancy, 253

Premenstrual Syndrome (PMS), 257

Prostate Issues, 261

Psoriasis, 263

Reflux, 266

Rosacea, 268

Sinusitis, 271

Sore Throat, 274

Stress, 276

Thyroid, 284

Varicose Veins, 288

Warts, 290

Appendices

A. Essential Oil Therapeutic Properties, 293

B. Bach Flowers, 295

C. Making Remedies, 301

D. Food Sources, 307

E. Acid-Forming Foods, 316

F. Buteyko Breathing, 319

G. Carrier Oils, 323

Index, 325

About the Author, 343

This book is dedicated to
my friend and esteemed colleague
Jennifer Price.

ACKNOWLEDGMENTS

Jen, to whom *Natural Remedies* is dedicated, has also been an incredible help and support in the writing of this book. Thank you to my agent Benython Oldfield (Zeitgeistmediagroup.com) for finding this book its first home at Rockpool Publishing. Thank you, Carol Killman Rosenberg and the team at Basic Health Publications, for Americanizing this book for U.S. readers. Thank you to Lisa Hanrahan and Paul Dennett from Rockpool Publishing and to editor Jody Lee for pulling the beast together and for the timely recommendations of Rescue Remedy and/or red wine. Megan Drinnan also, thanks for plowing through the millions of words and turning them into a readable form. A gifted aromatherapist and all-around gorgeous gal, Fiona (Fifi l'amour) Carr (Fiona Carr at Bodyworks): a huge thank-you for your fragrant contribution from such a wealth of knowledge. Thanks to Patrick McKeown (buteykoclinic.com), my Buteyko guru and generous teacher. Fellow naturopaths Bek Hall and Lisa Burnham; I appreciate your contributions. Thanks to my wonderful patients and friends for your valuable feedback—Amy Claire Kich, Christine Betros, Sarah Byrne, Katherine Carroll, and Sue Greta. A special thank-you to Dr. Tess van Duuren, a remarkable and compassionate doctor. Friends Linda van Niekerk and Greg Ockenden; I always trust your opinions. I thank my wonderful patients and students from whom I learn all the important bits; and lastly, my husband and friend, Billy Boy.

Introduction

Natural Remedies was initially meant to be a *simple* rewrite of my section of the popular book *Help Yourself: The A–Z of Natural Cures for Common Complaints,* which I coauthored with Jan Castorina way back in the last century. However, *simple* didn't happen, as I had not accounted for three factors. First was the appearance of Doctor Google, who was not born when I wrote the first book, but whose presence is now ubiquitous. Doctor Google has a Doctor Jekyll and Mister Hyde persona. The positive Doctor Google allows a wealth of access to medical information for the average bear that was previously the closely guarded possession of medical professionals. The negative Doctor Google allows a wealth of access to misguided and possibly dangerous health information that the average untrained bear may not realize is incorrect.

Secondly, evidence-based medicine has arisen as the practice *du jour* for both mainstream and naturopathic medicine. Basically it means "show me the research," with large randomized control trials being the preferred research tool. Trouble is, these trials are expensive to undertake, and few have been done on herbal remedies (with a couple of notable exceptions including St. John's wort, which came up very nicely when compared to prescription antidepressants), and it's extremely difficult to "placebo" lifestyle changes such as increasing exercise, avoiding sugar, or practicing belly breathing. The cynic would say that the larger trials are mostly funded by wealthy pharmaceutical companies that are looking to patent and sell medicines, as you can't patent an herb or a vitamin or a breathing technique. But that would be cynical. The remedies and suggestions in this book include some evidence-based natural remedies, treatments that have been used by herbalists and natural therapists for centuries, in addition to the things I have found work well for my patients, evidence based or not.

And finally, the third factor was that I had not realized how much, in the preceding sixteen years since writing the previous book, I had changed as a naturopath and a person. I have had sixteen extra years of treating patients, learning more about the rapidly expanding world of nutrition and natural medicine, and gaining more life experience, the greatest teacher of all.

However, even with these massive changes in the medical landscape, many of the dietary recommendations and remedies I suggested long ago remain the same, which is comforting, as are the basic rules of good health, which also remain the same—namely, eat well, exercise, be happy, and take time to rest and relax.

HOW TO USE THIS BOOK

Natural Remedies is not meant to be read from cover to cover; rather it is intended as a reference guide to help you know what to do if you, or a family member, has a particular ailment. In each entry, "What Is It?" gives an overview of how this condition affects the body. "Symptoms" outlines some of the more common signs you can expect to see with this complaint, and "What Causes It?" talks about the possible causes. Sometimes a complaint relates to the food you eat or environmental factors—or it may come down to a poor choice of parents, namely, the condition is inherited.

"What to Do" is divided into three parts, "Diet," "Remedies," and "Other," and gives practical advice on natural treatment. It is recommended that, rather than attempting every suggestion, you choose just two or three from each part of "What to Do."

If you wish to treat yourself with any natural remedies, it is important that you do not self-diagnose, but rather consult a good practitioner, orthodox or alternative, for a professional diagnosis, and then keep them informed of any therapies you undertake or wish to undertake.

A GENERAL GUIDE
TO USING REMEDIES

REMEDY AVAILABILITY

With a widened acceptance of natural remedies, herbs, and supplements available in many shops in cities and towns together with the Internet you have access to obtaining most remedies, wherever you live. Always choose the highest quality and most trustworthy brand you can afford. There are many health food shops and reputable companies that also sell online that employ naturopaths to advise people. Use them! Ask what herbal or supplement combination is best for you.

If you are keen to make your own remedies, see Appendix C.

WHICH REMEDY TO CHOOSE?

With many of the ailments, there will be many remedies and lifestyle changes recommended, too many for you to consider taking or doing. Ideally, according to naturopathic principles, go with the basics first; that is diet and exercise. If your diet is not supporting your health and there are foods that you are eating that should be eliminated, this would be the best first step before considering supplements.

Very often several vitamins, minerals, and herbs are suggested. Rather than buying each one separately, very often you will be able to buy a formula in tablet or other form that already con-

tains a combination of some of the remedies. Don't worry if it doesn't contain all of the remedies. Wherever possible choose a tablet or remedy that is recommended by naturopaths as this will usually be of higher quality and have the most efficacious combination of remedies.

DOSAGES

You will find that I give few specific dosages. There are several reasons for this. Firstly, some people are incredibly sensitive to medication, natural or pharmaceutical. For example, vitamin C or ascorbic acid: in the very sensitive individual as little as 500 milligrams (mg) will cause diarrhea, whereas another person could take 10 grams (10,000 mg) without any ill effect.

Be guided by the label; however, be aware label dosages are often on the low side as a safety precaution. If, after a reasonable amount of time, you are not noticing any benefits from the remedy, it might be the wrong dosage. The best course of action is to ask a trained practitioner who is aware of the safety and dosage range of the remedy.

A Word on Dosage

Any medicine, natural or not, can have side effects. It is always wise to err on too little than too much, and even wiser to consult a health practitioner who is trained in this area.

How much of a medicinal plant to give varies. Small doses over a long period of time may suit a chronic condition like arthritis or eczema, whereas larger doses given frequently may be more appropriate for an acute condition like a cold.

Herbal medicine has refined the art of dosage, which can be as important as the very herbs that are chosen. Understanding dosage is part of the training of any herbalist. Western herbalists rely on references, including the *British Herbal Pharmacopoeia* and German Commission E for guidance.

Generally, herbal teas are to be taken 3 cups a day, and tinctures from 12 drops to 5 milliliters (mls), 1–3 times daily, diluted in some water. Apply cream, compresses, poultices, and baths as required.

REMEDIES AND CHILDREN

Many of the remedies are safe for children to take. This is signified by the † symbol. All of the dietary recommendations are appropriate for children.

However, if the diet is too restrictive this may have implications for obtaining the correct nutrients necessary for growth. Check with your healthcare practitioner.

Children from as young as six months can take herbs. Children under eight or nine generally will not swallow capsules or tablets, so crushed tablets, powders, or tinctures can be used. Australian herbalist Rob Santich (and father of five children) has a nifty idea for delivery for less palatable remedies. In an old-fashioned ice cube tray, pour some natural jelly into each cube, leaving enough room for the appropriate dose of herb, then set in fridge. Each jelly cube is a dose. Another way would be to put the crushed tablet or powder into a small amount of juice.

What Dosage?

Usually the appropriate dosage for children is mentioned on the label. However, below are the calculations herbalists use when prescribing for children. When in doubt, consult with your practitioner.

SUGGESTED DOSAGES FOR CHILDREN

UNDER TWO YEARS OF AGE — FRIED'S RULE

Age in months divided by 150 equals the fraction of adult's dose to use.

For example, for a twenty-month-old child:

20 divided by 150 = 0.006th of adult dose

If an adult dose is 5 ml, the child's dose equals .03 ml per dose

OVER TWO YEARS OF AGE — AUSBERGER'S RULE

1.5 times weight in kilograms (kg)* is percentage of adult's dose to use.

For example, for a 24 kg child:

1.5 multiplied by 24 equals 36

36 percent of an adult's dose for the child dosage, which equals 1.8 ml per dose.

*Use kilograms, not pounds. 1 kilogram equals approximately 2.2 pounds.

NATURAL REMEDIES DURING PREGNANCY

Although pregnant women have used herbs for hundreds, if not thousands, of years, it is usually recommended to err on the side of caution. However, most common herbal teas and a wide variety of vitamin and mineral supplements are safe. Always seek advice from a healthcare practitioner before you take the herbs.

INTERACTIONS WITH OTHER MEDICATIONS

If you are taking prescription medication, there is the potential that herbs and nutritional supplements may interact with your pharmaceutical medicine. Although this is comparatively rare, it can happen. There is more and more research into this area, and most naturopathic practitioners have access to regularly updated databases that determine what goes with what, and what does not. Drugs like warfarin, with narrow dosage parameters, tend to be the more difficult drugs to team with natural remedies.

REACTIONS

Just because a remedy is natural doesn't mean it is necessarily safe. If you develop a reaction to, or simply do not feel good on any food, herb, supplement, or therapy suggested, stop it immediately. The best thing would be for you to consult your trusted practitioner to check out whether it might be the remedy or something totally unrelated. Sometimes the problem may be that you have done too much too soon. If this is the case, slow down and start with small amounts of one thing before moving on. As with any medicine, there is a chance that it simply does not suit your body. Fortunately, there are many roads to Rome —another remedy or therapy may better suit your needs.

HOW LONG BEFORE I FEEL BETTER?

A general rule of thumb for natural therapies is that it takes up to one month of treatment for every year of an ailment. Usually you will notice improvement within days of starting a remedy or change in diet, but it helps to be patient. My guiding principle in treatment is that natural therapies should not be a hardship. Hopefully the road to healing will be a pleasurable and enlightening experience.

ACNE

WHAT IS IT?

Pimples en masse are called acne or officially *acne vulgaris, vulgar(is)* here meaning common rather than *vulgar*, meaning uncouth. Common or uncouth, acne is better absent than present. Acne occurs when the sebaceous glands, which provide the skin's naturally protective skin oil known as sebum, become blocked. Sebum hardens and oxidizes, forming a blackhead. The familiar pustule associated with acne occurs when debris collects in the sebaceous gland and a small infection occurs creating a pus-filled pimple.

Fifty percent of teenage girls and 75 percent of teenage boys suffer from acne; however, many people suffer this ignominious condition well into their twenties and thirties. Any condition, like acne, that appears on the face can have an impact on your sense of self-esteem, and for the very sensitive, may create secondary psychological problems, including social phobia, anxiety, and depression.

SYMPTOMS

- ☑ Most commonly found on the face, acne can occur on the shoulders, neck, throat, back, and buttocks.
- ☑ Blackheads
- ☑ Whiteheads
- ☑ Papules (small red bumps)
- ☑ Pustules (pus-filled bumps)
- ☑ Redness around the bumps
- ☑ Scarring
- ☑ Cysts

WHAT CAUSES IT?

- ❏ Hormones. Acne often occurs at the time of puberty when hormones surge through young bodies. Hormonal pimples are often blind or cyst-like, lying under the surface, causing the skin to look red and painful. In women, hormonal acne is often located along the jawline and may extend to shoulders, neck, and back. An outbreak prior to the menstrual period is another giveaway of hormonal hijinks. For young men, hormonal acne can be especially bad, covering the entire face, as well as chest, shoulders, and back.

- ❏ Sugar. Bacteria are involved in the pimple process, and bacteria (like the rest of us) just love sugar. Avoid sugar in your diet, and your pimples will disappear. Interestingly, acne has been called skin diabetes and may herald a problem with metabolizing sugar and possible future diabetes. Avoiding sugar is a great start to avoiding a diagnosis of diabetes down the track.

- ❏ Dairy sensitivity. Although chocolate may sometimes cause an outbreak of pimples, by far the most common food culprit, apart from sugar, is dairy.

- ❏ Stress. An outbreak that occurs at or after exams or times of high emotions is most likely stress related.

- ❏ Constipation or a slow bowel transit time allows toxins from the bowel to circulate in the bloodstream and trigger an outbreak on the surface of the skin.

WHAT TO DO

Identifying the cause of the problem will lead to the appropriate treatment. Regardless of the cause, the general rules of skin care still apply, that is, regular cleansing and moisturizing, drinking plenty of water, and eating a healthy diet.

Diet

❏ If dairy products are the cause, it is most likely due to a sensitivity to casein, the protein component of milk rather than lactose (milk sugar), which usually results in tummy problems. The best way to tell if your acne is due to a dairy sensitivity is to avoid all dairy foods for one month, including milk (skim or full cream), cheese, yogurt, cream, butter, chocolate, and any processed food with added milk protein. One month is enough time to witness significant improvement. If this does not occur—happy days—reintroduce dairy into your diet. If dairy has proved to be the problem, either continue to avoid dairy foods completely, or if you are a dairy food fan, reintroduce dairy products gradually, as is it may be a question of quantity. The first dairy product to reintroduce is a good unsweetened probiotic yogurt, half a cup daily. If this seems to be okay, then keep adding dairy foods until the first pimple appears—a sign you've reached your daily limit. The nutritional impact of eliminating or reducing dairy foods is not dire; after all, the majority of people on the planet have not traditionally eaten dairy products. However, if dairy is off the menu, you do need to ensure you are consuming sufficient protein and calcium from dairy-free sources.

❏ Avoid cakes, biscuits, soft drinks, and all processed foods with added sugar.

❏ Water. Skin needs to be hydrated, and water helps to flush toxins away. Drink at least 1.2 liters, preferably 2 liters, of water daily in addition to other fluids such as the herbal teas mentioned below.

❏ Fiber. If your acne coincides with a sluggish bowel, make sure you eat plenty of fiber. Fiber hastens transit time, taking toxins more quickly out of the body, with less time to be reabsorbed. High-fiber foods include nuts, seeds (particularly chia seeds), whole grains, legumes, vegetables, and fruit. If after adjusting your diet to include plenty of fiber and drinking at least 2 liters of water you still suffer from constipation, see page 104.

❏ Unless you eat prodigious amounts of chicken nuggets or other fried food, acne is unlikely to be caused by fat. In fact, the good fats found in nuts, seeds, avocadoes, and olive oil are important for healthy skin and are encouraged.

Remedies

❏ Hormonal imbalances take time to resolve. Be patient. You should notice some improvement in four to six weeks. The herb chaste tree (Vitex agnus-castus) is a lovely hormonal normalizer,

LOCATION, LOCATION, LOCATION

Just where your pimples are located may point to their cause. For instance, pimples on the cheeks are often the sign of a food intolerance such as dairy, whereas cyst-like pimples along the jawline are most likely to be hormonally triggered. Hormonal outbreaks also appear on the chest, back, and shoulders. Small pimples with red surrounds grouped closely together signify a localized infection just under the skin. Removing sugar from your diet will help in addition to taking the blood-purifying herbs that are mentioned below. Pimples on the forehead may be due to stress, or if there are bangs, excess sweating. Pimples on the chin reflect poor digestion or constipation.

perfect for boys, girls, men, and women. Chaste tree alone is excellent; however, in a particularly nasty case, two other herbs to help include nettles and saw palmetto. Two micronutrients that assist in hormone balance include zinc and vitamin B_6. Evening primrose oil contains substances that are anti-inflammatory for the skin and act to regulate hormones. Take at least 4 grams daily.

❏ Blood-purifying herbs. In the tradition of natural medicine, skin is seen as one of the major organs of detoxification alongside the liver, bowels, lungs, and kidneys. Any affliction of the skin, including acne, is a signal that the body needs help with detoxifying. A group of herbs with special affinity for the skin are known as blood purifiers, alteratives, and depuratives and have been used for centuries. These herbs include clover, yellow dock, calendula, burdock, sarsaparilla, dandelion, and echinacea. Usually taken in a combination of two or more, these herbs can be taken in extract, tincture, tablet, or tea form; however, for skin conditions, a water-based tea is preferred. Drink at least 3 cups daily. When cooled, this tisane (infusion) makes a fine toner or spray to apply after cleansing and before applying moisturizer.

❏ Vitamin A and zinc. This vitamin and mineral combination is excellent for the skin. Vitamin A has an important role in the maintenance of healthy epithelial cells, the cells that line the body inside and out. Zinc is used by hundreds of enzymes, including those that regulate hormones and sugar metabolism. Zinc is also important for healing. The two micronutrients are often found together in skin-focused supplements.

❏ If sugar is the culprit, and you have eliminated sugar from your diet (as you must) and you still experience sweet cravings, then take a tablet that contains a combination of zinc, gymnema, and chromium with each meal.

Remedies

❏ Cleanse and moisturize. A common misconception among acne sufferers is that skin should be squeaky clean, the squeakier the better. In fact, the skin actually likes to have a slightly oily protective covering and produces sebum for this purpose. If the outer layers of the skin become dry, more sebum is produced to compensate for this, adding to the pimply problem. Wash the skin with a mild cleanser. If you wish, this cleansing can be followed with a toning wash of a cold tea of the blood-purifying herbs mentioned above. Then use a light, low-allergen moisturizer perhaps containing aloe vera, calendula, or tea tree. The best antipimple program will not work unless you follow a regular routine of cleansing and moisturizing the skin.

❏ Tea tree oil or gel applied directly onto the pimple helps to reduce reddening and further infection. Tea tree oil helps skin regenerate and has antibacterial properties, making it an excellent ingredient in any cleanser, gel, or moisturizer in your acne-treatment program.

❏ A little sunshine and seawater can work miracles.

❏ Don't pick! Beauty therapists suggest you leave squeezing to them rather than attempt this potentially disfiguring procedure yourself. Try a course of facials as a start on clearing the skin, and while you're there ask about basic skin care. This is particularly pertinent to boys and men who may lack skin-care knowledge. Generally, maintaining good personal hygiene is also a great way to prevent breakouts. Picking, scratching, and touching spreads infection and will contribute to scarring. Desist.

❏ From an emotional perspective, acne may represent inner conflicts and disharmony. If you feel this applies to you, speak to a friend or try counseling to help understand and resolve these internal difficulties.

AROMATHERAPY

The following blend will have a calming, soothing, cleansing, and purifying effect on the skin. It can be used in a blend of 20 ml calendula and 10 ml rosehipbase oils—pressed onto a cleansed face in the evening. It can also be mixed into 30 grams of an unscented cream base and used each morning on a cleansed face.

- ❏ 4 drops of lemon-scented tea tree—analgesic, anti-inflammatory, antiseptic, and bactericidal.

- ❏ 5 drops of lavender—has regenerative and soothing effects on irritated or damaged skin, along with being antibacterial.

- ❏ 2 drops of cypress—astringent and an antiseptic.

- ❏ 4 drops of sandalwood—antiseptic, astringent, anti-inflammatory, and antibacterial.

For a deep-cleansing face mask—reduce the number of drops of essential oils by half and add to a paste of green clay. For spot treatment use 2 drops lavender and 1 drop lemon-scented tea tree and use cotton swab to apply directly to the spot(s) in question. Lymphatic drainage facial massage will greatly assist in cleansing/purifying and decongesting the skin.

AT A GLANCE

DIET

- ➡ Dairy foods may be the cause of your pimples so avoid things like milk, cheese, yogurt, cream, butter, chocolate, and processed foods that contain milk protein. Try this for a month to see if there is any improvement.

- ➡ Sugar can be a culprit, and cutting out cakes, cookies, and soft drinks will help to clear up your skin.

- ➡ Water, lots of it, to flush away toxins. Aim to drink 2 liters a day.

- ➡ Include lots of high-fiber foods such as nuts, seeds, whole grains, legumes, fresh fruit, and vegetables.

- ➡ Minimize the bad fat in your diet such as deep-fried and fatty foods, but make sure you have the good fats found in nuts, seeds, avocados, and olive oil. The good fats are beneficial for your skin.

REMEDIES

- ➡ The herb chaste tree works well for hormonal acne. In more severe cases of acne, adding nettles and saw palmetto can help.

- ➡ Take zinc, vitamin B_6, and evening primrose oil supplements to strengthen your skin. Combining vitamin A with zinc is an excellent vitamin and mineral combination for the skin.

- ➡ Acne can be a sign that your body is not detoxifying. Traditional blood-purifying herbs such as clivers, calendula, yellow dock, burdock, sarsaparilla, dandelion, and echinacea come to the rescue—choose three or more to be taken in tablet, extract, or tea.

OTHER

- ➡ Adopt a daily practice of cleansing and moisturizing. Choose gentle low-allergy skin products.

- ➡ Dab a drop of tea tree gel or neat oil onto any spots as they appear.

- ➡ Live near the beach? Splash some seawater onto your face and body, and soak up (a few) rays.

- ➡ Don't pick! Treat yourself to a monthly facial.

ANEMIA

WHAT IS IT?

Are you exhausted? I mean really exhausted. On a scale of 1 to 10, with 10 being jumping-full-of-beans, do your energy levels hover around 2 or 3? It could be iron-deficiency anemia. Iron-deficiency anemia is the most common nutritional deficiency in the world.

SYMPTOMS

☑ Common symptoms of anemia include fatigue, yawning, bruising easily, irritability, poor concentration, muscle weakness, dizziness, spots before the eyes, looking very pale, headaches, palpitations, and increased tendency for infections.

☑ Other signs include a red shiny tongue, brittle nails with longitudinal ridges, pale nail beds, or slightly concave nails (the opposite of normal). Pull down the lower eyelid; many tiny blood vessels live there, so if it is very pale, anemia is a possibility. The signs and symptoms mentioned above all indicate anemia, but the best way to make sure is a blood test arranged by your doctor.

WHAT CAUSES IT?

❏ A diet deficient in iron. Those at special risk include vegetarians and vegans.

❏ Poor absorption of iron. Iron is a tricky mineral to absorb at the best of times; having a condition such as celiac disease or gluten intolerance compounds the issue. Other causes of poor absorption include the removal of the stomach or parts of the small intestine and inflammatory bowel disease. Low stomach acid (hypochlorhydria) where there is insufficient production of hydrochloric acid (stomach juice) decreases iron absorption. People taking antacid medication will have lower levels of hydrochloric acid, which may impact iron absorption. This is not a reason to stop taking your medication, but may explain why your iron levels are low.

❏ Blood loss. Women who experience heavy menstrual periods can lose 100 ml of blood each cycle. This equates to a significant loss of 150 mg iron. To add insult to injury, low iron levels may be the cause of heavy periods. An injury or surgery often incurs blood loss. More insidious causes of blood loss include a slowly bleeding ulcer, hemorrhoids, polyps, and inflammatory bowel disorders.

❏ Various medications as well as tea and coffee may impact iron absorption.

❏ Some health conditions, including low thyroid function and kidney disease, may increase your risk of anemia.

Although the most common cause of anemia is iron deficiency, other forms of anemia include pernicious or megaloblastic anemia—a deficiency of vitamin B_{12}, macrocytic anemia—a deficiency of folic acid (vitamin B_9), and sickle cell anemia—a hereditary disease where red blood cells are abnormally shaped and their ability to carry oxygen is impaired.

WHAT TO DO

If your blood tests show you are anemic, then the best remedy is to take an iron supplement. Once iron levels are in range, you should be able to maintain this by eating iron-rich foods. Your blood tests should reveal a positive change after a month. The following dietary advice will help prevent future recurrence.

Diet

❏ Increase iron-rich food. Choose from both heme and non-heme foods. See list on page 310.

❏ If you prefer to eat less animal food or are a vegetarian or vegan, add some vitamin C–rich foods to your meal to increase absorption of non-heme iron. For example, squeeze some lemon juice over your meal, add raw capsicum or cabbage, or enjoy some vitamin C–rich fruit for dessert, such as kiwi fruit, guava, strawberries, papaya, and any citrus.

❏ The liver is where iron is stored, so it makes sense to eat liver if you are anemic (and are not a vegetarian). The liver is where toxins can be stored also, so if paté, liverwurst, or sautéed liver appeals, please make sure the animal from whose liver you are eating has been raised on an organic farm.

❏ Avoid drinking tea or coffee half an hour before and one hour after meals. One study showed that drinking a cup of coffee after a meal containing minced meat reduced the absorption of iron by 39 percent, whereas drinking a cup of tea reduced absorption by a whopping 64 percent.

❏ All is not lost; a glass or two of alcohol consumed during a meal increases iron absorption.

❏ Uncooked bran is another iron antagonist due to the phytates in the whole grain. However, phytates are inactivated by heat, so cooked cereals, such as oatmeal, are safe.

❏ Bitter foods improve functioning of all digestive organs, including production of hydrochloric acid from the stomach. Bitter foods include grapefruit, rocket, olives, and

BEHIND THE SCENES

The mineral iron is vital for human life. Iron forms part of hemoglobin, the molecule that imparts the red color to red blood cells and is responsible for capturing oxygen inhaled by the lungs. Hemoglobin attached to red blood cells transports and delivers this oxygen around the body via the bloodstream. No iron; no hemoglobin. No hemoglobin; no oxygen. No oxygen; no life. Despite the importance of iron, the entire body stores are a measly 2–4 grams, less than a teaspoon. Good things do indeed come in small packages. However, unlike some other nutrients, iron is stored in the body and does not need to be eaten daily. As well, the body is pretty stingy with its iron, constantly recycling it, and unless there is blood loss via menstruation or other bleeding, iron levels can be maintained by eating a regular diet.

Dietary iron occurs in two forms: "heme" iron and "non-heme" iron. Heme iron is found in animal food and while absorption is not fabulous (e.g., only 25 percent of the iron present in red meat is actually absorbed), it is superior to non-heme iron found in the vegetable kingdom (only 2 to 15 percent of iron found in plant food is absorbed). Factors that decrease non-heme iron absorption include vegetable protein (which makes things worse for the iron-deficient vegetarian), oxalic acid (found in rhubarb and tea), phytic acid (found in grains but deactivated when cooked), zinc and calcium (so don't take these supplements at the same time as an iron supplement or an iron-rich meal), and tea and coffee. Factors that increase non-heme iron absorption include animal protein (sorry, vegetarians), vitamin C (squeeze lemon juice over your vegetables), and copper (cook in copper pans).

radicchio. Or enjoy a bitter aperitif or digestive aid before or after your meal.

Iron-rich foods include:

- Dried fruit—prunes, raisins, dates
- Dark, leafy, green vegetables—kale, bok choy, gai lan (also known as Chinese broccoli or Chinese kale), spinach
- Legumes—lentils, kidney beans, soybeans
- Seaweed
- Parsley
- Blackstrap molasses
- Mollusks—oysters, clams, mussels
- Red meat—beef, lamb, venison, goat
- Egg yolks

Remedies

NOTE: Before you go charging into the pharmacy and scoff down iron tablets, it is best to be certain you are iron-deficient as taking iron in excess to your body's needs is not a good thing. Excess iron in the body will oxidize, or rust. Additionally, iron and zinc compete in the body, so excess iron may create a zinc deficiency. Although iron deficiency is relatively common, it is worth bearing in mind that the opposite can happen too. This is most often caused by hereditary conditions such as hemochromatosis (see page 187). Treatment for this condition is giving blood. Interestingly, the symptoms of excess iron can mirror those of a deficiency, feeling tired, and so forth—another reason to obtain a correct diagnosis before taking an iron supplement.

- Iron supplementation is the obvious and most effective course of treatment. As is the case with many minerals, iron needs to be chelated (pronounced *kee-late-ed*) or bound with something in order to cross the barrier from belly to blood. There are several forms of chelated iron available, including ferrous (ferrous means iron) fumarate, ferrous amino acid chelate, ferrous succinate, ferrous carbonate, and ferrous sulfate. The latter sometimes leads to tummy upsets or constipation. If this happens to you, don't persevere. Just swap to another form. If possible, take your iron supplement in divided doses, as absorption will be increased this way.

- Liquid iron preparations made from herbs and fruits may offer less iron per dose, but are generally well tolerated and a good choice if you are "topping up" your iron levels, say after a heavy menstrual period.

- Iron-rich herbs include nettles, yellow dock, and dandelion root.

- Traditional Chinese medicine has a group of herbal remedies that help to "build" the blood, working as general tonics and assisting the body to absorb more of this precious metal. These are nice to take if anemia is "your thing." By this I mean you have a history of low iron levels. These herbs include codonopsis, rehmannia, and dong quai. Withania, from the Ayurvedic *materia medica,* has similar properties.

- Vitamin C assists in iron absorption. Take 500 mg with your iron supplement, if it doesn't already contain vitamin C. Take vitamin C with meals containing non-heme iron-rich foods—for example, leafy greens.

Other

- If you are low in iron, there is absolutely nothing else you can do for this condition except eat food that contains iron and/or take an iron supplement.

Diet

⟹ Eat iron-rich foods including red meat, liver, green leafy vegetables, dried fruit, and legumes.

⟹ Squeeze lemon juice over your green vegetables to increase iron absorption.

⟹ Avoid drinking tea or coffee half an hour before and one hour after meals, as they interfere with iron absorption.

Remedies

⟹ If iron levels are low, take an iron supplement. Some forms of iron can cause constipation or tummy upsets. If this is the case, don't give up on iron; choose another form.

⟹ Herbs that contain iron and help with iron absorption include nettles, yellow dock, dandelion root, codonopsis, rehmannia, dong quai, and withania.

Other

If you are low in iron, you are low in iron. There is nothing else to be done except eat foods containing iron, take an iron supplement, or worst-case scenario, have a blood transfusion.

ANOREXIA NERVOSA

WHAT IS IT?

Any eating disorder, including anorexia nervosa, is special torment for both the sufferer and those who care for them. Anyone who has not experienced this condition has difficulty understanding how completely it takes over your life and happiness. The word "anorexia" simply means loss of appetite. Anorexia nervosa, however, is a more complicated disorder, as much psychological as physical. Anorexia nervosa is a condition marked by reduced eating and loss of body weight, and can lead to tragic consequences. It usually begins in adolescence, but can start as early as nine years old, and sadly, can continue throughout life. Only about 5 percent of anorexia nervosa cases are male, although this figure is on the increase; men tend to develop exercise addiction, particularly weight training, rather than anorexia. A high percentage of patients are from the middle- and upper-socioeconomic stratum and are typically high-academic achievers.

SYMPTOMS

☑ Marked weight loss. At least 15 percent below normal weight is a warning sign.

☑ Disordered body image (dysmorphia). Anorexics believe they are fat or overweight even when they are clearly not.

☑ Preoccupied with food and further weight loss.

☑ Loss of menstrual cycle in women

☑ May also exercise to excess. Continuing to exercise even when injured.

☑ May also be taking diuretics (increase urination), laxatives, and appetite suppressants

☑ Will often feel uncomfortable eating with others

☑ Have a fear of gaining weight or becoming fat

☑ Fine long hair on arms and legs and face

Complications of long-term anorexia may include:

- ❑ Osteoporosis. Below a certain percentage of body fat, women cease menstruating and estrogen levels drop. Estrogen increases bone strength, and so women who have been anorexic for some time will have a greater risk of osteoporosis.

- ❑ For those who have recovered from eating disorders such as bulimia and anorexia nervosa, a large percentage will suffer from ongoing gastrointestinal problems such as irritable bowel syndrome and constipation.

- ❑ Thyroid hormone problems.

- ❑ The mortality rate of anorexia is 10 percent. This is a scary disease, particularly for family members who can do little but watch and worry.

WHAT CAUSES IT?

There is rarely just one simple "cause." However, the following may offer some explanation for anorexia nervosa:

- ❑ Addiction. Anorexia nervosa is similar to, and may coincide with, other sorts of addictive behavior such as overeating, bulimia, laxative abuse, overexercising, and alcohol and drug abuse. Many anorexics are children of parents who have addictions such as alcohol and gambling.

- ❑ Control. Many adolescents feel that they have little or no control over their life and are not yet old enough to have gained perspective. Issues such as divorce or separation of parents, moving to a new home, changing school, jealousy of a sibling, illness or death of a parent, are all hard for an adolescent or child to understand and beyond their control. However, the amount of food you eat is something you can control.

- ❑ Loss. Anorexia nervosa can be viewed as an insidious form of suicide. The anorexic may be expressing a wish to "not be here" or fade away, after suffering a traumatic loss. The death of a parent, particularly the father, can have this effect. However, the loss through death or separation of parent, sibling, pet, or close friend may trigger the onset of anorexia.

- ❑ Fear of fat. A study that confirmed our society's morbid fear of fat revealed that most of the school-aged children surveyed would prefer to be confined to a wheelchair for life than be fat. Many anorexics feel disgust when looking at their body. Even when pathetically thin, they can still pull a loose piece of skin as proof that they need to lose even more weight.

- ❑ Sexuality. One theory is that anorexia nervosa may be an expression of fear of maturing sexually, of what it might mean. Anorexia often first appears around puberty, and it will often delay or stop the monthly cycle of hormones. After all, the poor little body is struggling to survive, let alone breed! The change from girl to woman is difficult, and society has many unreasonable expectations of what "the sexual woman" should be and look like.

- ❑ At puberty, a girl's role in the family changes, and it has been suggested that some parents might subconsciously fear the signs of their child becoming a woman and want to keep her a "little girl" for as long as possible. Children are pretty good at picking up on their parents' subconscious thoughts.

- ❑ Another theory suggests that the onset of sexual maturity may cause immense subconscious anxiety in any child who has experienced sexual abuse.

- ❑ An overwrought sense of perfectionism may be driving anorexia nervosa.

WHAT TO DO

Successful treatment depends entirely on whether you have had enough of being obsessed with food and weight. If the anorexia nervosa has become life-threatening, then medical intervention including intravenous feeding will be necessary. Many people fighting anorexia substitute this addiction with another, such as bulimia or exercise addiction. If this happens, don't judge yourself harshly. As long as you are committed to addressing the underlying issues, and learn to like then love yourself, all will be well. For the family and friends of an anorexic person, you have a tricky path to tread. Show concern but try not to be overbearing or controlling. It's almost impossible to say the right words, but your love and acceptance for them no matter what is vitally important.

Diet

❏ Do *not* under any circumstances fall prey to any diet, however "healthy" it is meant to be. It will only serve to bring your focus back on food. After you feel you are "over" the anorexia, you might wish to explore such diets, although my advice to all my patients who have suffered from eating disorders in the past is *don't.* The same goes for "diet" foods and drinks; buying them is buying into the same psychological game that you are trying to get out of.

❏ Eat whatever *you* want. At the beginning of your recovery, it doesn't matter if it is bean sprouts or hamburgers. Any food is better than no food. Many anorexics tend to eat from only a small range of "safe" foods—generally low fat or vegetarian. It is best not to try to force the issue. In your own good time, new foods can be introduced gradually, one at a time.

❏ The body needs at least 50 grams of protein every day. In anorexia nervosa, the body starts to "eat" its own muscle because not enough protein is provided in the diet. Because high-protein foods often contain fat, many anorexics avoid protein foods. Some low-fat protein options include fish, egg white, tofu, legumes, cottage and ricotta cheese, low-fat yogurt, and protein powders.

Remedies

❏ By definition, an anorexic is deficient in all nutrients. At the very least a multivitamin and mineral supplement should be taken every day.

❏ Absorption of nutrients is often poor, so the best supplement is in a liquid form.

❏ Serotonin, the happy neurotransmitter, is often low in this condition. St. John's wort is an excellent choice of herb to help counteract this.

❏ Several studies show that anorexics' zinc levels are especially low. A liquid zinc supplement is the best option, to be taken daily in conjunction with a multivitamin.

❏ Bach flower remedies that may help include crab apple for "dislike of self," mimulus for fear (of putting on weight), walnut for "times of change," rock water for those who are hard taskmasters of themselves, and white chestnut for incessant thoughts (usually about food and body image).

Other

❏ There is no one correct way to treat anorexia nervosa. Each patient must find his or her own unique path.

❏ Anorexia nervosa is very much a psychological condition. Good counseling is a must. It may help if the therapist is familiar with eating disorders; however, an "eating disorder therapist" may not always be the best choice, as this condition is a symptom of inner troubles. Choose a therapist you feel comfortable with and who "gets" you.

- Accept the fact you probably have a disordered image of yourself. This can be helpful as you start to fill in some curves. Accepting you are not the best judge of what is a healthy or attractive body takes some heat off.

- The images of women perpetuated in the media show that society's standards can be devastating to those who are anything but stick-thin. But consider this: Grace, a slim woman who recently returned from India, spoke of her visit to a village where she met a woman with a very full, rounded figure, whom she described as luscious, and extremely feminine. Grace said, "Standing next to this woman, I felt malnourished, somehow not quite ripe."

- Meditation. Anorexics often find it hard to "switch off" and relax. Learning meditation will help.

- Gentle exercise is all that is needed. Not punishing gym schedules or marathons.

- The inner child. During the 1980s, the concept of the "inner child" was popular. The idea being that at some level, we all react to situations initially as a small child, and then our "adult" self intervenes with the appropriate reaction to the situation. This can be taken a step further if you ask yourself how would you feel if your small child (imagined if you don't have children) was suffering in this way because anorexia nervosa is a condition of great suffering. Would you be stern with her or him? Or would you be kind and gentle? The anorexic is usually their own harshest critic, so imagining "another" may allow some sorely needed compassion in.

AT A GLANCE

Diet

- Any food is good food initially.

- Trying to increase protein is important, as the body will use muscle if there are not enough calories. Lean meats, legumes, egg whites, and ricotta cheese are all low fat and low in calories, so are more likely to be acceptable. Protein powders are a good compromise until "real" food is eaten with joy.

Remedies

- A good quality multivitamin will go some way to replacing nutrients not consumed in food. A liquid supplement is a good choice for quicker absorption.

- St. John's wort helps to increase serotonin, the happy neurotransmitter, which is often low in anorexia nervosa.

Other

- Each person must find their own way. The journey to healing will most likely give you skills and a depth of life knowledge that will serve you later in life.

- A good therapist is invaluable. Be prepared to kiss a few frogs before you find your therapeutic match.

- Learn to meditate. Find respite from that busy, judgmental mind.

ANXIETY

WHAT IS IT?

Anxiety is a marriage between body and mind—an unhappy marriage. The more anxious you feel, the more symptoms your body exhibits—from diarrhea and nausea to heart-gripping chest pains. Defined as a "generalized pervasive fear," some people suffer anxiety all day, every day. Feeling frightened all the time is not a pleasant way to live. An anxiety or panic attack is an episode of anxiety ramped up dramatically. The pain and fear are so extreme, panic attacks are often mistaken for a heart attack.

SYMPTOMS

- ☑ Muscle tension, especially around neck, shoulders, and jaw
- ☑ Insomnia
- ☑ Trembling or shaking
- ☑ Sweating, particularly on the palms and underarms
- ☑ Feelings of apprehension, helplessness, and uncertainty
- ☑ Palpitations
- ☑ Chest pain
- ☑ Hyperventilation, fast and shallow breathing
- ☑ Dizziness
- ☑ Diarrhea
- ☑ Nausea
- ☑ Reflux

WHAT CAUSES IT?

- ❏ The biochemical driver of anxiety is the hormone adrenaline (and its silent but equally dangerous sidekick cortisol, also created by the adrenal glands), which is released in response to a stressor. A stressor may be the irrational demands of a sociopathic business partner, but it can also be something as blame free as an infection, sports injury, or even an excessively hot day.

- ❏ Genes may be a factor. Anxious parents beget anxious children, though whether this is nature or nurture is open for debate.

- ❏ Lack of sleep, whether due to insomnia, shift work, or burning the candle at both ends, can cause or exacerbate anxiety.

- ❏ Anxiety may be a symptom of a physical or mental illness or a side effect of medication.

- ❏ Trauma such as a car accident or death of a close friend or family member can instigate anxiety.

- ❏ Hormonal changes, including premenstrual tension and menopause, may increase feelings of anxiety.

- ❏ Anxiety is often experienced by people who are withdrawing from drugs of addiction, including alcohol and tobacco.

WHAT TO DO

While it is important to manage the diet to reduce stimulants and settle the nerves, the most important thing of all is to find a way for your body to calm down. When your physical body is calm, your mind will follow suit. This is fundamental to helping ease the awfulness that is anxiety. Find a technique or method that works for you, and faithfully and consistently use it.

Diet

❏ Avoid eating when emotionally upset. During a bout of anxiety, the body is placed on red alert, with stress hormones flooding the body. Nonessential activities such as digesting food are shut down. Obviously, if the anxiety continues for days you need to eat. In this case, it is best to eat small meals that are easy on the stomach, such as soup, smoothies, or even baby food.

❏ Avoid caffeine. Caffeine increases the release of adrenaline, the hormone already in abundance.

❏ Reduce or avoid alcohol. Alcohol may quell the feelings of anxiety momentarily, but the next day you will be back on the roller coaster. A glass or two may be fine, more will make things worse.

❏ Sweet foods will help at the time of an anxiety attack, particularly a hot cup of herbal tea with honey. Stop the presses! This is the *only* time this particular little black duck is ever likely to recommend something sweet. However, of course, there is a proviso. For the longer-term anxiety sufferer, the highs and lows of blood sugar levels only serve to make matters worse as they impact on the stress hormones adrenaline and cortisol, so reserve sweet drinks for crisis times only.

❏ Choose calming foods like brown rice, oatmeal, miso soup, stews, casseroles, soups, and baked root vegetables, including carrots, parsnips, turnips, and potatoes.

Remedies

❏ Herbs are outstanding for anxiety. They really take the edge off feelings of panic and fear. Choose from the following: kava, zizyphus, withania, passionflower, magnolia, valerian, hops, and lemon balm. If you are prone to anxiety, take herbs daily as a preventative measure. Although not sedative (except valerian), these herbs will help you to sleep, as anxiety is most likely the cause of your sleeplessness.

❏ The two minerals calcium and magnesium are a good combination. Calcium is vital for steady nerves and magnesium helps take the tension out of anxious muscles. Take a tablet or powder combining both twice daily.

❏ If your muscles take the brunt of your anxiety, more magnesium is required. Take 400 mg 2 to 3 times daily.

❏ The tissue salts mag. phos. (magnesium phosphate) and kali. phos. (potassium phosphate) taken together are another excellent combination, particularly for children, the extra-sensitive, and the easily startled. These can be taken every hour or so in anxious times.

❏ The Bach Flower Rescue Remedy is tailor-made for quelling anxiety. Whenever you feel anxious, add a few drops to water and sip frequently. A couple of drops of Rescue Remedy can also be taken under the tongue, or rub a drop onto your temple or inside wrist where it will be absorbed by the body. If you suffer from anxiety attacks, have a vial of Rescue Remedy handy at all times.

Other

Anxiety is a state of mind and body, but begins in the mind. The best and sometimes only way to quiet the anxious mind is to access it via the body. Choose one or more techniques suggested below. If you are a constant worrywart, try to incorporate the method daily so that your body slowly adjusts to a steadier, less anxious state. After a prolonged period of anxiety the adrenal glands become "trigger happy," releasing stress hormones well after the initial cause of anxiety has disappeared. For instance, becoming excessively and inappropriately stressed or anxious at loud noises or the annoying habits of your partner or children.

The Buddhist phrase "The body is slower than the mind" fits this scenario. Although your mind has consciously processed the stressful situation, your body is still reacting.

❏ Next time you feel anxious, notice where you are breathing. Most likely it is the upper chest. Hyperventilation (overbreathing) associated with anxiety and panic attacks leads to a decrease in blood carbon dioxide levels, which in turn causes symptoms of dizziness, fatigue, and nervousness. Decreased carbon dioxide levels in turn trigger the release of stress hormones. This is known as a vicious circle. The old-fashioned remedy was to breathe into a paper bag, thereby restoring carbon dioxide levels. The following Buteyko breathing technique (see Appendix F), known as "small breath holds," has the same effect and will help restore calm any time you feel anxious, and may prevent a panic attack. Sit comfortably, both feet flat on the ground. Take a small breath in, followed by a small breath out. Close your mouth throughout the exercise. Hold your nose for a slow count of five. Release your nose, breathing normally for a count of ten, repeat holding your nose for five and relax for ten. Continue for four to five minutes or until calm is restored. The slight increase in carbon dioxide activates the relaxing parasympathetic nervous system, good for calm and peace.

❏ Belly (abdominal or diaphragmatic) breathing is the way we were meant to breathe. Over time, and especially for anxious people, breathing travels further up the body. Look at a dog or young child at rest—belly breathing. Initially, lie on your bed with a pillow beneath your head and knees. Place your hands palm down on your lower belly. Breathe in through your nose, counting slowly to three or four. Feel your tummy rise with the breath. Breathe out just as slowly, allowing the belly to drop. Once you feel comfortable with this, progress to doing this seated, and eventually you will feel so calm, you can belly breathe as you fight your boss for a pay rise.

❏ Aerobic exercise, swimming, walking, jogging, and cycling all increase serotonin levels, which is good medicine for anxiety. Incorporate exercise three or more times in your week.

❏ Yoga will calm your body and mind. In the height of anxiety it is impossible to settle down enough to learn the techniques. When you are in a calmer state of mind, make it a priority to sign up for a course. The following yoga pose can be used immediately. A classic yoga posture (asana) known as child's pose (Balasana) is excellent for anxiety. Kneeling on the floor, sit on your heels, knees as wide as your hips. Exhale and lay your tummy over your thighs. Rest your head on the floor or pillow. Keep arms alongside each leg, palms facing up. Relax in this pose for at least three minutes daily.

❏ For the long-term sufferer of anxiety, counseling or therapy might be useful to explore and treat deeper causes.

❏ Massage. The healing power of another's caring touch may be what is required. Now is not the time for a bruising deep-tissue muscle massage; seek out a gentle-souled massage therapist with the hands of an angel.

❏ Hypnotherapy has a good track record for treating those who suffer from anxiety.

❏ Avoid movies, books, and computer games that increase adrenaline; even the nightly news may cause you to feel stressed.

❏ "Music hath charms to soothe the savage breast, to soften rocks, or bend a knotted oak" (William Congreve). Think Bach, not Black Sabbath.

- Add a few drops of lavender or chamomile oil to an oil diffuser to create a calm atmosphere.

- Affirmations can be an effective way to calm your thoughts when anxious. Repeat to yourself, "all is well" or "calm", over and over until the feelings of anxiety subside.

- Cocooning. Feelings of vulnerability and being exposed often accompany anxiety. Cocooning is a technique that creates a sense of much needed peace. Gently place both hands either side of your face. Close eyes and mouth. Rest both little and ring fingers on eye lids, forefingers closing ears, thumbs cradling your jaw. Be still and breathe.

- Avoid Facebook, Twitter, and social media for a while. You don't need to be connected all the time.

- Think like Spock. Fans of *Star Trek* (mea culpa) know that Spock and all Vulcans (a race of pointy-eared humanoids) control their emotions by the mastery of logic. Logic is the enemy of anxiety. Anxiety sufferers are prone to "catastrophizing"—that is, exaggerating a small worry into a catastrophe. Cognitive behavioral therapy (CBT), a school of psychology, suggests one question one's thoughts in a logical and pragmatic way. For example, if running late triggers anxiety, question what is the worst that can happen if you are late? Will you die? Will the sky fall in? Or could you ring the babysitter, and ask them to stay an extra half hour?

CHILDREN

Anxiety is certainly not the domain of adults. In fact, the luxury of perspective that only years on the planet can give you, and the ability to reason that most of your fears are unreasonable, are outside the intellectual ambit of the young child. Your child may have an anxious personality or could be picking up on a stressful situation in the home or school environment. No matter the origin of the anxiety, the following are some gentle remedies that will calm and soothe.

- The tissue salts kali. phos. and mag. phos. combined have the nervous system–calming and muscle-relaxing action of potassium and magnesium. The tablets can be crushed and added to a child's drink or food. A tablet every hour if necessary, or as a precaution twice daily.

- The Bach flower Rock Rose is recommended for terror and is especially for night terrors. Rock Rose is one of the Bach flowers in Rescue Remedy, the all-purpose emergency remedy. If Rock Rose doesn't work try some Rescue Remedy. The flower essences can be applied on the skin or in bathwater as well as the traditional method of drops under the tongue or in water. Use a couple of drops before bed or whenever necessary.

- Depending on the age of your child, teaching them the breathing techniques mentioned above (small breath holds and belly breathing) will bring almost instant relief. It will serve them well if you can practice this daily, so they can soothe themselves whenever they start to feel anxious.

- Herbs for anxiety include chamomile, zizyphus, lemon balm, withania, skullcap, and passionflower.

AROMATHERAPY

- ❑ 3 drops of frankincense—has the ability to slow and deepen the breath; is carminative, tonic, sedative.

- ❑ 1 drop of ylang ylang—sedative, soothing, and calming.

- ❑ 2 drops of vetiver—calming, soothing, and sedating, and a great tonic to the nervous system.

- ❑ 4 drops of Roman chamomile—soothing, balancing, calming, restorative, and sedating.

5 drops of bergamot—revitalizing, uplifting, regulating, balancing, and antidepressant.

Once mixed together, 6 to 8 drops of this wonderfully relaxing, soothing, and uplifting blend can be used in a room vaporizer. Mixed with jojoba oil it can be worn as a personal perfume. Placed in a 30 ml spray bottle with an essential oil dispersant and rose or orange blossom water—it can be used as a personal spray. Mixed into 125 grams Epsom salts makes for the most relaxing bath. Use as a massage blend in sweet almond oil for a full-body, relaxing Swedish massage.

AT A GLANCE

Diet

- ➦ Eat sparingly if you are very anxious. Eat small meals regularly to maintain blood sugar levels.

- ➦ Stick to easy-to-digest foods such as soups, stews, even baby food.

- ➦ Avoid caffeine as it stimulates adrenaline, the hormone you are trying to diminish.

Remedies

- ➦ Herbs are very effective for reducing anxiety. Choose from kava, passionflower, magnolia, valerian, and lemon balm.

- ➦ Take magnesium for your tense muscles.

- ➦ Rescue Remedy, the most famous of the Bach flowers, works wonders. Take a few drops under your tongue whenever you are feeling anxious.

Other

Calming your body is the quickest and most effective way to calm an anxious mind.

- ➦ Small breath holds. Keeping your mouth closed throughout the exercise, hold your nose closed for five seconds, release and breath gently for another ten seconds. Repeat for four minutes.

- ➦ Have a gentle massage, preferably followed by a warm bath.

- ➦ Repeat calming affirmations to yourself to override the anxious thoughts. Simple phrases such as "all will be well" or "calm" can be very settling.

ARTHRITIS (OSTEOARTHRITIS)

WHAT IS IT?

By the time we reach fifty years of age, most of us will have some degree of osteoarthritis (OA). Almost all vertebrates are affected, even whales and fish. Osteoarthritis is not a newfangled disease; skeletons of mummified Egyptians and bones of brontosauruses have revealed arthritic changes. The only vertebrates who don't get OA are bats and sloths; the one activity they share is hanging upside down.

Also known as degenerative joint disease, OA occurs when the cartilage between bones degenerates. Cartilage acts like a shock absorber between the bones of joints such as the hip, knee, fingers, and between the vertebrae of the back. As cartilage degenerates, the poor old bones will grind against each other causing inflammation and pain. As a protective measure, the bones get a little thicker and can even form bony spurs. This, in turn, inhibits mobility and makes movement painful.

SYMPTOMS

☑ Pain and/or tenderness

☑ Stiffness, particularly in the morning or after not moving for a while

☑ Limitation of movement around the affected joint

☑ Swelling

☑ Crepitus, a creaking, grinding sound and feeling

☑ Deformed joints

WHAT CAUSES IT?

❏ Overuse or injury to a joint can lead to arthritis later in life, including football and other sports injuries or work-related injuries, especially from heavy lifting, repetitive factory line work, or an accident. Operations on the joints may also prove to be trouble spots in the years to come.

❏ Genetics plays a role. If your parents or grandparents were troubled with arthritis, your chances of OA are higher. The time to be treating OA is at the first sign of pain or stiffness or if arthritic changes have been revealed in an x-ray. Treat before more damage occurs.

❏ Overweight. Carrying extra pounds places extra strain on the joints.

❏ Joint misalignment. A genetically out of place joint will lead to extra wear-and-tear and ultimately OA will set in.

❏ Naturopathically, arthritis is considered as an "acidic" condition. This slight change in the body chemistry toward acidity can be caused by the food we eat, injury, or stress. The acidity here does not refer to heartburn, but a slight change in the tissue pH. Treating the acidity is treating the arthritis.

❏ Food allergy is rarely a cause, but it may make matters worse. The three main culprits are wheat, oranges, and tomatoes.

WHAT TO DO

Osteoarthritis takes its time to appear, and treatment may also take a while. The success of treatment depends on the extent of the arthritis. If your joints are very damaged (this can be seen by x-ray), recovery will be slower than if damage is minimal. If degeneration is severe, full movement of the afflicted joint will probably not be restored, but hopefully there will be less pain and further damage may be halted.

Aspirin and NSAIDs (nonsteroidal anti-inflammatory drugs) such as ibuprofen and indomethacin are often given to ease the pain of arthritis. Although NSAIDs may be effective in easing pain, be wary of them for three reasons. Firstly, they commonly cause gastritis and stomach ulcers. Secondly, a little known side effect of gastritis and stomach ulcers is that the lining of the gut becomes more permeable or "leaky," increasing the risk of food allergy. And thirdly, NSAIDs accelerate cartilage destruction. This means that by buying temporary relief with these drugs now, you are paying for future damage. Natural pain relievers are mentioned below.

Diet

❏ Eat fish three to four times a week. The omega-3 fatty acid EPA, found in fish, is anti-inflammatory. Fish containing the most EPA are the fattier fish such as sardines, salmon, mullet, halibut, trout, and tuna.

❏ Increase fluid intake. Cartilage consists of about 80 percent water, which partially explains its cushioning effect. Even without OA, after a day in the vertical position we are all about 1 cm shorter than when we left our beds in the morning. This is because the cartilage has been squashed. Drink plenty of fluids, at least 1.5 liters each day.

❏ Reduce acid-forming foods and increase alkaline-forming foods (see Appendix E). Acid-forming foods include grains, meat, sugar, egg yolk, and prawns/shrimp. Alkalizing foods include all fruits and vegetables. Vegetable juices are very alkalizing as they concentrate all the alkalizing minerals. Drink one to two juices daily: one carrot and ginger juice and one "green" juice made from all the green vegeta-bles you can find, such as beetroot tops, celery, parsley, and cucumber.

❏ Best foods for OA include alfalfa, wheatgrass, watercress, potatoes, yams, celery, parsley, garlic, comfrey, endive, pineapple, bananas, cherries, blackcurrants, mango, kiwi fruit, and blueberries.

❏ Avoid allergens. The tomato is often cited as a culprit in arthritis. The theory about the evils of tomatoes was first promulgated in the 1950s by an American, Norman F. Childers. Tomatoes, and to a lesser extent, other members of the Solanaceae family (potatoes, eggplants, chilies, capsicum), contain alkaloids that promote degeneration of the joint and inhibit repair of mucopolysaccharides. To test whether tomatoes are a problem for you, avoid them completely for one month, then have a tomato feast, with tomatoes at every meal for one day. If your joints are more painful a couple of days after this, chances are tomatoes should be avoided forever. However, if you feel no different by avoiding tomatoes then they are not a problem for you. The same goes for other potential allergens such as oranges and wheat. If the shoe does not fit, do not wear it.

❏ Turmeric, the yellow spice, has anti-inflammatory properties. If you already love curry, further your passion.

❏ Mucopolysaccharides. Substances known as mucopolysaccharides (also known as proteoglycans and glucosamines) increase the elasticity and bounce in cartilage. With encroaching osteoarthritis, mucopolysaccharides in the body can diminish by half. Foods containing mucopolysaccharides include tripe, oysters, oats, Irish moss, mussels, calf trachea, aloe, and okra. If these foods don't rock your culinary boat, don't fret; supplements of the active ingredient are available.

Remedies

❑ Fish oil contains the omega-3 fatty acid EPA, and is brilliant for relieving the symptoms of arthritis. However, you need to take a fair bit—that is, 10 to 15 ml daily to make an impact. Given the quantity you need to consume, liquid supplementation makes better economic and psychological sense. After all, that's 10 to 15 capsules you need to swallow.

❑ Glucosamine is the other supplement that is really very good for osteoarthritis. Most often prescribed as glucosamine sulfate, it reduces pain and increases movement, as importantly (and in contrast to pharmaceutical medication), glucosamine helps to regrow cartilage, which is damaged in osteoarthritis. You need to take around 2 grams daily. Chondroitin (a similar compound to glucosamine) is often used alongside glucosamine.

❑ Curcumin is a constituent of turmeric, the yellow curry spice. It has many properties including being antioxidant and anti-inflammatory.

❑ Herbal remedies can be transformative for the OA sufferer. However, every case of OA is unique, and the herb one person finds helpful may not help another's pain. The following herbs are worth trying alone or in combination. Take the highest recommended dose for one month before making a judgment: ginger, turmeric, boswellia, devil's claw, celery seed, guaiacum, and willow bark

❑ An oldie and still a goodie, this traditional Vermont remedy will help digestion and hopefully your arthritis. Drink one teaspoon of apple cider vinegar and one teaspoon of honey in hot water first thing each morning before breakfast.

❑ Silica and nat. phos.—these tissue salts are recommended for OA. Silica (and its big brother mineral silicon) is known as a calcium reorganizer, helping to break down bony spurs at the same time as strengthening cartilage. Nat. phos. is the alkalizing tissue salt.

❑ Take a decent multivitamin tablet daily to provide the micronutrients necessary for the synthesis of collagen and maintenance of normal cartilage. These micronutrients include zinc; manganese; copper; boron; bioflavonoids; and vitamins A, E, and B_6.

❑ Methionine is a sulfur-containing amino acid that maintains cartilage structures. It is both analgesic (pain relieving) and anti-inflammatory. Studies have shown when administered in the form S-adenosylmethionine (SAM), this amino acid has been found to be superior to ibuprofen in the treatment of OA.

Other

❑ Hot compresses and poultices give immediate relief, so use when pain is bad. Choose from one or more of the following:

• Ginger compresses. Grate a cupful of ginger on the middle of a kitchen wipe or muslin cloth, and fold to form a ginger parcel. Place in a shallow bowl and pour half a cup of boiling water over it. Leave until bearably hot. Gently squeeze and place on the painful area, then wrap the body part and ginger parcel with plastic wrap. Wrap again in a towel, then relax and keep warm for twenty minutes before unpeeling.

• Castor oil packs. Heat 3 to 4 tablespoons castor oil, then saturate a face cloth with the oil. Place cloth on the affected area and cover with plastic wrap, then a towel, and rest for thirty minutes. Stick a hot water bottle or heating pad over the towel.

• Heat paraffin wax until it is above blood temperature, but not hot enough to burn—up to about 51°C (about 124°F). Dip the affected joint in the warm wax, remove when cooled. The wax may be reused. This treatment is especially good for OA of the hands.

❏ Acupuncture can be excellent for OA, particularly to relieve the inflammation and improve mobility.

❏ The subtle bodywork methods such as Alexander Technique and Feldenkrais will improve mobility and teach how to move your body with less strain.

❏ Copper is necessary for collagen and cartilage synthesis. Try rubbing a little copper chelate ointment onto the affected joints. This may be why copper bracelets help some people.

❏ Exercise is vital for the person living with OA. However, any jolting exercise such as jogging should be avoided. It's a case of use it or lose it. It is necessary to move every joint as the cartilage degenerates if there is no movement in a particular joint. Swimming or aquarobics are particularly recommended as being joint-friendly exercises.

❏ It is worth spending the money on a pair of good, cushioned shoes to prevent jarring the joints.

❏ Rest. When we are active, the cartilage compresses and a good rest in the horizontal position allows it to rehydrate.

❏ Act like a bat (or sloth). Try out an inversion table.

❏ If you are carrying excess pounds, get rid of them, as extra weight increases stress on the joints.

AROMATHERAPY

❏ 2 drops of sweet fennel—anti-inflammatory, detoxifying, stimulating.

❏ 3 drops of ginger—analgesic, antispasmodic, warming.

❏ 4 drops of German chamomile—excellent for inflamed joints, analgesic, anti-inflammatory.

❏ 6 drops of lavender spike—analgesic, decongestant.

To use this wonderful soothing blend, mix with 15 ml sweet almond oil and 5 ml St. John's wort and apply to the affected area as needed. You can also sprinkle 8 drops of the essential oil blend into some cool water and use as a cool compress as needed. Use 10 drops of the essential oil blend in 125 grams Epsom salts in a hand, foot, or full-body bath.

Diet

- Eat fish three to four times a week, especially the high omega-3 fatty acid kinds such as salmon, mackerel, halibut, trout, and tuna.

- Foods that improve OA include alfalfa, wheatgrass, watercress, potatoes, yams, celery, parsley, garlic, comfrey, pineapple, bananas, cherries, blueberries, cherries, and apples.

- Reduce acid-forming foods in the diet, such as red meat, sugar, and grains, and increase alkalizing foods—fruit and vegetables.

Remedies

- Fish oil is fab. You need to take at least 10 ml daily to see the benefits.

- Glucosamine has anti-inflammatory properties and helps to maintain the synovial membrane that protects the joint.

- Herbs to try include boswellia, turmeric, white willow, ginger, and celery seed.

Other

- Gentle exercise that improves muscle strength and preserves mobility, such as swimming or tai chi.

- Acupuncture can be very effective, particularly for pain.

- Lose weight if you are carrying extra pounds; excess weight only makes arthritis worse.

ARTHRITIS (RHEUMATOID ARTHRITIS)

WHAT IS IT?

Rheumatoid arthritis (RA) is the vicious cousin of osteoarthritis (OA). Rheumatoid arthritis is often excruciatingly painful, more so than OA. Whereas OA goes about its business of slow degeneration over time, making a first appearance after fifty years of age, RA attacks often with no prior warning, afflicting a younger cohort aged between twenty to forty years. Rheumatoid arthritis (RA) is an autoimmune condition that affects synovial membranes. Synovial membranes surround free-moving joints, secreting fluid that lubricates joints for easy movement. In RA, the synovial membrane becomes inflamed and damaged, and the lubricating fluid dries up, causing the joint to become tender and swollen. Diagnosis is usually made via a blood test looking for rheumatoid factor and other inflammatory markers.

SYMPTOMS

- ☑ Painful joints. Joints typically involved in RA are those of the fingers, toes, wrists, ankles, and knees. Joints are often affected bilaterally, that is, both sides of the body.

- ☑ Swollen joints

- ☑ The joints can look red and feel hot to touch.

- ☑ Nodules may appear on the affected joints.

- ☑ As the disease progresses, deformities develop in the joint, causing more pain and restricting movement.

- ☑ Fatigue

WHAT CAUSES IT?

❑ No one really knows why autoimmune conditions such as RA occur. We do know that there is a strong hereditary component, but why it affects one person and not another is still open to speculation. Any great shock, whether physical, such as a car accident, or emotional, such as divorce or death of a loved one, can unhinge the immune system, unlocking the genetic potential of a disease such as RA.

❑ Stress is nearly always a factor in the onset of RA.

❑ Septic loci theory. This is an old medical diagnosis not often mentioned, but every now and then it perfectly explains a mysterious condition such as RA. A septic loci is a small, encapsulated ball of infection, usually bacterial in nature. This tiny mass is not large enough to cause the full spectrum of fever and chills normally associated with a systemic infection, but it is enough to wear down the immune system and cause mysterious low-grade symptoms, including fatigue, headaches, eczema, and sinusitis. In fact, it's not the infection per se, but the by-products of the bacteria within the capsule that are being released into the bloodstream, that offends the immune system. Common pockets for septic loci include tooth abscesses, sinuses, tonsils, appendix, and within the bowel. These septic loci can brood for years. In the event of a shock or stress, the immune system will suddenly take umbrage, and instead of brooding, create havoc, attacking its own tissue.

❑ Studies have shown that RA has been linked to prior infections involving a variety of possible suspects, including Epstein-Barr, rubella, and a species of amoeba.

❑ Food allergy, if not a cause, may trigger and aggravate RA. Possible allergens include wheat, corn, dairy, and the Solanaceae (tomato) family.

❑ RA is more common among smokers.

WHAT TO DO

The goal is to stop pain and inflammation and halt the condition before it causes permanent damage to the affected joints. Many sufferers take cortisone and immune-suppressing drugs to deal with the pain. As always, don't stop your prescribed medication without first talking to your doctor. Natural remedies can generally be taken in conjunction with your prescribed medication, but check with your practitioner first.

Diet

❑ Go vegan. Rheumatoid arthritis is a full-on disease that requires a full-on therapeutic diet. If you are willing, try a vegan diet, as profound results can be obtained on this admittedly rather restrictive regime. If, after eight weeks, there are no significant improvements, discontinue, unless you are enjoying other benefits. A vegan diet forgoes all animal products—dairy, fish, eggs, animal flesh—all are verboten. Protein is obtained from legumes, nuts, and seeds.

AUTOIMMUNE CONDITIONS

There are over eighty autoimmune conditions, including multiple sclerosis (MS), ulcerative colitis, and RA. An autoimmune condition is one where the immune system, whose role ordinarily is to defend against outside invaders such as bacteria and viruses, all of a sudden gets its knickers in a knot and begins to destroy the body's own tissue or "self ." Specifically, the myelin sheath surrounding nerves in the case of MS, the bowel wall in the case of ulcerative colitis, and synovial membranes in the case of RA.

If veganism does not appeal or has not proved helpful, pursue some of the following suggestions. You may notice the dietary recommendations below are the same as for OA. Both conditions involve inflammation, so similar dietary changes will help.

❑ Eat fish three to four times a week. The omega-3 fatty acid EPA, found in fish, is anti-inflammatory. Fish containing the most EPA are the fattier fish, such as sardines, salmon, mullet, halibut, trout, and tuna.

❑ Reduce acid-forming foods and increase alkaline-forming foods (see Appendix E). Acid-forming foods include grains, meat, sugar, egg yolk, and prawns/shrimp. Alkalizing foods include all fruits and vegetables. Vegetable juices are very alkalizing as they concentrate all the alkalizing minerals. Drink one to two juices daily: one carrot and ginger juice, and one "green" juice made from all the green vegetables you can find, such as beetroot tops, celery, parsley, and cucumber.

❑ Good foods for RA include alfalfa, wheatgrass, watercress, potatoes, yams, celery, parsley, garlic, comfrey, endive, pineapple, bananas, cherries, blackcurrants, mango, kiwi fruit, and blueberries.

❑ Avoid allergens. The tomato is often cited as a culprit in arthritis. The theory about the evils of tomatoes was first promulgated in the 1950s by American Norman F. Childers. Tomatoes, and to a lesser extent, other members of the Solanaceae family (potatoes, eggplants, chilies, capsicum), contain alkaloids that promote degeneration of the joint and inhibit repair of mucopolysaccharides. To test whether tomatoes are a problem for you, avoid them completely for one month, then have a tomato fest, with tomatoes at every meal for one day. If your joints are more painful a couple of days after this, chances are tomatoes should be avoided forever. However, if you feel no different by avoiding tomatoes then they are not a problem for you. The same goes for other potential allergens such as oranges and wheat. If the shoe does not fit, do not wear it.

❑ Turmeric, the yellow spice, has anti-inflammatory properties. If you already love curry, further your passion.

❑ Various natural substances have the potential to stop the expression of certain genes. If you want to prevent a gene's expression of RA (along with many other conditions), then taking these elements in food or supplements may prove helpful. These substances include the micronutrients zinc and folic acid and phytochemicals such as EGCG (found in green tea), curcumin (found in turmeric), resveratrol (found in red grapes, peanuts, pistachios, pomegranates, berries), and oligomeric proanthocyanidin complexes (OPCs) from grapeseed and maritime pine bark.

Remedies

You will notice that some of the remedies are the same for OA and RA, particularly in the case when you are reducing inflammation. With RA, remedies differ when they are addressing the underlying cause—that is, a defective immune response.

❑ Fish oil contains the omega-3 fatty acid EPA, and is brilliant for relieving the symptoms of arthritis. However, you need to take a fair bit—that is, 10 to15 ml daily to make an impact. Given the quantity you need to consume, liquid supplementation makes better economic and psychological sense. After all, that's ten to fifteen capsules you need to swallow.

❑ Herbal remedies that dampen inflammation are useful for RA as well as for OA. These include ginger, willow bark, devil's claw, boswellia, and turmeric.

❏ There are several herbs that are useful in any autoimmune condition, including RA. Rather than stimulating the immune response, which you want to avoid when the immune system is hyped up anyway, these herbs help to modulate and regulate immune function. They include echinacea, Rehmannia, bupluerum, cat's claw, and astragalus. A bevy of some of these herbs together with one or more of the anti-inflammatory herbs mentioned above will work well for RA.

❏ If you suspect a "septic loci" may have been the originating trigger, investigate. Go to the dentist and get that bad tooth pulled if necessary. Even if you can't locate the loci, it is worthwhile taking some of the antibiotic herbs, many of which are also immune modulating. The herbs include: echinacea, calendula, cat's claw, baptisia, and goldenseal. Top these up with a dollop of vitamin C, say 500 mg three times daily.

❏ Selenium, vitamin D, vitamin E, zinc, manganese, potassium, copper, and boron have proved to be helpful in the treatment of RA. Take a combination daily.

❏ Vitamin B_9 (folic acid), in the dosage found in a good B complex, can help protect against side effects of immune-suppressing medications that are sometimes prescribed for RA.

❏ Homoeopathic remedies, which may offer relief, include apis, bryonia, and ledum.

Other

❏ Hot compresses and poultices give immediate relief, so use when pain is bad. Choose from one or more of the following:

• Ginger compresses. Grate a cupful of ginger on the middle of a kitchen wipe or muslin cloth, and fold to form a ginger parcel. Place in a shallow bowl and pour half a cup of boiling water over it. Leave until bearably hot. Gently squeeze and place on the painful area, then wrap the body part and ginger parcel with plastic wrap. Wrap again in a towel, then relax and keep warm for twenty minutes before unpeeling.

• Castor oil packs. Heat three to four tablespoons castor oil, then saturate a face cloth with the oil. Place cloth on the affected area and cover with plastic wrap then a towel and rest for thirty minutes. Place a hot water bottle or heating pad over the towel.

• Heat paraffin wax until it is above blood temperature, but not hot enough to burn—up to about 51°C (about 124°F). Dip the affected joint in the warm wax, remove when cooled. The wax may be reused. This treatment is especially good for RA of the hands.

❏ Acupuncture can be excellent for RA, particularly to relieve the inflammation and improve mobility.

❏ Gentle exercise is important to maintain mobility of the joints. Choose an activity such as swimming or tai chi that will not aggravate this painful condition.

❏ Get pregnant! The change of hormones during pregnancy often creates a time of remission for autoimmune conditions such as RA.

❏ Sometimes illness can teach us valuable lessons. Patience, for example. RA often affects self-sacrificing, unassertive types. If this sounds like you, perhaps the lesson on this occasion is to voice your needs and stand up for yourself. Go get 'em, tiger.

- Sometimes, in a ruthless condition like RA, it is well worth pursuing a line of inquiry that may result in cure or cessation of symptoms. If you believe the RA came on after a "shock" to the body or mind, re-examine that event. Treat it as if it has just occurred. For example, if the incident was a car accident, you may like to try homoeopathic arnica or the Bach flower Star of Bethlehem, both indicated for shock. Hypnotherapy or kinesiology may also prove fruitful.

AROMATHERAPY

- 4 drops of eucalyptus—analgesic, antirheumatic.

- 4 drops of juniper—antirheumatic, antioxidative, depurative.

- 5 drops of lavender spike—analgesic, decongestant.

- 5 drops of sweet marjoram—analgesic, antispasmodic, diuretic.

To use this wonderful soothing blend, mix with 15 ml sweet almond oil and 5 ml St. John's wort and apply to the affected area as needed. You can also sprinkle 8 drops of the essential oil blend into some cool water and use as a cool compress as needed. Use 10 drops of the essential oil blend in 125 grams Epsom salts in a hand, foot, or full-body bath.

AT A GLANCE

DIET

- Go vegan. A vegan diet is a plant-based one free of any animal products including dairy and eggs.

- Eat more fish. The omega-3 fatty acid EPA, found in fish, helps to reduce inflammation. Choose fatty fishes such as salmon, sardines, herring, mackerel, and tuna.

- Decrease acid-forming foods including grains, sugar, and meat. Increase alkalizing foods—fruits and vegetables.

- Avoid the Solanaceae family—tomatoes, eggplants, capsicum, potatoes, chilies.

REMEDIES

- At least 10 to 15 ml of fish oil daily will help with inflammation. The oil is easier and more economical than capsules.

- Herbs for inflammation include ginger, turmeric, willow bark, and boswellia.

- Herbs to modulate the immune system include echinacea, Rehmannia, cat's claw, and bupleurum.

OTHER

- Hot compresses made with ginger or castor oil may relieve symptoms.

- Try a course of acupuncture for pain relief.

- Keep moving. Do gentle exercise to maintain mobility of the joints. Use it or lose it.

ASTHMA

WHAT IS IT?

A Treatise of Asthma was written by Moses Maimonides, rabbi, philosopher, and medico. In this text, written more than 1,000 years ago, Maimonides clearly describes how asthma symptoms often start as a common cold during the wet months, with the patient coughing and gasping for air. Recommended treatments included seeking a dry climate, plenty of sleep, fluids, moderation of sexual activity, *and* chicken soup. *Oy vey.* Moses must have made his mother proud.

Asthma occurs when the airways, in reaction to a trigger, become inflamed and swollen. In response, cells lining the airways release sticky mucus and inflammatory substances such as histamine, causing the airways to constrict, reducing airflow. The wheezing sound common to asthma is created by air attempting to leave the narrowed airways, and coughing occurs when the lungs try to get rid of the aforementioned mucus. Not being able to breathe is frightening, and this fear makes the muscles around the chest, throat, neck, and shoulders tense and tight, restricting airflow even more. Chronic asthmatics often have tight muscles in these areas, even when their breathing is normal.

SYMPTOMS

☑ Coughing—with or without phlegm

☑ Shortness of breath—often worse with activity or exercise

☑ Wheezing

☑ Tightness in chest

WHAT CAUSES IT?

❏ An episode of asthma is often set off by an accumulation of several triggers. Like the straw that breaks the camel's back, one little extra thing is enough to tip the balance. If you look after your asthma, you can probably tolerate a little of an allergic substance or trigger. However, if you are under stress or getting over a cold, that same trigger could cause an attack.

The following are some common triggers for asthma:

❏ Environmental triggers. Including pollen, animal dander (fur and other pet trimmings), cockroach droppings, cigarette smoke (children of smokers are more prone to asthma), household chemicals such as oven cleaners, change of season, mold, weather conditions, such as humidity, wind, and cold air, petrol fumes, some pets, and dust mites.

❏ Food allergies and sensitivities. Common food allergens in asthma include milk, chocolate, peanuts, wheat, and citrus. Other sensitivities include monosodium glutamate (MSG), sulfites (common in beer, wine, and dried fruit), histamines (which occur in red wine, blue cheese, and tuna), tartrazine (red food coloring number 102), salicylates, chocolate, and yeast.

❏ Exercise.

❏ Respiratory infections such as a cold, bronchitis, or sinus infection.

❏ Sudden temperature or barometric changes.

❏ Back problems and poor posture may also trigger asthma. Pressure on the nerves that nourish the lungs may be affected by a stooped posture.

- As it is for so many conditions, stress is often a precursor for asthma.
- Even laughing and crying may initiate an attack.

WHAT TO DO

Asthma is potentially fatal, so don't meddle with any prescribed medication. Cortisone, in particular, must be phased out slowly and under medical supervision. If it is stopped abruptly, asthma is very likely to rebound, with symptoms worse than ever.

The following natural therapies may be used in conjunction with conventional medical asthma treatment. Do not discontinue your medication before consulting with your practitioner, even if you show positive results from the interventions suggested below.

Diet

- Avoid known allergens and sensitivities. Foods to look out for include dairy, wheat, preservatives, and colorings.

- Eat one onion a day, cooked or raw, red, white, or brown. Onions are not only antibiotic, they reduce the viscosity of mucus, freeing the wheeze. Garlic shares similar properties with onions in the prevention and treatment of asthma. Eat liberally.

- Drink at least 2 liters of fluid daily, keeping that mucus from becoming too viscid and sticky, and preventing the airways from drying out.

- Fish contains the omega-3 fatty acid EPA, which is particularly anti-inflammatory and good for asthma. Eat four to five servings of fish or seafood (canned, frozen, or fresh) each week.

- Decrease salt. High levels can increase your reaction to histamine, an inflammatory substance released by the cells during an asthma attack.

- A cup of strong black tea may stop an attack. The theophylline (one of a group of chemicals called xanthines) in tea is a bronchodilator; that is, it widens the airways, allowing more air in and out. Tea may relieve the temporary symptom of wheezing, but is not a long-term preventative treatment. A cup of strong black coffee may have a similar effect because of its caffeine, another xanthine that dilates the bronchi.

- Chicken soup with the addition of plenty of garlic is just what Maimonides ordered.

Remedies

- Immune herbs. Asthma is often triggered by respiratory tract infections such as head colds, coughs, and sinusitis. It pays to keep your immune system in tip-top shape. Herbs that improve the immune system can help with asthma, including astragalus, Siberian ginseng, and echinacea. Some people fear taking echinacea if they have asthma; this is only the case if you are allergic to echinacea. An allergy to echinacea is actually quite rare; the symptoms are immediate and include a rash and wheezing. So if you are an asthmatic and have tried echinacea in the past with no reaction, you are extremely unlikely to be allergic to it and so can add it to your immune system repertoire. Herbs to take during a respiratory infection include thyme, goldenseal, white horehound, elecampane, licorice, and mullein. These herbs are also good to take in the longer term if your lungs have been weakened by years of asthma or previous infections such as pneumonia.

- Herbs that reduce the spasming of the airways include grindelia, adhatoda vasica, elecampane, and valerian. Use these if you are a chronic asthmatic.

- ❏ Vitamin A is important for the health of lung tissue. Take daily, or in the form of a cod liver oil capsule, which will also provide a little vitamin D and EPA.

- ❏ Vitamin D levels are often low in asthmatics; take a supplement of vitamin D if so, and then maintain your vitamin D levels with daily cod liver oil supplementation.

- ❏ Quercetin, a bioflavonoid, helps modulate the inflammatory nature of asthma. Take daily.

- ❏ Vitamin C has natural antihistamine powers. Take 500 mg daily. One teaspoon of vitamin C powder in some water may abort an attack if imminent. Adjust the dose for children (see page 4).

BUTEYKO BREATHING

While researching heart disease in the 1950s, Konstantin Buteyko, a Russian doctor, developed a breathing technique that helped reduce not only high blood pressure, but also a variety of conditions including asthma. The premise of the technique is that many conditions, including asthma, are the result of overbreathing or chronic hyperventilation. Completely at odds to the popular view that taking big, deep breaths of air is "good" breathing, the Buteyko way is to minimize intake, reducing and calming the breath. Not so different from ancient yogic pranayama breathing. Signs of overbreathing include mouth breathing, frequent yawning, sighing, sniffing, heavy breathing at night, loud breathing, and snoring.

A study reported in the *Medical Journal of Australia* showed that after three months, people practicing the Buteyko technique had decreased their requirement for asthma-relieving medication by 90 percent and the use of inhaled corticosteroids by 49 percent. Buteyko believed that we need to increase carbon dioxide levels in the body. Mostly considered a "waste" gas, carbon dioxide is vital to life. A slight rise in carbon dioxide opens airways and blood vessels, improving air and blood flow to the body. The way oxygen travels around the body is to "stick" to hemoglobin molecules, themselves attached to red blood cells scooting through the bloodstream. It is actually an increase in carbon dioxide that "tells" hemoglobin to let go of the oxygen molecules, ensuring the precious oxygen cargo gets delivered to the organs and tissues where it is most needed. This is a basic physiological concept known as the Bohr effect. Buteyko breathing, using relaxation and minimal breathing volume, works to reset the carbon dioxide levels. By reducing the breath, carbon dioxide levels increase, switching on the parasympathetic nervous system, which acts to soothe and calm. The Buteyko technique incorporates several carbon dioxide–lowering breathing exercises.

Small breath holds is one of the exercises taught in the Buteyko technique. To do this, close your mouth. Take a small breath in, then out. With thumb and forefinger of one hand, gently hold your nose closed for five seconds. Release and relax for ten seconds, breathing gently through your nose. Repeat ten times or until you feel calmer. For those with acute breathing difficulties, such as the beginning of an asthma attack, close your nose for only a couple of seconds, and allow a longer interval of relaxed breathing in between, up to fifteen breaths.

❑ Magnesium supplementation is a must for anyone suffering from asthma. Magnesium relaxes the tiny breathing passages—bronchioles—reversing any tendency for them to tighten. Take 200 mg, two to three times a day. For children, the tissue salt mag. phos. may be sufficient.

Other

❑ Breathe through your nose, not your mouth. This will be easier if you keep your tongue positioned at the roof of your mouth, just behind the front teeth. Nose breathing is the way we were designed to breath.

❑ Buteyko breathing is a proven technique for reducing the symptoms of and preventing asthma. Recommended for children over the age of seven. It can be literally a lifesaving course to take. Practice the small breath holds exercise. See breakout box on page 35.

❑ An extremely useful tool is desensitization. The trigger allergen(s) are determined either by a blood test or skin prick test and a program of desensitizing, using drops under the tongue or injections, is implemented for a number of months. Various doctors and natural practitioners specialize in this area.

❑ If your breathing becomes strained, try standing under a steaming-hot shower. The steam will help open the airways. Employing the same logic, if you are tight chested during the night, place a humidifier beside your bed. They are available from most pharmacies. You could add a couple of drops of thyme, eucalyptus, or lavender oil to the water.

❑ If stress is a big trigger for you, it is imperative you learn some effective techniques for managing stress. Then use them, whether it be meditation, yoga, or embroidery. Asthma is not a condition to be toyed with. Everyone who has experienced an asthma attack (including onlookers) knows how frightening it is. If you can possibly remain calm, best achieved by the breathing technique mentioned above, this will reduce the severity of the attack.

❑ Dust mites and molds are a very common asthma trigger. Here are some ideas for keeping them under control. If possible, have wooden floors or tiles instead of carpet, and remove heavy curtains. Dust mites love beds; use mattress and pillow cover protectors, and wash them every week. Vacuum your mattress every month or so and then spray with weak black tea to deactivate dust mites. Let the sun shine on your mattress and as much of the room as possible. Every month get someone else to scrub moldy bathrooms with bleach and wipe over with tea tree oil. If this task cannot be delegated, make sure you wear a mask. Wash shower curtains regularly; they are fervent collectors of mold. Let fresh, dry air and sunshine flood the house. If all else fails, move to a drier abode. If mold is a trigger, consider removing mold and yeast foods from your diet to see whether this relieves your asthma. (See also Candida on page 73.)

❑ Is your back out? If there is any problem with the thoracic or middle part of the back, this can affect the nerves that feed the lungs. A problem with the back can in turn cause or trigger your asthma. Go to a chiropractor, osteopath, or physiotherapist for assessment.

❑ Activities that improve posture and strengthen the back, correcting asthmatic tendencies, include yoga, Pilates, the Alexander Technique, and the Feldenkrais method.

❑ Regular massage may help with particular attention to shoulder, upper back, and chest.

❑ In the emotional anatomy of the body, the lungs are the organs of grief. Asthma has been described by some as a "silent scream" and may be an expression of feeling claustrophobic in relationships, often with family.

AROMATHERAPY

❑ 6 drops of cajeput—analgesic, febrifuge, antiseptic, expectorant, antispasmodic.

❑ 6 drops of eucalyptus or peppermint—decongestant, expectorant, mucolytic, balsamic.

❑ 4 drops of sweet fennel—antispasmodic, carminative, expectorant.

Combined, this is a gentle, calming, and breathe-easy blend. Use in a balm or gel rubbed into the lung area of the body. Mix with sweet almond oil for a massage oil. Use 6 drops of this blend in a vaporizer or sprinkled onto a tissue for a dry inhalation.

At a Glance

Diet

➡ Eat onions and garlic every day. Not only are they naturally antibiotic to ward off coughs and colds, but they also help keep mucus fluid, important for the asthma sufferer.

➡ Fish contains the omega-3 fatty acid EPA, which is anti-inflammatory. Eat fish such as salmon, tuna, herrings, and mackerel three to four times a week.

➡ Reduce salt as a high-salt diet is associated with asthma.

➡ Avoid any known food sensitivities that may trigger your asthma. Common triggering foods are dairy, wheat, preservatives, and colorings.

Remedies

➡ Magnesium is a muscle relaxant, helping to keep the airways relaxed and open.

➡ Vitamin C and the bioflavonoid quercetin have antihistamine and anti-inflammatory properties.

➡ Cod liver oil capsules (or for the brave, cod liver oil) contains vitamins A and D, both excellent for the health of the lungs.

➡ Take lung tonic herbs including mullein, licorice, thyme, and elecampane.

Other

➡ Learn Buteyko breathing. It is amazing for treating and preventing asthma. (See also Appendix F.)

➡ Go to a chiropractor, osteopath, or physiotherapist to assess your back for misalignment.

➡ Always breathe through your nose.

ATHEROSCLEROSIS

WHAT IS IT?

Atherosclerosis, the hardening and thickening of artery walls that restricts blood flow, is not a disease in its own right, yet its presence invites all the heavy hitters, including coronary heart disease, congestive heart failure, stroke, and peripheral vascular disease. The word is derived from the Greek *athero*—for an "atheroma" or plaque—and *skle-ro-sis*—for "sclerosis"—a hardening of the artery wall.

SYMPTOMS

☑ Very often there are no symptoms that your arteries are closing up.

☑ Chest pain or discomfort. But the pain can also be felt in the upper back, arms, and neck.

☑ Shortness of breath

☑ Fatigue with activity or light exercise

WHAT CAUSES IT?

❏ Age. The older you get, in the industrialized West, the greater the chance of having atherosclerosis.

❏ Being male. Men have a greater risk of atherosclerosis. Women are more protected, especially prior to menopause.

❏ Family history. As always, there is a genetic predisposition to this disease also.

❏ High blood pressure is both a cause and symptom of atherosclerosis. High blood pressure can cause the initial injury to the lining of the artery (epithelium), and can make matters worse by dislodging the cap and causing a thrombus to form.

THE PRITIKIN DIET

Nathan Pritikin, an American engineer, started the ball rolling in 1955, when a specialist told him that his arteries were in bad shape and that if he wanted to avoid dying from a heart attack, he would have to take cholesterol-lowering drugs and stop exercising for the rest of his life. Pritikin, who was only 43, decided this was not for him and immersed himself in research about his condition. He put himself on a strict low-fat, high-carbohydrate, vegetarian diet modeled on that of the Tarahumara Indians in northwest Mexico and the hill tribes in Papua New Guinea and began a wicked exercise regime. His book, *The Pritikin Diet*, became a best seller.

Nathan Pritikin died in 1985, by his own hand, after finding out that he was suffering a relapse of leukemia. However, an autopsy found that his arteries were free of any sign of atherosclerosis, upholding the validity of his life's

work. Ironically, the high-carbohydrate diet adopted by government agencies and heart foundations of the United States, United Kingdom, and Australia have inadvertently created further public health epidemics of obesity and diabetes. Nice one, Nathan.

Pritikin took fat reduction too far. Recent studies have shown that extremely low cholesterol levels have been linked to increased risk of suicide. If we decrease fat in our diet excessively, we risk the chance of hormonal disturbances, immune system problems, deficiency of the fat-soluble vitamins A, D, E, and K, and nervous system dysfunction. Since the Pritikin days, fat is the new black, and we now know that certain fats are positively protective against heart disease, particularly the kinds of fats found in fish, coconuts, avocadoes, nuts, and seeds.

- Obesity and diabetes. Altered fats and sugars in the bloodstream.

- Physical inactivity. People who don't exercise are twice as likely to die of heart attacks as people who do. Regular exercise strengthens the heart muscle, reduces blood pressure, and helps to lower body weight.

- Cigarette smoking. Cigarette smoking constricts blood vessels, and the chemicals inhaled cause damage to the artery wall.

- Alcohol. A couple of drinks a day lowers your risk, more than this increases your chances of atherosclerosis.

- Stress. Hostility outrates other risk factors, including smoking, high blood pressure, and high cholesterol. The classic type A stress personality is more aggressive, achievement oriented, and a "go-getter." In addition, stress decreases HDL levels and increases blood fats, making the blood stickier.

WHAT TO DO

Diet

- Vegetarians are less prone to heart disease. Vegetable protein, found in legumes, grains, nuts, and seeds, appears to be more protective for the artery wall than animal flesh protein.

- Garlic is a beaut for atherosclerosis as well as for the all aspects of heart disease. It is proven to help prevent atherosclerotic changes from occurring; it also reduces blood fats and improves blood flow. Cooked garlic is as helpful as raw on this occasion.

- Nitric oxide helps to dilate blood vessels. Foods that increase natural nitric oxide production and are jam-packed full of antioxidants include grapes and berries, red wine, garlic, soy beans, cocoa, tea (green and black), olive oil, and pomegranate.

> ### EARLOBE CREASE
>
> A strange little sign, which is an early warning of atherosclerosis, is the "earlobe crease": a slightly curved vertical crease on the lower, fleshy part of the earlobe. If your earlobe looks a little creased, have a checkup. Another predictive sign of cardiovascular disease is found in the eye, known as *arcus senilis*, *arcus cornealis*, or among iridologists as a cholesterol ring—a grayish-white arc around the upper segment of the iris. Don't freak out if you find these signs; rather, be thankful for a sign to step up your exercise and spruce up your diet.

- Reduce sodium. Sodium is linked with high blood pressure, and high blood pressure is linked to atherosclerosis. Don't add salt (sodium chloride) to your meals and eat as little processed food (where most salt is found in the diet) as you can.

- Alcohol. One to two drinks daily is protective against heart disease. More is not. Desist.

Remedies

- Herbs found to help prevent and treat atherosclerosis include astragalus, ginkgo, tea (green and black), turmeric, globe artichoke, and American ginseng.

- If you don't regularly include garlic in your diet, rethink that. Or take a daily freeze-dried whole garlic supplement.

- Magnesium allows muscles to relax, including the smooth muscle that surrounds arteries.

- Niacin—vitamin B_3—has been successful in helping to treat atherosclerosis. However, the doses required are quite high (2 to 3 grams day) and can cause uncomfortable flushing. There are slower-release tablets available.

Other

- You must start managing your stress. Don't just think about it. Do something for it every day, such as walking, tapestry, knitting, singing, meditation, rock climbing, yoga, dancing, and/or counseling.
- Lose weight if necessary.

- Stop smoking. Another reason.
- Exercise. Regular aerobic exercise (jogging, cycling, fast walking) decreases the "bad" cholesterol levels or LDL levels and most atherosclerosis risk factors.
- Buteyko breathing helps lower blood pressure and increase nitric oxide levels (see Appendix F).

AT A GLANCE

DIET

- Increase garlic in your diet as it reduces blood fats and improves blood flow, a heart-winning combination.
- Eat foods high in antioxidants and nitric oxide, both of which help prevent atherosclerosis— grapes and berries, red wine, garlic, soy beans, cocoa, tea (green and black), olive oil, and pomegranate.
- Decrease salt. Sodium increases blood pressure, not a good thing if your arteries are already compromised.
- Have a cup of tea or two. Tea, whether it be green or black (oolong or white) helps prevent damage to the artery walls.

REMEDIES

- Herbs helpful in the treatment of atherosclerosis include astragalus, ginkgo, turmeric, globe artichoke, and American ginseng.
- Magnesium is a muscle relaxant. Arteries walls are made of muscle. Magnesium will help to dilate and relax them.

OTHER

- Regular aerobic exercise is vital, whether it be cycling, jogging, or gym classes.
- Stress is a major factor in heart disease. Find ways with which to reduce and handle your stress.
- Lose weight if you are carrying excess pounds.
- Still smoking? Stop being a twit.

HISTORY OF A HEART ATTACK

Lining each artery is the epithelium. As a result of high blood pressure, diabetes, smoking, or free-radical damage, the epithelium becomes damaged. As a kind of Band-Aid, cholesterol molecules and other fats patch over the wound, creating a fatty streak. Smooth muscle cells smooth over the fatty streak, creating an often unstable cap. If and when the cap is dislodged, platelets gather forming a clot, much like a scab on the skin. This internal clot is called a thrombus. This thrombus can completely block the artery, or start flowing down the arteries, causing blockage further along. No cell in the body can live without blood providing oxygen and nutrients. If the artery supplying the heart (coronary artery) becomes blocked, this results in a heart attack or myocardial infarct. Blocked arteries to the brain result in a stroke.

BAD BREATH (HALITOSIS)

WHAT IS IT?

Is your breath on the doggy side? Do colleagues reel back and dry heave when you ask where the stapler is? Even if things aren't this dire, bad breath or halitosis is a condition that is a source of embarrassment and self-consciousness.

SYMPTOMS

✓ Bad breath is usually a symptom of an underlying cause.

✓ The tongue, particularly toward the back of the mouth, may have a thick coating that is cream-colored through to green and brown.

✓ Bad taste in your mouth

✓ Friends who now prefer to Skype and text when you used to meet up for coffee.

WHAT CAUSES IT?

❏ Blocked sinuses. If sinuses become clogged with mucus after a cold, sinusitis, or an allergy, bad breath may result. (See also Sinusitis on page 271.)

❏ Postnasal drip (PND) is when mucus draining from the sinuses, drips down the back of the throat. (See also Sinusitis on page 271.)

❏ *Helicobacter pylori,* the stomach bacteria responsible for stomach ulcers can also result in bad breath.

❏ Reflux, also known as gastroesophageal reflux disorder (GERD), is where stomach acid and undigested food are regurgitated up into the throat. Although many people are aware of the symptoms of GERD or heartburn, you can also have silent reflux where there are no symptoms. (See also Reflux on page 266.)

❏ Constipation. A lengthened transit time means feces takes a long time to travel the length of the colon. As a result, products of fermentation and putrefaction are released into the bloodstream and eliminated via the lungs, causing bad breath. (See also Constipation on page 104.)

❏ Bad bugs. The entire gastrointestinal tract, from mouth to anus, is home to about 3 pounds of microflora, collectively known as the microbiome. Most of these resident bugs are bacteria. The metabolic by-products of bacteria are often gas, and depending on the variety of bacteria, smelly gas that may be the cause of your smelly breath.

❏ Gingivitis (gum disease) is a common cause of bad breath. Gums may look red and swollen and bleed during tooth brushing. The bacteria that cause gum disease are very likely also causing your bad breath. (See also Gingivitis on page 175.)

❏ The other dental cause of bad breath is inadequate cleaning of dentures, braces, and plates.

❏ Water. Simply not drinking enough fluids can cause bad breath.

❏ Medicine. Particularly if you have an "odd" or metallic taste in your mouth along with the bad breath, it could be a side effect of medication. It's worth asking your doctor about.

❏ Stress. Bad breath can be a symptom of stress.

❏ Coffee. For some people, drinking coffee (and sometimes tea) causes bad breath.

❏ Dairy sensitivity. Lactose intolerance (intolerance to milk sugar) and/or dairy sensitivity (allergy to milk protein) may cause bad breath.

□ A throat or tonsil infection may be the source of the problem.

□ Dry mouth. Insufficient saliva impacts on good bacteria that may result in bad breath. Insufficient saliva can be due to Sjögren's syndrome, some medications, and mouth breathing.

□ Smoking tobacco or marijuana.

WHAT TO DO

Bad breath is not a disease but a symptom of something awry. Finding out why your breath is on the stinky side may take a bit of detective work, but the alternatives such as sucking on peppermints or using mouthwash will just give you minty bad breath.

Diet

□ The following foods may cause bad breath, but only for a few hours after consumption: cheese, particularly blue cheese, deli meats such as salami, strong curry spices, garlic, and onions.

□ Eat prebiotic and probiotic foods. Prebiotics encourage the growth of beneficial microflora in the mouth and all points south. Prebiotic foods include: asparagus, Jerusalem artichokes, leeks, and onions, legumes such as baked beans, chickpeas, and lentils, and supplementary fibers including psyllium, pectin, guar gum, and slippery elm. Probiotic foods include fermented foods: yogurt, miso, sauerkraut, kefir, natto, tempeh, and the Korean delicacy kimchi.

□ Avoid sugar as sugar feeds bad-breath bacteria.

□ Avoid dairy foods for one week including milk, cream, cheese, ice cream, chocolate, and yogurt. If your bad breath disappears then reduce these foods in your diet, and make sure you eat plenty of calcium-rich foods to make up for any deficiency. High calcium foods include nuts (especially almonds) and seeds, green leafy vegetables, tofu, parsley, salmon and sardines (canned), and dried figs.

□ Drink 2 liters of water daily in addition to other fluids.

□ Avoid coffee and tea for one week. Again these might be the cause. Resume if your bad breath is still with you after the week-long abstinence.

□ If you are constipated, make sure you are eating plenty of fiber-rich foods including vegetables, whole grains, and legumes. (See also Constipation on page 104.)

NETI POT

Very much like a takeout version of wiping out while bodysurfing in the Pacific, the Neti pot (an Indian invention) is used to treat and prevent sinusitis. Looking like a small teapot with a phallic-shaped spout, the Neti is used for an intranasal douche. Into a Neti, pour about 250 ml warm water (about blood temperature) and one teaspoon of sea salt. Stand over the sink holding your head to the left side. Slowly pour a little of the warm, salty water up your right nostril. Within a couple of moments your left nostril should drip, then flow. Gently blow through the nose to clear out water and mucus. Then swap sides. Using a Neti pot is a pleasant experience—trust me. Neti pots can be bought from yoga studios, some pharmacies, and online. A small teapot may be used in the absence of an authentic Neti pot. At your next tea party, just don't let your guests know what you do with the pot when you are not serving them tea.

Remedies

❏ The specific probiotic for good oral health and sweet-smelling breath is *Lactobacillus salivarius*. If you cannot find a supplement containing this specific bug, choose a good multiprobiotic containing other lactobacillus strains. Take a dose before breakfast each day.

❏ Herbs for sinusitis or postnasal drip include eyebright, goldenseal, echinacea, elder, andrographis, goldenrod, horseradish, and garlic. Vitamin C is also good.

❏ Gum disease. Once a day, squeeze out the contents of a 100 mg coenzyme Q_{10} (CoQ_{10}) capsule onto the gums, and massage it in with a soft toothbrush. In addition, swill and gargle a mixture of one or more of the following herbs, made from tincture or tea, making sure mixture stays in contact with the gum tissue for at least a minute: calendula, goldenseal, echinacea, myrrh, and/or propolis (bee product). You can also swallow the mixture, as it is good for the immune system as well as healing to gums, but be warned, the taste is deadly. Suck on vitamin C and zinc tablets, taking one three times a day.

❏ If *Helicobacter pylori* is the culprit, take the appropriate antibiotics, and follow up with a course of probiotics.

❏ For constipation, take digestive bitter herbs before meals—bitter herbs include artichoke leaf, angelica, dandelion, and gentian root, among others and are available as a liquid tonic—and dietary supplements such as psyllium husks and chia seeds.

❏ Reflux. Take a teaspoon of slippery elm powder in water, mashed banana, or yogurt with each meal. (See page 266.)

Other

❏ If you suffer from sinusitis or postnasal drip use a Neti pot each morning.

❏ If you have insufficient saliva, chew on sugarless gum, particularly after meals.

❏ Breathe through your nose. Mouth breathing contributes to a dry mouth and bad breath.

❏ If your bad breath is due to gum disease, be diligent about regular visits to the dentist, dental hygienist, and periodontist. Save your teeth and gums while sweetening your breath. Brush and floss regularly.

❏ Buteyko breathing helps reduce gum disease, mouth breathing, and reflux, all potential causes of bad breath. (See also Appendix F: Buteyko Breathing.)

❏ Use a tongue scraper in addition to brushing and flossing. Tongue scrapers have been used for centuries and are recommended in the Ayurvedic approach to health and well-being. They are ergonomically designed to scrape away bacteria, plaque, and fungi, all of which may cause bad breath.

❏ Stop smoking.

DIET

→ Drink 2 liters of water daily.

→ Avoid dairy foods, coffee, and tea, or at least try a week without them to see if they are contributing to your bad breath.

→ Eat prebiotic and probiotic foods: prebiotic—asparagus, Jerusalem artichokes, leeks and onions, and legumes; probiotic—yogurt, miso, sauerkraut, kefir, natto, tempeh, and kimchi.

REMEDIES

→ Take probiotics daily.

→ For sinus problems and postnasal drip, take the following herbs: eyebright, goldenseal, echinacea, elder, andrographis, goldenrod, horseradish, and garlic.

→ For gum disease: rub in the contents of a 100 mg CoQ_{10} capsule each day, and gargle and swallow one or more of the following herbs from a tea or tincture—calendula, goldenseal, echinacea, myrrh, and/or propolis.

OTHER

→ Regularly use a Neti pot and tongue scraper.

→ Regularly visit the dentist and periodontist—and don't forget to floss.

BALDNESS (ALOPECIA)

WHAT IS IT?

A paper entitled "Shorn Scalps and Perceptions of Male Dominance" revealed that bald or closely shaven men were perceived to be stronger and taller than their hairier colleagues. Despite these findings, squillions of dollars and thousands of counseling hours are spent in the pursuit of cranial hirsuitism. Perhaps it's because hair adorns the face, the bit we show the world, or the sexual connotations bestowed by freely flowing locks, that hair and its loss is the focus of many. If you are losing your hair, try the methods below. If all else fails, take solace in baseballer Joe Garagiola's quote, "I'd rather be bald on top than bald inside."

SYMPTOMS

☑ Alopecia areata. Hair is lost in small, often circular patches from the scalp and beard.

☑ Male-pattern baldness. Hair recedes from the temples and top of the scalp.

☑ Alopecia universalis. Rarely, hair is lost from all parts of the body—scalp, arms, legs, pubic area, and eyebrows.

WHAT CAUSES IT?

❑ You are male. The male hormone, testosterone, is responsible for male-pattern baldness where the hair starts to recede first at the temples, and keeps receding until it's a little shaggy thing, perching precariously low, at the back of the head, between the ears.

The average scalp boasts 100,000 hairs. Each day sees the loss of approximately 100 of these hairs. The bit that we preen and perm is the shaft of the hair, protruding from the surface of the skin and made of keratin, a type of protein. Beneath the skin lies the hair root, sometimes called the bulb, encased by the hair follicle. It is from within the hair follicle that the yet unheralded hair is nurtured. The follicle provides all nutrients for healthy growth as well as producing sebum, the natural oil that keeps the skin healthy and hair glossy.

❏ Alopecia areata, distinct round pale patches of baldness, is nearly always stress-related.

❏ Medication (or ceasing medication), including oral contraceptive pills or cortisone, may be the cause of your hair loss.

❏ A sudden emotional or physical stress including high fever, major surgery, illness, or a crash diet can cause hair loss. It may take weeks to a couple of months for the hair to fall out after such an event.

❏ Chemotherapy—while not all chemotherapy drugs cause hair to fall out, it is a relatively common side effect of treatment. Hair will grow back, but may have a different texture or color.

❏ Postmenopause, many women find their hair thinning. This may be due to a relative increase in the male hormone, testosterone, after estrogen levels have dropped.

❏ Polycystic ovarian syndrome (PCOS) may cause a male-pattern hair loss due to an imbalance of hormones. Quite unfairly, hair on the scalp may reduce, while facial and other body hair increases.

❏ After baby. During pregnancy women tend not to lose their allotted 100 hairs a day. Postbirth, a massive molt takes place two to three months after birth where all the saved-up hairs fall out. This is perfectly normal, and within a year your luxurious pelt will return.

❏ Iron-deficiency anemia is the most common nutritional reason for hair loss.

❏ Ringworm of the scalp may appear as circular, bare red patches very similar to alopecia areata, but this is due to this fungal infection.

❏ Certain illnesses may cause hair loss, including low thyroid and the autoimmune condition lupus erythematosus.

WHAT TO DO

Be patient with treatment. It may take months for hair to regrow.

Diet

❏ Iron deficiency is the most common nutritional cause for hair loss, followed by iodine deficiency. Foods high in iron include prunes, raisins, and dates; dark leafy green vegetables—kale, bok choy, gai lan, spinach; legumes—lentils, kidney beans, soy beans; seaweed; parsley; blackstrap molasses; mollusks—oysters, clams, mussels; red meat—beef, lamb, venison, goat; and egg yolks. Foods high in iodine include seaweed, seafood, and iodized salt.

❏ Circulation to the hair follicle is important for hair growth. Foods that improve circulation include ginger, chili, pepper, and garlic

❏ To grow strong and healthy hair, it is important to consume plenty of good fats. Good essential fatty acids for hair are found in seeds, nuts, fish, avocadoes, coconut, and olive oil.

Remedies

❏ If hormonal imbalance is the reason for hair loss, particularly for women, then the herb vitex agnus-castus may prove beneficial. If hair loss is due to polycystic ovarian syndrome (PCOS), the herbs licorice and peony are an excellent combination.

❏ Herbs to improve circulation to the peripheries, fingers, toes, and scalp include prickly ash, ginkgo biloba, ginger, bilberry, and cayenne.

❏ If your hair is brittle and poor quality as well as thinning, the mineral silica will help. Take in liquid or tablet form. Eat alfalfa sprouts and drink horsetail tea.

❏ If iron deficiency appears to be the problem, take an iron supplement. (For more on iron-deficiency anemia see page 10.)

❏ If stress initiated the hair loss, take a B-complex supplement, as well as nervous system restorative herbs such as St. John's wort, passionflower, lemon balm, and the appropriately named skullcap.

Other

❏ Massaging the scalp improves circulation, bringing oxygen and nutrients to help hair growth. Plant the pads of your fingers on your scalp, press firmly as you rotate the fingers, shifting the skin over the scalp. Massage with the essential oil combination mentioned below or traditional Indian neem tree oil.

❏ A combination of the following essential oils is effective for hair growth—2 to 3 drops each of thyme, rosemary, lavender, and cedarwood. Rub into the scalp at night two to three times a week. Leave in, or wash out in the morning.

❏ Nettle has been traditionally used as a hair tonic. Make up some nettle tea, let it cool, and use as a rinse after shampooing.

❏ Give up cigarettes—they restrict blood supply.

❏ Inverted postures are useful exercises because placing the head lower than the rest of the body increases blood flow to the scalp. Lie for fifteen minutes on a slant board, or with your legs up the wall and your bottom on a firm pillow. If you practice yoga regularly, try a ten-minute shoulder stand daily.

❏ Accept it. For men who suffer from hair loss, the news is bleak—male pattern baldness is hereditary. Please, please, please do not resort to the comb-over.

AROMATHERAPY

Some essential oils that are helpful for hair health:

❏ 8 drops of rosemary—stimulating, restorative, rubefacient.

❏ 6 drops of juniper—tonic, rubefacient.

❏ 3 drops of clary sage—rejuvenating, revitalizing, and balancing.

❏ 4 drops of ginger—tonic, stimulating, rubefacient, antioxidant.

❏ 4 drops of bay—revitalizing, hair tonic, warming.

Use this blend in a stimulating head massage blend using coconut oil as a base—add the blend to 50 ml of coconut oil. The hair can be wrapped in a warm towel and left for an hour—wash out after removing the towel as hair will be oily. Repeat weekly.

This blend can also be used as a shampoo when mixed with 50 ml pure castile soap. If you want 100 ml, double the amount of drops.

DIET

➡ Baldness may be due to a deficiency in iron or iodine. Iron-rich foods include red meat, dark leafy greens, and dried fruit. Iodine-rich foods include seaweed, seafood, and iodized salt.

➡ Foods to increase circulation to the scalp include ginger and chili.

REMEDIES

➡ Take an iron supplement if you are deficient in this mineral.

➡ If hormones are behind the balding process, take vitex agnus-castus for men or women. If you are a woman with PCOS, take licorice and peony and treat the underlying condition.

OTHER

➡ Massage the scalp with a combination of 2 to 3 drops of each of the following essential oils: juniper, rosemary, clary sage, and bay.

BODY ODOR

WHAT IS IT?

Bromhidrosis, body odor or BO, occurs when resident skin bacteria get their hands (or comparable bacterial body parts) on proteins that are excreted when we sweat. The bacteria convert these proteins into a variety of pungent chemicals including propionic acid, which smells sour, and isovaleric acid, which has a cheesy odor. Other substances from food or the body's own processes can be released from the skin and also smell ugly.

A quick scrub in the shower is usually all that is required to banish body odor; however, sometimes body odor can be more persistent and may be a sign of ill health or a poor diet.

SYMPTOMS

☑ A bad and noticeable strong smell that can occur anywhere on the body.

WHAT CAUSES IT?

❑ Various proteins excreted in sweat are broken down into odiferous chemicals by bacteria that reside on the skin.

❑ Meat and animal fats, particularly dairy fat such as butter and cream, are associated with body odor.

❑ Natural chemicals in certain foods are more inclined to exit via the skin; these foods include garlic, asparagus, cumin, aged cheese, deli meats, onion, alcohol, and fenugreek. Depending on the nose, these smells are either inviting or offensive.

❑ An overgrowth of the common yeast *Candida albicans* can sometimes result in body odor.

❑ Nonsmokers often complain of the smell of smokers.

❑ Sometimes an unusual body odor indicates an

illness, including untreated diabetes and kidney or liver disease.

❏ Times of great hormonal changes, particularly puberty, can cause body odor.

❏ Some medications can contribute to body odor.

WHAT TO DO

Diet

❏ Drink 2 to 3 liters of fluid daily. Spring water is best.

❏ Try six weeks on a vegan diet. Animal protein and fat are the main smelly offenders.

❏ Avoid red meat, deep-fried food, deli meats, milk products (except yogurt), sugar, and alcohol.

❏ Chlorophyll is nature's deodorizer. Drink chlorophyll-rich green vegetable juice daily; mix several of the following in a base of green apple: parsley, alfalfa, cucumber, spinach, kale, beetroot tops, and celery.

❏ Burdock, one of the blood-purifying herbs mentioned below, can also be eaten as a vegetable; it is particularly popular in Japan, where it is known as "gobo."

❏ If you think you may have an overgrowth of *Candida albicans* see page 73; the candida diet may prove beneficial.

Remedies

❏ At bedtime, wipe your body with a cloth saturated with lemon juice or vinegar (white or malt). Allow to dry before going to bed. Wash off in the shower in the morning. The reasoning behind this unusual bedtime ritual is that the acid from the lemon juice or vinegar changes the skin's pH, thus inactivating the bacteria responsible for the odor.

BEHIND THE SCENES

The two major types of sweat glands are eccrine and apocrine. Eccrine glands are located everywhere and are primarily concerned with cooling the body during exercise and hot weather. The apocrine glands are situated in armpits, feet, groin, genitals, and behind the ears. These glands are more sensitive to emotions such as fear and stress, and the sweat from these areas has a stronger scent.

❏ If anxiety is the reason you are sweating, take anxiety-relieving herbs, including valerian, zizyphus, St. John's wort, passionflower, and kava. The minerals magnesium and potassium are also helpful.

❏ Bach Flower Rescue Remedy will help if fear is prevalent.

❏ Traditional blood-purifying herbs are indicated for body odor. Brew several of the following into a tea, and drink two to three cups daily as part of your water rations: burdock, red clover, echinacea, clivers, nettle, calendula, and dandelion root.

❏ The tissue salt silica, or the mineral silica helps excessive perspiration, particularly if you are cold and sweaty, whereas the homoeopathic remedy sulfur suits the hot and sweaty individual. Take a dose of whichever is indicated each morning.

❏ Chlorophyll supplements help to deodorize from within. Choose from one or a combination of the following, available in tablet or powder form: barley grass, spirulina, chlorella, and wheatgrass.

Other

❏ Naturopathic advice is to recommend against antiperspirants as the body is designed to sweat, and the skin is our largest organ of elimination. As it is bacteria that is responsible for the odor, choose a deodorant with antibacterial properties such as colloidal silver or tea tree oil. Natural crystal deodorants made from potassium alum also work as a local antibacterial agent. Many people find them effective. They do contain aluminum, but there is no evidence this is absorbed into the body.

❏ Avoid clothing made from synthetics as this will trap sweat. Choose natural fibers—cotton, hemp, wool. There are sports fabrics designed to absorb body sweat. In all cases, wash clothing in hot water using bactericidal detergent, or one containing tea tree oil. Dry clothes out in the sunshine.

❏ Bathe frequently. Use soap and deodorants containing antiseptic essential oils and herbs including tea tree, lavender, rosemary, calendula, or thyme.

❏ Wax or shave your armpits; the hair traps the smell.

❏ If your feet are particularly smelly, regularly pumice rough heels and areas of dead skin.

This is where bacteria breed. Wipe the insides of your shoes with surgical spirit, and steer clear of plastics and synthetic textiles, except specially designed smell-free sportswear.

❏ If you are chronically constipated, a series of colonic irrigations may be useful.

❏ The apocrine sweat glands are governed by fear. If you are particularly anxious or fearful, explore avenues to reduce this distressing state. Learn and practice meditation or seek counseling.

AROMATHERAPY

❏ 4 drops of pine scotch—bactericidal, deodorant, refreshing, and cleansing.

❏ 5 drops of cypress—antiperspirant, antiseptic, astringent, purifying, and protective.

❏ 3 drops of lemongrass—antiperspirant, deodorant, astringent, antimicrobial, refreshing, penetrating, and active.

❏ 2 drops of rosewood—antimicrobial, antibacterial, deodorant, and fresh.

This blend can be made into a soap using a melt-and-pour soap base, or with castile soap and used as a soft soap. For using as a body powder, blend with 125 grams white clay or corn flour—put in a shaker and use accordingly.

DIET

➧ Avoid meat and dairy (except yogurt). Animal protein and fat are linked to body odor.

➧ Drink at least 2 liters of water daily.

➧ Drink a juice made from chlorophyll-rich herbs and vegetables, such as wheatgrass, parsley, spinach, and kale, beet tops. Chlorophyll is nature's deodorant.

REMEDIES

➧ Take chlorophyll supplements such as barley grass and spirulina.

➧ If anxiety is the reason why you perspire, take kava, valerian, passionflower, and zizyphus. Magnesium and potassium are also helpful.

➧ Take the following herbs as a herbal tea or tincture: burdock, calendula, nettles, red clover, clivers, and dandelion root.

OTHER

➧ Before going to bed, wipe body with a cloth saturated with either lemon juice or vinegar. This changes the skin's pH, thus inactivating the odor-producing bacteria.

➧ Use deodorant containing antibacterial agents such as colloidal silver, tea tree oil, or calendula.

➧ Wash regularly.

➧ Use natural fibers and wash clothes in hot water.

➧ If anxiety is the reason for excessive perspiration, take up meditation.

BOILS

WHAT IS IT?

A boil is an infected hair follicle in which the infection (usually the bacteria *Staphylococcus aureus*) has spread to surrounding tissue. Groins and armpits are common locations for boils, but they may also grace face, neck, breasts, and bottoms. A stye is a tiny boil within the eyelash hair follicle.

SYMPTOMS

☑ Red painful lump(s) in which a pocket of pus may appear in the center.

☑ Swollen lymph nodes can occur near the location of the boil.

☑ A red streak may appear from the boil, signifying a spread of infection.

☑ Fever and generally feeling ill

WHAT CAUSES IT?

❑ Hair follicles become clogged and infected from sweat, creams, or dirt.

❑ Poor hygiene

❑ Excessive sugar in the bloodstream caused by a high-sugar diet or possibly undiagnosed diabetes.

❑ If your immune system is under par, you are more prone to infections, including boils.

❏ People with eczema have an increased risk of developing boils, especially if affected areas are particularly itchy and inflamed. Try not to scratch, or at least make sure nails and hands are scrupulously clean.

WHAT TO DO

If the boil is on your face, neck, or spine, you are experiencing a fever or chills, or there is a red streak emanating from the boil, best see your doctor and take a course of antibiotics if recommended. The advice below is for a minor boil and are preventative strategies if you are susceptible to boils.

Diet

❏ Avoid fatty and fried foods, alcohol, recreational drugs, and refined carbohydrates.

❏ Avoid red meat, chicken, and pork. Fish is fine.

❏ Avoid sugar.

❏ Increase vegetables and fruit. Raw is best, otherwise lightly steam, stir-fry, or bake.

❏ Drink 2 to 3 liters of water daily.

❏ Eat three to six cloves of raw garlic daily. Garlic is an excellent antibiotic. Swallow a clove whole, pointy end down first. Take after food. If you think six cloves of garlic sounds radical, so does the boil.

❏ Drink the juice of half a lemon or two teaspoons apple cider vinegar in hot water before breakfast.

Remedies

❏ Traditional blood-purifying herbs that work wonderfully well for boils include burdock, red clover, echinacea, clivers, nettle, and dandelion root and can be taken in combination with antibiotic herbs including calendula, andrographis, echinacea (in another role), and goldenseal. Drink three cups of herbal tea, made from one or a combination of these herbs each day, included as part of your water intake.

❏ If you have a stye, wash the eye using an eyebath, or saturate cotton wipes and rinse the eye twice a day with the herbs calendula, goldenseal, and echinacea as a strong cooled tea or diluted tincture.

❏ *Phytolacca decandra,* which goes by the less fancy name of poke root, is quite specific for the treatment of boils. It is very strong, so best dispensed by a herbalist.

❏ Take one teaspoon of a vitamin C and zinc supplement in powder form, three times a day.

❏ Take a dose of the tissue salt calc. sulph. three times daily, to ripen the boil to a head.

Other

❏ Wash your hands. Keep your grubby mitts away from it. Don't touch!

❏ Apply tea tree oil or colloidal silver to the boil as an antiseptic and to reduce infection when the boil bursts.

❏ Apply colloidal silver to the boil twice a day as an antiseptic.

❏ Hot compresses or poultices will bring the boil to a pointy "ripe" head so that it can be drained. Don't help it along with a pin; the boil will burst when it's good and ready. The following can be used for poultices or compresses—essential oils such as slippery elm powder, strong calendula tea or a diluted tincture, mashed cooked potato with some raw garlic, and calc. sulph. The calc. sulph. tablet can be dissolved in hot water and used to soak a cloth for a compress. Remember to keep a clean muslin or kitchen cloth between the boil and the poultice material.

AROMATHERAPY

The following healing blend has these therapeutic properties—analgesic, antiseptic, antibacterial, antimicrobial, antineuralgic, astringent, cytophylactic (increases white blood cells to fight infection), and depurative (supports the body to clean toxins out of the body, making it excellent for treating boils).

❏ 2 drops of bergamot

❏ 3 drops of roman or German chamomile

❏ 3 drops of lavender

❏ 2 drops of grapefruit

This blend can be used as a hot compress on the area up to three times a daily.

Add a few drops to the bath water with a dispersant to use as a general disinfectant.

Add a few drops to a warm clay poultice and apply to an already formed boil. The blend can also be made into a soothing balm or gel.

AT A GLANCE

DIET

⇒ Avoid sugar, red meat, alcohol, and refined carbohydrates.

⇒ Eat six cloves of raw garlic daily.

⇒ Drink 2 to 3 liters water daily.

⇒ Increase vegetables and fruit.

REMEDIES

⇒ Take blood-purifying herbs such as red clover, nettle, and clivers, in addition to antibiotic herbs such as echinacea, calendula, and goldenseal.

⇒ Take vitamin C and zinc three times a day.

OTHER

⇒ Hot compresses will bring the boil to a head so it can burst and drain. Use essential oils, mashed potato, and raw garlic, calendula, or slippery elm powder.

⇒ Wash hands and clean nails.

⇒ Apply tea tree oil or colloidal silver.

BRONCHITIS

WHAT IS IT?

Any word ending in "-itis" means something is inflamed; in the case of bronchitis, it is the bronchi, the air passages that lead to the lungs. Shaped like an upside-down tree, the trunk of the bronchi is your trachea or throat, then it bisects into two, one for each lung, thereafter becoming a network of smaller branches or passageways known as the bronchioles that eventually end in alveoli, the small sacs where oxygen moves from the air we breathe into the bloodstream. You can have just one attack of acute bronchitis or suffer symptoms that last more than three months, whereupon you have chronic bronchitis. If an attack of bronchitis is not managed, it can lead to pneumonia where the lungs themselves are affected. Chronic bronchitis may recur annually and if left untreated can result in emphysema when the damage has become irreversible.

SYMPTOMS

- ☑ Initial symptoms of acute bronchitis may be a chill, slight fever, back and muscle pain, and a sore throat.

- ☑ Gradually a cough develops, starting as dry and nonproductive progressing to productive.

- ☑ Acute bronchitis improves within three to five days, although the cough may linger for weeks.

- ☑ Chronic bronchitis involves excess secretion of mucus and eventually a thickening of the bronchial wall. When this happens, the wall becomes less flexible and prone to further infections, difficulty breathing, pneumonia, and ultimately heart failure—a path no one wants to tread.

WHAT CAUSES IT?

- ❑ Viral infection similar to a cold and flu virus.

- ❑ Bacterial infection, usually secondary to a viral infection.

- ❑ A reaction to an allergen or an irritating substance in the air such as dust, smoke, and ammonia.

WHAT TO DO

Diet

- ❑ Drink 2 to 3 liters of clear liquids daily. Fluid makes the mucus less sticky, enabling easy elimination. Hot clear fluids are good too, such as hot honey and lemon, herbal teas, broths, miso soup, spicy soup, and chicken soup.

- ❑ Try the following tea, which is excellent for any inflammation and infection of the respiratory tract, including bronchitis. Combine:
  - Juice of one lemon
  - Rind of half the lemon, chopped
  - 1 stick of cinnamon (optional)
  - 1 handful of fresh thyme, crushed
  - 3 cm of fresh ginger root, grated
  - 2 to 3 tablespoons of honey

  Pour 1 liter of boiling water over ingredients and let stand for five minutes.

- ❑ Avoid dairy products if they increase mucus. For some people they do, others not.

- ❑ Eat fresh pineapples and drink pineapple juice. Pineapples contain bromelain, a substance that helps to break down mucus.

- ❑ Foods that are good for the lungs and bronchi include onion, garlic, pepper, aniseed, and cinnamon.

Remedies

❏ Onion syrup helps to soothe the mucous membranes lining throat and lungs, and is also helpful if you are coughing a lot. Take one tablespoon of syrup every hour or so. This remedy is excellent for children with bronchitis—decrease the dose to one teaspoon.

To make onion cough syrup: roughly chop an onion (red, brown, or white) and place into a bowl. Pour over some runny honey until covered. Leave in warm place for a few hours or overnight. Onions are part of the Allium family, as is garlic, and they both have bug-killing and mucus-thinning properties.

❏ Herbs that help soothe the airways and boost immunity include mullein, grindelia, licorice, thyme, marshmallow, sundew, euphorbia, elder, white horehound, and garlic.

❏ Quercetin is known for its ability to reduce inflammation often associated with allergies and respiratory complaints.

❏ Cod liver oil, containing vitamin A (for mucous membrane support) and vitamin D (for immunity) is helpful for preventing coughs. Good for children too. Now available in capsule form, rather than the psychologically scarring spoonful dosage of yesteryear.

Other

❏ Humidifiers, available from pharmacies, help to moisten the airways and allow for a peaceful night's sleep. Add a dab of Vicks or a few drops of essential oil to the water in the humidifier: eucalyptus and/or thyme oil for an infection, lavender for a calming effect.

❏ If your cough is driving you (and those around you) mad, try the following breathing exercise. Coughing can be caused by a spasm in the smooth muscles that line the airway. Switching on the parasympathetic nervous system by a slight increase in carbon dioxide relaxes the smooth muscle and stops the coughing. Sounds simple? It is. Try this. Close your mouth. Take a small breath in, then out. With thumb and forefinger of one hand gently hold your nose closed for five seconds. Release and relax for ten seconds, breathing gently through your nose. Repeat ten times or until the coughing stops.

❏ The Buteyko technique will help reduce coughing. (See page 319.)

❏ Steam inhalation. Once or twice a day, and definitely before bed, have a steam inhalation to relax the airways and help elimination of mucus. Bring a pot of water to the boil. Add a teaspoon of Vicks or eucalyptus oil. Place the pot of water on a table. Sit close by, draping a towel over your head and the pot. Keeping some distance from the water to prevent burning, breathe the vapors in through your nose. Stay in this position for as long as comfortable.

AROMATHERAPY

❏ 2 drops of everlasting has cough-relieving and mucus-thinning properties as well as being anti-inflammatory.

❏ 4 drops of sandalwood—anti-inflammatory, antiseptic, antispasmodic, and anticongestive.

❏ 4 drops of cajeput—analgesic, febrifuge (fever reducing), antiseptic, expectorant, and antispasmodic.

❏ 6 drops of ravensara—antimicrobial, antiviral, antiseptic, immune stimulant, and expectorant.

Use this blend as a chest rub mixed into a neutral balm or gel, applying to the chest and back as needed. Use 6 drops of the essential oil blend on a tissue as a dry inhalation or in a bowl of steaming water as a steam inhalation. The essential oil blend can also be used as a room vaporizer.

DIET

➭ Drink at least 2 liters of clear fluid to allow for easy elimination of mucus. Hot fluids are best. Drink 3 cups of the lemon brew in the section on Diet above.

➭ Lung- and bronchi-friendly foods include pineapple, onion, garlic, pepper, aniseed, and cinnamon.

REMEDIES

➭ Onion cough syrup is soothing for the mucous membranes lining the airways. See recipe in section on Remedies above.

➭ Herbs for a cough include mullein, grindelia, licorice, thyme, marshmallow, sundew, euphorbia, elder, white horehound, and garlic. Take as tablet, tincture, or tea form.

OTHER

➭ A steam inhalation, especially at night, will help clear the airways and allow for a restful cough-free sleep. Bring a pot of water to the boil. Add a teaspoon of Vicks or eucalyptus oil. Place the pot of water on a table. Sit close by, draping a towel over your head and the pot. Keeping some distance from the water to prevent burning, breathe the vapors in through your nose.

BRUISING

WHAT IS IT?

Even if you invest in puffer jackets and padded pants, it is impossible to avoid life's sharp edges. The best you can do is to put on a brave face and hope the bruise looks impressive enough to win you a seat on the bus.

A bruise is blood that has accumulated under unbroken skin due to damage to underlying small blood vessels. Medically, a bruise is called a contusion. The area becomes deprived of oxygen for a short while, causing the bruise to change color due to oxidation, from initially red, purple, and blue to green, yellow, and brown. All the colors of the rainbow displayed on your very own leg.

SYMPTOMS

☑ After a knock or fall, the affected area soon becomes discolored due to the bleeding beneath the surface.

☑ The area will feel tender to touch and may be swollen.

☑ If a muscle is involved, movement will be restricted.

WHAT CAUSES IT?

❑ If something bumps you hard enough, it is perfectly normal to bruise, but some people bruise more easily than others.

❑ Blood-thinning drugs such as warfarin, aspirin, and even large doses of vitamin E (over 1,000 IU daily) may increase your tendency to bruise.

❑ Certain medications including steroid drugs will expedite bruising.

- The older you are, the more fragile your skin, the easier it bruises.

- Vitamin K helps clotting. A deficiency may increase your tendency to bruise.

- A deficiency of vitamin B_{12} (pernicious anemia) may result in bruising easily. Additionally, those with inflammatory bowel conditions or celiac disease often have difficulty absorbing vitamin B_{12} and as a result may bruise easily.

- Easy bruising is one of the early symptoms of the classic vitamin-C deficiency disease scurvy. While scurvy is reserved for eighteenth-century sailors, many twenty-first-century landlubbers eat no fruit and fewer vegetables, leaving them at risk of vitamin C deficiency.

- Excess alcohol intake increases bruising.

- Certain autoimmune, blood clotting, or liver conditions can cause easy bruising.

WHAT TO DO

Diet

- Eat plenty of vitamin C and bioflavonoid-rich foods: citrus fruits (eat the white pith as well), buckwheat, rye, berries, rosehip tea, rhubarb, chilies, and capsicum.

- Eat pineapples and drink pineapple juice. Pineapples contain bromelain, which helps to reduce bruising.

- Avoid alcohol, other than a glass or two of quality red.

- Vitamin K–rich foods include all green leafy vegetables and alfalfa sprouts.

- Vitamin B_{12} is found in meat and eggs.

Remedies

- Arnica. No home first-aid cupboard should be without the homoeopathic remedy arnica. As soon as you knock yourself, or after surgery, in fact any time your body takes a bruising, take some drops (spray or pillules) under the tongue. The more recent the bruising, the more often you take the remedy. Arnica cream (made from the herbal or homoeopathic arnica) can be applied to the bruise; avoid applying to broken skin. Arnica as a herb is toxic, so only homoeopathic arnica is recommended to take orally.

- The homoeopathic remedy Ruta will help for a bone bruise.

- A group of plant pigments or bioflavonoids are effective for strengthening blood vessel walls. These include: quercetin, rutin, and resveratrol. If you can find one or more combined with vitamin C, another substance that strengthens connective tissue, this would be an excellent supplement to take in the short term for one bruise, or longer term if you frequently suffer bruises or have another connective tissue condition such as varicose veins.

- Herbs that help treat and prevent capillary fragility include horse chestnut, ginkgo biloba, bilberry, grapeseed, butcher's broom, and pine bark.

- If you are found to be vitamin B_{12} deficient via a blood test, take a supplement or injection.

Other

- For the first few hours after the bruising, apply cold compresses. A bag of frozen peas wrapped in a towel is perfect. Compress for ten minutes, rest for twenty minutes; keep going until you get sick of it. In between, rub in some arnica or other herbal cream mentioned above.

- If you are bumping into things more than normal, and there is no other underlying health reason for your bruising, take a look inside your head. Are you rushing too much, or is your world going too fast? The bruising may be a warning sign to slow down. Collect your thoughts and move forward with grace and dignity.

AROMATHERAPY

❏ 2 drops of yarrow—a great hemostatic and astringent.

❏ 2 drops of German chamomile—has anti-inflammatory and analgesic properties.

❏ 3 drops of lavender—excellent as an analgesic and antispasmodic.

❏ 3 drops of geranium—hemostatic, anti-inflammatory, and astringent.

The blend is most effective in 15 ml sweet almond oil mixed with 5 ml arnica-infused oil. Apply gently to the bruised area as needed. You can also make it into a balm or gel. This blend is a beautiful blue, so don't be alarmed if the bruised area appears to be darker—it's ok!

AT A GLANCE

DIET

➠ Increase vitamin C and bioflavonoid foods, including oranges, lemons, mandarins (eat the white pith as well), buckwheat, rye, berries, rosehip tea, rhubarb, chilies, and capsicum.

➠ Enjoy pineapples and pineapple juice as they contain bromelain—very good for reducing swelling and bruising.

➠ Drink no more than one or two alcoholic drinks a day, otherwise you'll bruise more than your leg.

➠ Vitamin K–rich foods include all green leafy vegetables and alfalfa sprouts.

REMEDIES

➠ Arnica spray under the tongue as soon as the bruise happens.

➠ Bioflavonoids, quercetin, vitamin C, rutin, resveratrol, pine bark, and grapeseed extract.

➠ If you are a frequent bruiser, then go on a course of herbs to help strengthen blood vessel walls; these include horse chestnut, ginkgo biloba, bilberry, grapeseed, and butcher's broom.

OTHER

➠ Compress with ice or something cold.

➠ Are you trying to fit too much into your day?

BULIMIA

WHAT IS IT?

Meaning "great hunger," bulimia is marked by episodes of excessive eating and/or bingeing. After a binge, in an attempt to avoid putting on weight or as a punishment for eating in the first place, the sufferer will often induce vomiting or purge with laxatives. Binge foods are often high in starches and fat, such as sweet biscuits, ice cream, chips, cake, and diet soda, but vary from person to person. Bulimia is often a hidden condition, where your family and/or partner are unaware you are driven by such torment. The shame, guilt, and despair can be overwhelming. No one on the outside would suspect a bulimic has an eating disorder as their body shape often appears normal, unlike anorexia and exercise addiction—conditions with which bulimia shares similarities. All three disorders may coexist or alternate. It's a miserable and lonely existence. Often weekends revolve around a planned eating and purging alone, and an invitation out to a restaurant with friends can be fraught with foreboding because such an event, however innocuous to nonsufferers, can be a potential trigger.

SYMPTOMS

☑ Frequent induced vomiting causes inflammation and eventually may result in ulceration of the esophagus.

☑ The lining of the stomach will possibly be inflamed.

☑ Hydrochloric acid from the stomach contents can damage tooth enamel.

☑ If laxatives are overused, the bowel may ultimately become reliant on them, resulting in a lazy bowel.

☑ Frequent diarrhea means the loss of nutrients.

☑ Longer term side effects of bulimia (and anorexia) often result in bowel conditions such as irritable bowel syndrome.

☑ Due to the coinciding psychological aspect of this condition, anxiety and/or depression is often present.

☑ Vomiting will disrupt blood sugar levels. The erratic blood sugar levels may in turn trigger another binge/purge cycle.

☑ Excessive eating, vomiting, and purging affect neurotransmitters including serotonin (the calming chemical). In turn, this exacerbates mood disturbances.

☑ Low potassium (hypokalemia) and other micronutrient deficiencies can result from frequent vomiting and purging. This can affect the heart, and in extreme cases, may be fatal.

☑ Vomiting and diarrhea often result in dehydration.

☑ Fatigue and exhaustion can result as the binges can go on for hours.

WHAT CAUSES IT?

❑ The issues underlying bulimia are often similar to those of anorexia nervosa, and involve a host of emotional and psychological issues, sometimes relating to body image, sometimes not.

❑ An emotional shock in adolescence.

❑ Not feeling understood by emotionally remote and/or controlling parents.

❑ A radical change in diet during childhood, such as a food allergy diet or converting to vegetarianism, may predispose you to bulimia later in life.

WHAT TO DO

Although it sounds counterintuitive, it is more helpful *not* to focus on the bingeing. Bulimia is merely a symptom, overeating is the manifestation of an underlying cause. So, don't shoot the messenger. If you suffer from bulimia, the most important lesson you can learn is compassion. Compassion for yourself. When a binge happens, instead of beating up on yourself, and promising to be even stricter, try to forgive yourself. Know that you are doing what you can to get better, and it is a slow journey, with many ups and downs along the way. If it's hard to show compassion to yourself, try to imagine how you would respond to your best friend or someone you love if they were in a similar situation. While the journey toward wellness may take some time, the following advice is to help your body recover so that you can enjoy years of good health and well-deserved happiness. Interestingly, for many people, their eating disorder develops alongside a passion for cooking and feeding others.

Diet

Bulimia often feels like an addiction, but unlike those with an alcohol or drug addiction, the person with an eating disorder cannot avoid their drug of choice . . . food.

❏ Try to avoid becoming excessively hungry.

❏ It is wisest to avoid foods that you associate with overeating such as chips or chocolate. This varies from person to person.

❏ Now is not the time to become a gourmet chef. Stick to simple meals that contain some protein—for example, fish, eggs, legumes, and meat—with vegetables and carbohydrate such as rice, bread, and pasta.

❏ If you have had an eating disorder for some time, your appetite control mechanism will be out of kilter, and you will need to relearn how and when to eat. Learn what a "normal" portion of food looks like. Some people have never acquired these skills from their family of origin.

❏ An eating plan that involves eating several small simple meals throughout the day may be the best model to follow because it will not make you feel deprived, and your blood sugar levels will remain constant, reducing a tendency for craving. However, the road to recovery is all about learning what suits your body. If three meals a day is more appropriate, then go with that. However, once you have decided, you need to maintain your chosen routine.

❏ Don't judge yourself harshly if you do slip. You are not perfect. No one is. Forgive yourself and hop back in the saddle straight away . . . don't wait until tomorrow.

❏ Eat plain yogurt made with acidophilus or bifidus daily to help re-establish your intestinal microflora.

❏ If you are vomiting and using laxatives, make sure you drink plenty of water or you risk becoming dehydrated.

How Do You See Yourself?

Bombarded by media images of Botoxed celebrities and perfect models, it's not surprising those of us not blessed with such comeliness may feel inadequate. For some, this may lead to a disordered view of their body shape (body dysmorphia) and confusion about what food to eat—disordered eating. When does this disordered way of thinking morph into an eating disorder? When it takes over a large percentage of your thoughts and affects you on a day-to-day basis—coloring what you eat and wear, and how you exercise, which can change your perception of who you really are.

Remedies

❏ Slippery elm powder helps to line the stomach, is helpful after vomiting, and soothes the bowel after diarrhea caused by laxatives. Take one teaspoon of slippery elm powder in yogurt, mashed banana, or warm water morning and night.

❏ Take a multivitamin supplement. Powdered or liquid supplements may be better absorbed. Depending on frequency of vomiting and purging, you are quite likely deficient in a variety of micronutrients, in particular zinc and potassium. If vomiting is very frequent, an extra potassium supplement is recommended.

❏ The Bach flower remedy crab apple is recommended for those who have moments of self-loathing and disgust.

❏ The herbs meadowsweet, chamomile, lemon balm, ginger, and peppermint are kind to the digestive system. Have them in tincture or tea form daily.

❏ Glutamine is an amino acid that helps repair damaged gut cells. Take regularly. Often glutamine is found in supplements combined with other healing substances, including aloe vera, gotu cola, and zinc.

❏ Neurotransmitters, including the calming serotonin, are disrupted by bingeing and purging. Various herbs, including St. John's wort, passionflower, zizyphus, and magnolia will help to regulate this.

❏ The microflora in your digestive system will be traumatized by all the commotion going on with vomiting and/or frequent bowel movements. Take a teaspoon or three capsules of a good mixed probiotic each morning.

❏ Stomach acid is harsh on tooth enamel. After vomiting, rinse out your mouth with a tea- spoon of soda bicarbonate in water to buffer the acid; spit out the soda bicarbonate after rinsing so as not to disrupt the normal pH of the stomach.

❏ If your tummy bloats after eating a normal meal, take a digestive enzyme/hydrochloric acid tablet with every meal.

Other

❏ Seek counseling. The therapist you choose does not necessarily need to specialize in eating disorders; the eating disorder is merely a symptom of underlying issues. Make sure you feel understood by your counselor. You might need to kiss a few frogs before you find your therapist prince/princess. Once you feel understood, connected, and safe, stick with them.

❏ Bingeing may be an attempt to stuff down bad feelings. When you feel likely to binge, sit quietly for a moment and try to identify what you are feeling: you don't necessarily have to understand why. Write down these feelings, or draw them, or describe them to a good friend.

❏ There are support groups for eating disorders. Bulimia is an isolating condition, so it is good to connect with others who share similar experiences. All states have a foundation for eating disorders that can provide valuable resources and information.

❏ If neurotransmitters (like serotonin) are out of whack, it is much harder to gain equilibrium. If natural methods are not working for you, it may prove fruitful to talk to your doctor about taking a course of antidepressant medication, just until the chemical imbalance is sorted. Once you feel better and the behavior has receded, the medication can be reduced.

❏ Find the courage to confide in your dentist. They will be able to place a protective covering on your teeth each visit and suggest the right kind of toothpaste.

❏ Do something you love every day. As many people with eating disorders also happen to be perfectionists, this something should be a simple activity with no level of skill; for instance, lying on the grass in the sunshine, listening to a piece of music, petting a purring pussycat.

At a Glance

Diet

➠ Avoid known binge trigger foods. These may include biscuits, ice cream, or chips. It will vary with each person.

➠ Find which eating plan suits you; either small meals five times a day or three meals a day.

➠ Each meal needs to contain some protein and carbohydrate.

Remedies

➠ Take 1 teaspoon of slippery elm powder twice daily to protect stomach and esophagus lining from excessive vomiting.

➠ After vomiting, rinse the mouth with soda bicarbonate in water to minimize damage to teeth enamel.

➠ Take a multivitamin daily as you are most likely deficient in nutrients.

➠ The Bach flower remedy crab apple will help if you have moments of self-loathing, a common feeling with this condition.

➠ If you are bloated after meals, take a digestive enzyme and hydrochloric acid tablet with food.

➠ Lemon balm, meadowsweet, chamomile, ginger, and peppermint are all good calming herbs for the digestive system. Take them in tea or tincture form daily.

➠ St. John's wort, passionflower, and zizyphus will help restore nervous system equilibrium.

Other

➠ Find a good therapist. The journey to recovery can be hastened with good friends and wise counsel.

➠ Every day do something simple you enjoy such as listening to birdsong or walking your dog in the park.

➠ Join a support group. Bulimia is an isolating condition and you are not alone.

➠ As the wise Taoist philosopher Lao Tse (circa 600 B.C.) wrote, "The snow goose need not bathe to make itself white, / Neither need you do anything but be yourself."

CANCER

WHAT IS IT?

Cancer is not a new disease. Evidence of it appears in the skeletons of prehistoric man, and Galen, the prominent Greek physician of the second century AD, observed that "melancholic" women appeared to be especially susceptible to cancer of the breast, demonstrating an early recognition of the relationship between mind and body, as well as confirming the long history of a cancer that today affects one in eight women.

Most cells in the body are designed to die after they have achieved their cellular duties, a natural process known as apoptosis. Cancer cells do not follow this law of nature. Cancer cells are immortal; they do not die, they just keep dividing and dividing until their host organism falls off the perch. The DNA or genetic recipe in cancer cells has become mutated or damaged, so that the apoptosis message is not encoded into the dividing cells.

Cancer generally takes years to develop, a gradual progression rather than a spontaneous formation of a tumor. Viewing cancer as a chronic (long-term) disease encourages you to make appropriate changes such as decreasing stress, improving diet, and losing weight, all of which reduce your risk of developing cancer.

Cancer is the second most common cause of death in the United States, accounting for about one in four deaths. More than 1.6 million new cancer cases were diagnosed in 2013 in the United States, and over 580,000 people died of cancer—nearly 1,600 people daily. There are over 100 different kinds of cancers. In the United States, the most commonly diagnosed cancers (in order) are prostate, breast, lung, and colorectal cancers. Although cancer diagnoses are becoming more commonplace, the good news is that as knowledge about cancer is increasing exponential-

ly, there is earlier detection and treatments are proving more successful and less injurious to the rest of one's health. Being diagnosed with cancer is no longer the death sentence it used to be, but it's still not a diagnosis anyone wants.

Cancers are named according to the tissue in which they originate:

❑ Carcinoma. Eighty to ninety percent of all cancers are this type. It develops from epithelial tissue, which is the tissue that covers and lines the body, so this can affect the bowel, the skin, the lungs, and the ducts of breast tissue.

❑ Leukemia is a blood cancer that develops from bone marrow.

❑ Lymphoma develops from lymph tissue.

❑ Sarcoma develops in connective tissue including muscle and bone.

Cancer cells commonly grow into a mass known as a tumor. Some cells from the tumor may disseminate (metastasize) and colonize other parts of the body, ultimately interfering with the functioning of other tissues and organs. The tumor is capable of creating its own blood supply (known as angiogenesis).

WHAT CAUSES IT?

❑ Obesity. More often viewed as associated with heart disease and diabetes (which it is) or an aesthetic issue (in our culture it is), being overweight is also a significant risk factor for cancer. A number of mechanisms explain the link between being overweight and getting cancer. For starters, fat, particularly belly (visceral) fat, does not just create difficulty squeezing into skinny jeans, it is metabolically active in a bad way, sending out substances that are inflammatory. Inflammation has been found to be a risk factor for cancer, possibly by switching on the gene (mentioned above). Additionally, being overweight also increases secretion of the hormone insulin. Insulin is a growth factor, an agent that increases cell growth, which is exactly what we don't want with cancer cells that are already growing out of control. And finally, increased body fat increases sex hormones, linked with certain cancers including breast and prostate. All in all, losing weight is an excellent cancer prevention strategy.

❏ Genetics is the cause of only 5 to 10 percent of cancers. The influence of lifestyle and diet is much greater. A good example of this is the story of Japanese migrants to Hawaii. Japanese living in Japan have a relatively low rate of breast and colon cancer; however, within one generation, Japanese migrants who moved to Hawaii developed the same risk of these cancers as their American compatriots, making an unhealthy transition from sushi and soy to burgers and fries.

❏ Lowered immunity. The formation of cancer cells is a moment-to-moment occurrence in the body, but a healthy immune system, with adequate antioxidants, enzymes, and nutrients, is able to disarm them. If the immune system is compromised—for instance, by an ongoing infection or chronic stress—it is less likely to rise to the challenge of eliminating errant cancer cells. Certain drugs (e.g., cortisone) can also jeopardize your immune response, creating a weaker defense against cancer cells. Research has shown a link between viruses and some cancers. For example, the HIV virus often precedes Kaposi's sarcoma. The same seems to be true for the hepatitis B virus and liver cancer, and the papilloma virus (genital warts) predisposes women to cervical cancer.

❏ Stress. Many people with cancer can recall an episode of great stress or shock that preceded their diagnosis, sometimes by many years. The stress could have been a bankruptcy, the death of a relative, spouse, or close friend, or a relationship breakup. The science of psychoneuroimmunology (psycho–mind; neuro–nervous and endocrine systems; immunology–immune system) verifies the link between our emotions, nervous system, and immune system. Nonpsychological stressors also impact the body, including shift work, poor sleep, infections, accidents, and pain. Stress, acute or chronic, takes its toll on the immune system, leaving you more vulnerable to cancer.

❏ Excess alcohol. Alcohol itself is carcinogenic. Additionally, alcohol increases the activity of enzymes that convert precarcinogens into carcinogens. And finally, heavy drinkers often have a poor diet, deficient in protective nutrients found in vegetables and fruit.

❏ Smoking. There is a significant correlation between smoking cigarettes and many kinds of cancer, particularly lung cancer.

CANCER: GENETICS VERSUS LIFESTYLE

The genes we inherit from our mother and father in the form of DNA encodes our potential. However, not every gene is expressed or turned on. Even if you inherit a gene for a particular cancer, it doesn't mean you will necessarily get that cancer. Enter the new science of epigenetics that states that a gene needs first to be turned on before it can be expressed. Poor lifestyle and diet choices turn on that switch. Many of the foods and remedies mentioned below appear to work by stopping the expression of cancer-related genes.

- Inflammation in the body is thought to be one of the triggers for cancer. Inflammation can come from many sources, including being overweight, stressed, and having infections, arthritis, and autoimmune conditions.

- Excess sun exposure and exposure to other forms of radiation.

- Exposure to toxins from within the body (such as viruses) and the environment (such as pollution, heavy metals).

- Diabetes. With diabetes there is an increase in blood sugar and insulin levels, which can translate as food for the cancer cells, fueling them to grow. (See Diet below.)

WHAT TO DO

Diet

- Avoid all refined sugar as cancer cells are addicted to sugar. It's not that normal cells don't love glucose (the major blood sugar) as fuel, but cancer cells can't live without it. Other body cells (except nerve and brain cells) are happy enough to get their energy from other sources, predominantly fatty acids. A diet that reduces sugar and insulin in the body will go far toward the goals of reducing fuel and growth factors for cancer cells. The low-starch eating plan outlined on page 245 is a good place to start.

- Alcohol. More than a glass of alcohol a day increases your risk of cancer.

- Eating more than 500 grams of red meat weekly increases your risk of cancer.

- Avoid processed meats. Studies have shown a link with eating deli or processed meats and cancer, so it is advisable to cut down on bacon, lunch meats such as bologna, ham, salami, prosciutto, and sausages.

- Avoid charred or overcooked meat as the charring creates two carcinogens: polycyclic aromatic hydrocarbons (PAHs) and heterocyclic amines (HCAs)

- Reduce animal fats. People who have a high animal fat intake have higher death rates from

---

STAGES OF CANCER

Rudolf Steiner (1861–1925), the Austrian philosopher and founder of anthroposophy (spiritual beliefs about education, agriculture, and health), believed that there are three stages of cancer. The first stage may be initiated by a physical, psychic, or psychological shock, after which the person becomes fatigued or an insomniac. The second stage is the appearance of the tumor itself, which may or may not be diagnosed then. The third stage is the metastases, whereby the cancer travels to other parts of the body and infiltrates tissues and organs.

Although Steiner's second and third stages coincide with the conventional medical model, his stage one description is interesting. It implies that something happens before the appearance of the cancer. If there was some way we could identify stage one, this would be the very best time to start treatment, before stages two and three progress. Unfortunately, the symptoms of fatigue, malaise, and sleep problems are vague, all too common, and too easy to attribute to other causes. Nevertheless, we should take notice of the messages our bodies give. If you feel tired, you should rest; if you have undergone a great shock or sadness, don't underestimate its effect on your body and do what you can to nourish your spirit.

cancer of the colon, breast, and prostate than populations with a low fat consumption. The type of fat is also important. One study showed a 200 percent increase in breast cancer when beef and pork were consumed five or six times per week. Animal fat (except fish) appears to be more of a risk than plant oils. The fat found in fish, avocado, nuts, and seeds is protective, so you don't need to scrimp on these fats.

❏ Reduce calories. Frugal gourmands live longer. Those who consistently undereat (not starve) are less likely to have cancer.

❏ Increase your fiber intake. Fiber is not a nutrient as it is not absorbed across the intestinal tract nor does it provide us with calories, vitamins, and so forth. Nevertheless, fiber plays a vital role in our health particularly in prevention of cancer. Fiber helps the stool move through the colon, decreasing the transit time from mouth to anus. This decreases the time in which carcinogenic substances are in contact with the bowel wall, being absorbed into the bloodstream or affecting the bowel wall itself. Although we don't digest fiber, various beneficial bacteria living within the colon do enjoy snacking on fiber. Increased dietary fiber also lowers circulating estrogen levels, a risk factor for breast cancer. The by-products of their feast include substances such as butyric acid, which has an anticancer effect. Additionally, these by-products change the pH of the bowel environment, pushing it in an anticancer direction. There are many types of fiber. Don't just shake a handful of bran over your Cocoa Puffs; eat food that has its original fiber intact, such as legumes, whole grains (oats, brown rice, quinoa), vegetables, and fruit including the peel and seeds.

❏ Given the previous few recommendations, eating a plant-based diet is sounding like a good move.

❏ Raw food. Eat at least half your vegetables and most of your fruit raw. All minerals, enzymes, and vitamins are more abundant in raw food. Additionally, raw food has an abundance of the elusive "life force." This naturopathic concept imbues certain foods with subtle vibrational or energetic, health-giving qualities. For instance, alfalfa sprouts have more life force than a sponge cake, and an apple picked and eaten from the tree has more life force than a frozen reheated apple pie. Some foods, such as legumes and grains, however, need a certain amount of cooking before they are digestible.

❏ Juicing is a clever way of getting a large amount of vitamins, minerals, and phytonutrients in one glass from raw vegetables and fruit. The two negatives with juicing is losing out on the fiber, and cleaning the juicer. One or two juices daily are recommended. Following are a couple of classic juices, but after a while you will develop your own favorites.

• Green juice: to a base of green apples add a variety of kale, parsley, celery, beetroot leaves, cucumber, and/or cabbage.

• Red juice: to a base of carrots add a variety of beetroot, ginger, and/or red cabbage.

• Drink a juice at meal times to prevent a rapid increase in blood sugar and insulin levels.

❏ Increase alkalizing foods in the diet. Cancer cells prefer a more acidic environment than normal cells. In fact, cancer cells, as a consequence of their diet of sugar only, create this acidic milieu themselves. The pH is a measure of acidity/alkalinity in a cell environment. Normal pH around cells is 7.4, whereas the pH around cancer cells is between 6.7 and 7.1.

In regards to proper pH balance, the dietary goal is quite simple—make sure that you have a higher intake of alkaline-producing foods than acid-producing foods. Basically, an alkaline diet is one rich in vegetables and fruit, while avoiding an excess of grains, meat, eggs, and dairy. There is a difference between acidic foods and acid-forming foods. For example, while foods like lemons and citrus fruits may taste acidic they actually have an alkalizing effect on the body. What determines the pH nature of the food in the body is the metabolic end products when it is digested (sometimes called "metabolic ash"). For example, the citric acid in citrus fruit is metabolized in the body to its alkaline form (citrate) and may even be converted to bicarbonate—also alkaline. It's important to remember that, like everything in life, it's about balance. We need to eat some acid-forming foods too. See list of acid/alkaline foods in Appendix E.

❑ Fasting can be powerful medicine. A supervised water fast of seven days or more may prove helpful. As cancer cells are obligatory glucose users, the lack of food on a fast will hopefully stop cancer cells from multiplying. After fasting for two days, your body biochemistry changes whereby your cells, in particular the brain and nervous tissue, are able to accept some fatty acids from stored fat, instead of relying totally on glucose. Very little glucose in the body leaves the cancer cells to starve. Another reason why fasting is recommended is that it frees the energy formerly used in digestion, making more of it available to our immune system. A true fast can be deeply meditative and many people fast for spiritual reasons. Do not fast if you have lost a lot of weight, are pregnant, or have kidney disease. Do not fast on your own without qualified supervision. It is vital to rest during a fast of this kind. There are centers that specialize in therapeutic fasting.

Remedies

A diagnosis of cancer strikes fear and desperation into patients, their friends, and family. Unfortu-nately, desperation can result in seeking desperate measures, including being at the mercy of peddlers of hope who are more interested in financial gain than true healing. This is unfortunately the case in the world of natural therapies too. My advice is to be deeply suspicious of anyone offering a cure. However, natural therapies have much to offer the person dealing with cancer—especially as a preventative measure, but also to support the body during and after conventional treatments of surgery, chemotherapy, and radiotherapy and to protect against future reoccurrence of cancer.

Vitamins and Minerals

When antioxidants and their protective role against cancer first gained prominence, many people starting taking megadoses of supplemental antioxidants. However, years down the track, it now appears that large amounts of single nutrients do not help, in fact they may be detrimental. The best advice is to focus on eating a good diet with a wide range of fresh unprocessed food. The following antioxidant nutrients have shown to be helpful in the prevention of cancer. Take in moderation, and where possible, increase the foods containing that nutrient (see food source table on page 307) in preference to taking a supplement: beta-carotene, coenzyme Q_{10} (CoQ_{10}), selenium, vitamins A, C, D, and E, and zinc.

Herbs

Thousands of herbs have anticancer properties, whether by virtue of containing antioxidants, improving immunity, or helping the body deal with stress. Following are a few that have some or all of these properties: andrographis, bilberry, chamomile, dong quai, echinacea, feverfew, garlic, Korean and Siberian ginseng, goldenseal, rhodiola, rosemary, thuja, turmeric, St. Mary's thistle, schizandra, and withania.

FOODS THAT HAVE BEEN SHOWN TO PREVENT CANCER

The best advice is to increase fresh vegetables and fruit in your diet, rather than devoting your diet to "anticancer" foods. However, the following foods have been shown to contain substances that reduce your risk of cancer. Include a range of them in your weekly diet.

❑ The *Brassica* family of vegetables, including broccoli, Brussels sprouts, cabbage, Chinese cabbage, collards, horseradish, kale, kohlrabi, mustard, radish, rutabaga, turnip, and watercress contain cancer-preventing substances called indoles and isothiocyanates, which stimulate coenzyme glutathione to bind and neutralize carcinogens. Indoles appear to have an estrogen-blocking effect similar to Tamoxifen, the drug often given to prevent recurrence of breast cancer.

❑ Garlic, onion, leeks, and other members of the *Allium* (lily) family contain concentrated sulfur compounds that activate glutathione, the detoxifying coenzyme, and have been shown to destroy cancer cells without damaging healthy cells. There have been over thirty anticancer properties identified in this delicious and odiferous group.

❑ Resveratrol is an excellent antioxidant for reducing the effects of carcinogens. It is mainly found in blueberries, cranberries, grapes (red and purple), peanuts (with skins on), pistachios, and rhubarb. Resveratrol appears to be able to switch on apoptosis (the process of natural cell death discussed earlier).

❑ Brazil nuts are a good source of selenium. Selenium is needed by the super antioxidants of the glutathione peroxidase enzyme family. Selenium also may help reduce angiogenesis, the process where tumors create their own system of blood vessels that provide nutrients for the cancer to further grow.

❑ Fermented foods such as miso, yogurt, sauerkraut, and pickles.

❑ Seaweed, which contains fucoidan; Japanese studies have shown fucoidan to be protective against cancer.

❑ Soy, which contains phytoestrogens. A diet high in phytoestrogens appears to prevent cancers that are influenced by estrogen, such as breast, uterine, and ovarian cancers. There is an extremely low incidence of breast cancer in Japan, where the diet is high in traditional soy foods. There is a lot of controversy about whether soy does indeed help prevent cancer. While the jury is still out, it may be best to include traditionally consumed soy products (such as tempeh, small amounts of tofu, miso, and natto), rather than drinking large amounts of soy milk and soy protein powders (not traditional foods).

❑ Tomatoes contain lycopene (as do guavas, rosehips, watermelon, papaya, and pink grapefruit) a carotenoid, a powerful antioxidant. Heating increases the presence of this antioxidant, which has proven to be beneficial in the prevention of prostate cancer.

❑ Mushrooms, including reishi, shiitake, maitake, coriolus, cordyceps, field mushroom, and porio cocos. These contain beta-glucan polysaccharides, which supports immune function and have an antitumor action.

❑ Turmeric is well known for its anti-inflammatory abilities. Curcumin, a compound found in this yellow spice, is found to influence apoptosis as well as reduce inflammation, a possible trigger for cancer.

❑ Green tea contains epigallocatechin gallate (EGCG), an antioxidant found to be useful in reducing the risk of heart disease, neurodegenerative disease, and cancer.

Other

☐ On first receiving a cancer diagnosis, most people go into a state of understandable shock. Although you may feel pressured to make hasty decisions about treatment options, try to keep a steady head and gather as much information as you can, even a second opinion. It is easy to be overwhelmed by all that is happening. Bad news makes us hard of hearing. You do not remember everything said during a consultation at the best of times. Take notes, ask questions, and if possible, bring along a (calm) friend or relative with you to consultations, so you don't get forget things.

☐ Exercise increases oxygen in the body. Try gentle exercise such as walking, swimming, or yoga—anything that promotes good breathing. Cancer cells are predominantly anaerobic, meaning they don't thrive on oxygen, like normal cells. Gentle exercise also supports the immune system.

☐ Meditation, positive thinking, deep relaxation, or prayer stills the body, allowing the immune system to grow stronger. Meditation also reduces anxiety, reducing the inhibitory effect that the stress hormone cortisol has on the immune system. Adrenaline, another stress hormone, is thought to increase free radical production. Anything that reduces stress is useful so consider relaxation tapes, meditation courses, yoga (which emphasizes meditation), chanting, or praying. Try to include whatever practice you decide to follow every day.

A particular type of meditation, creative visualization, is an excellent way of targeting cancer cells. Some people visualize their white blood cells as soldiers in an army, destroying any and all cancer cells. Others visualize the tumor slowly shrinking and shrinking until nothing is left. Create your own scenarios.

☐ Counseling and/or support groups may prove invaluable.

☐ Give up smoking.

☐ It is not uncommon to hear people say that they are grateful for the challenges that cancer has brought them. In hindsight, being diagnosed and dealing with cancer has been a catalyst in their lives, changing attitudes, relationships, and priorities. If it means leaving the job you have endured for the last twelve years, do it. If it means sitting on top of a mountain, do it. If it means leaving an unhappy relationship, do it.

DIET

➡ Increase fresh fruit and vegetables and whole grains as these whole foods contain substances that protect against cancer.

➡ Foods that have proven anticancer properties include those from the Allium family (onions, garlic, leeks), Brassica family (broccoli, Brussels sprouts, cauliflower), and berries.

➡ Avoid deli meats as they contain cancer-containing substances.

➡ Avoid sugar and added sugar in your diet.

➡ Eat less animal protein (red meat, chicken) and more plant-based protein (legumes, nuts, and seeds).

REMEDIES

➡ Focus more on your diet than supplements; however, the following in moderate doses may be helpful: vitamins A, C, D, and E, CoQ_{10}, selenium, and zinc.

➡ Herbal remedies that improve your ability to deal with stress (adaptogens) and enhance immunity (colds and flu) are recommended, including echinacea, rhodiola, Siberian ginseng, and withania.

OTHER

➡ Learning ways to minimize and handle stress is a major factor in reducing your risk of cancer.

➡ Meditate.

➡ Don't smoke.

➡ Lose weight if you are carrying excess pounds.

CANCER TREATMENTS (DEALING WITH)

I believe the role of a natural therapist is to support the patient in whatever path they choose to take with their cancer treatment. With the increase in cancer diagnoses, modern medicine has devoted many keen minds and not an insignificant number of dollars to the treatment of cancer, and depending on the cancer, by pursuing medical treatment, the prognosis is better than it ever has been. Sometimes, however, I am reminded of the quote by British philosopher Francis Bacon (1561–1626), "Cure the disease and kill the patient."

Natural remedies can be very effective in supporting you during this time, increasing energy and immunity and reducing side effects. The interaction of herbs and supplements with chemotherapy drugs is still being investigated, and some cancer specialists prefer their patients to desist from taking anything other than the chemotherapy drugs. Other specialists actually recommend taking some supplements. So all of this conflicted advice is confusing. I would suggest you ask the medical team looking after your case whether and what they are happy for you to take during your treatment. If they are not keen on natural medicine, don't fret. Eat a fabulous diet, knowing you will launch into your herbs when the treatment is over.

WHAT TO DO

Surgery

Surgery is often the first medical treatment for cancer. Its purpose is usually to remove the primary cancer. Sometimes it is also necessary in later stages to reduce the size of a tumor causing pain or obstruction.

Diet

❑ Avoid eating sugar as it dramatically decreases immune function (by affecting phagocyte activity) and slows healing.

❑ Protein is needed for repairing tissue. Protein needs increase twofold during this time. This does not necessarily mean eating double the amount of food, as most of us consume more than adequate protein for our day to day needs, but it does mean keeping an eye on including protein in each meal. Meat, chicken, fish, dairy, legumes, seeds, and nuts are all protein foods.

❑ Recovering from surgery is a time of convalescence. Suitable foods include chicken and vegetable soup, brown rice, miso soup, and steamed fish. The recovery diet should always be governed by the patient's appetite: a hearty one is a good sign.

Remedies

❑ Arnica is the first-aid homoeopathic remedy. Take a few drops or spray as soon as possible after the surgery. Arnica increases the rate of healing exponentially, reducing internal and external bruising. Take at least three times daily for the first week after the operation.

❑ Rescue Remedy (the Bach flower combination remedy), and specifically Star of Bethlehem, which is in Rescue Remedy, calms the psychological shock. Take before surgery and whenever you are feeling anxious to calm the nerves.

❑ Support the immune system with a course of immune-boosting herbs that may include one or more of the following: astragalus, echinacea, olive leaf, and cat's claw. Start taking these as soon as you know you need surgery, but stop five days before the operation. This is general advise for all herbs and supplements so that there is no chance of increased bleeding during and postsurgery. Start taking again as soon as possible after surgery.

❑ Vitamin C and zinc are a good team when it comes to boosting immunity and promoting healing. Take one-half to 1 gram of C twice daily and 22 mg of zinc once daily. Take up until the day of the surgery (these are okay to do so) and as soon as possible afterward.

❑ After the operation add some adaptogen herbs; these remarkable herbs help the body recover from any stress, including that of surgery. Choose from these beauties: withania, Siberian ginseng, licorice, and panax ginseng.

❑ If there is swelling and inflammation, and there probably will be, take a strong bioflavonoid supplement that contains quercetin twice daily.

❑ Anesthetics that knock us out for the count during the operation also knock the body around afterward, particularly the liver. Give it a little support by drinking dandelion root tea, lemon juice, and water in the morning, stay away from alcohol and take liver herbs for a week or so including St. Mary's thistle, dandelion root, bupleurum, globe artichoke, and turmeric.

❑ If antibiotics are prescribed postsurgery, re-establish healthy gut flora by taking a good probiotic supplement during and for a week after the course of antibiotics.

Other

Allow yourself sufficient time to recover; surgery is a shock to the body.

CHEMOTHERAPY

A derivative of mustard gas used in World War I, chemotherapy was first used in the 1940s. It became somewhat unpopular due to its common side effect, death. Thankfully, more effective and less traumatic chemotherapy agents have been discovered in the decades since. Chemotherapy is the use of drugs to kill cancer cells. It is often used as an adjunct to other treatments such as surgery and radiation therapy. There are more than sixty different drugs used for various forms of cancer. Generally given in combination to reduce the risk of cancer cells becoming resistant to them, nowadays chemotherapy is more and more specific to the cancer cells and less deadly to the rest of the body. Nevertheless, chemotherapy does suppress the immune system and has several nasty side effects. Chemotherapy drugs target the fast-dividing cells of cancer so other fast-dividing cells in the body, such as those lining the digestive tract, bone marrow, and hair follicles, also bear the brunt. This explains the common symptoms of digestive problems (mouth ulcers, heartburn, nausea, diarrhea), reduction of red and white blood cell production, and hair loss.

Common side effects of chemotherapy include:

❑ Mouth ulcers

❑ Unpleasant taste in mouth

❑ Constipation and/or diarrhea

❑ Nausea and vomiting

❑ Lack of appetite

❑ Nail damage

❑ Reflux

❑ Lack of concentration ("chemo brain")

❑ Fatigue

❑ Anemia

❑ Pins and needles

❑ Lowered immunity due to lowered white blood cells

❑ Hair loss

❑ Fluid retention

❑ Heart palpitations

❑ Depression and/or anxiety

Diet

❑ Chemotherapy is a grueling marathon that often takes weeks or months to complete. And like a marathon, to last the distance in tip-top form, it is vital your diet be the best it can be. Adopt the recommendations stated earlier.

❑ To deal with nausea, eat very small meals quite often.

❑ Try to drink one fresh green vegetable juice daily.

❑ Avoid sugar.

Remedies

❑ Slippery elm helps to heal and protect mucous membranes that line the intestines. The bowel is most often affected in chemotherapy. Keeping the intestines as healthy as possible allows the nutrients from your fabulous diet to be absorbed. Slippery elm is particularly helpful for reflux. Take one teaspoon of slippery elm powder (not the tablets as you want the healing to start from the throat down) twice daily, before meals. It can be mixed with warm water, mashed into a banana, added to oatmeal, or mixed with yogurt. Slippery elm is a fiber and is not absorbed across the intestinal wall. This means it cannot interact with chemotherapy drugs that are given intravenously. If the drugs are taken by mouth, take the slippery elm on another day or twelve hours away from the medicine.

❑ Probiotics. Chemotherapy targets the rapidly dividing cells of cancer; unfortunately, other rapidly dividing yet healthy cells are also affected, such as those lining the gastrointestinal tract. This will have a negative impacts on the gastrointestinal microflora. Taking a probiotic supplement during and after chemotherapy is recommended and may prevent diarrhea.

❑ Low iron is a common symptom of chemotherapy. This is because newly forming blood cells are affected by the medication. Your iron levels will be determined by a blood test. If you are low in iron, take a nonconstipating form of iron such as the liquid tonic irons available in health food stores. See Anemia on page 10.

❑ Vitamin C and zinc lozenges. Sucking on three to four lozenges daily will help prevent and treat mouth ulcers.

❑ Generally, antiemetic (antinausea) drugs are given along with chemotherapy. Ginger may help a little with any lingering nausea, but is not a replacement for the antiemetic medicine. Drink ginger tea throughout the day. Ginger tea is made by grating or finely slicing 2 to 3 cm of peeled fresh ginger root, adding to a teapot or plunger, and pouring on 1 liter of boiling water. Allow to seep for eight minutes. You can make a day's worth by placing the ginger in a thermos with hot water; it is more delicious and effective the stronger it gets.

❑ Manuka honey may help to heal mouth ulcers.

❑ Psyllium husks help treat both constipation and diarrhea. The water-soluble fiber helps to solidify the stool and slow down transit time in the case of diarrhea, and will increase the size of stool and increase transit time in the case of constipation. Take two tablespoons in water each day. Drink a glass of water afterward.

❑ Herbal bitters improve appetite and digestion. Take one teaspoon in a glass of water and sip before dinner.

❑ B complex. A B-complex supplement will help supply a little energy. Folic acid (part of the B complex) is of particular importance as it is often depleted by the chemotherapy drugs. Take one strong B-complex vitamin each morning.

❑ Echinacea. A good herb for boosting immunity. It is important to support the immune system during this time, and echinacea helps keep white blood cell (WBC) levels high. Before each chemotherapy bout, WBC levels are taken, and if they are too low the chemotherapy is delayed. Other immune-supporting herbs include cat's claw and andrographis,

❑ Ginkgo biloba helps improve concentration and memory, which often are affected by "chemo brain." Ginkgo is also good for the circulation and may be helpful for the side effect of pins and needles.

❑ Adaptogen herbs help the body deal with stress of any kind. They improve energy levels and maintain immunity—if not during chemotherapy, definitely afterward. They include: astragalus, Korean and Siberian ginseng, and withania.

Other

❑ Acupuncture can help improve energy and reduce many of the side effects of chemotherapy. As it is not ingested (very unwise if you choose to swallow the needles!) there is not the possibility of interaction with chemotherapy drugs.

❑ Regular massage helps any aches and pains and is a nurturing treat during this difficult time.

❑ Several countries allow the medical use of marijuana to help reduce nausea caused by chemotherapy, and also to relieve pain. Not presently legal in most U.S. states, although this may change in the future.

- You may not feel particularly perky, but exercise will help give you a little energy, improve your sleep, and help reduce constipation,

- Meditation is an important skill to acquire and cultivate. Chemotherapy affects both mind and mood, both of which meditation helps to calm.

POSTCHEMOTHERAPY

Diet

- Eat a predominantly plant-based diet.
- Follow suggestions for cancer prevention on page 65.

Remedies

- After the celebrations (a smidgeon of alcohol with bubbles is highly recommended to mark the end of the long, hard haul of chemo), now is the time to detox. The liver and kidneys have done a sterling job and need to recuperate after dealing with such heavy-duty medication. Herbs for the liver include St. Mary's thistle, turmeric, yellow dock, burdock, globe artichoke, and dandelion root, to be taken in a tincture or tablet form.

- Adaptogen herbs (discussed earlier) help to restore immunity and vitality. Take for at least two months after treatment has ceased. These include astragalus, Korean and Siberian ginseng, and withania.

Other

- Avoid exercise that may overstretch or strain surrounding tissue.

RADIOTHERAPY

Radiotherapy involves directing a series of gamma rays at a specific area. It may be applied as a solo therapy, an adjunct to surgery, or combined with chemotherapy. It can also be applied as palliative treatment to reduce the size of a tumor causing pain or obstruction.

The purpose of radiotherapy is to damage and destroy dividing cells, but it also destroys normal cells in the neighborhood. Side effects can include fatigue, nausea, and vomiting, loss of appetite, diarrhea, cystitis, sore, discolored ("burned") and peeling skin, lower immunity, and hemorrhage. Delayed side effects include loss of hair, nerve damage, and blood vessel fragility (easy bruising).

Diet

- Garlic and seaweed helps protect healthy cells from the effect of radiation. Garlic sushi anyone?
- Diet as for cancer on page 62.

Remedies

- If you don't like garlic, or don't eat it every day, take a garlic supplement throughout your treatment. Seaweed also has the same protective properties, so add to soups or salads, or take as a salad.

- Adaptogen herbs—astragalus, Korean and Siberian ginseng, rhodolia, and withania—help the body deal with effects the radiation.

- After radiation treatment, there are various topical applications that will help prevent burns and promote healing of the tissue. These include:
  - cold plain flour dusted across the radiated area
  - white or green clay powder, mixed with water into a paste
  - aloe vera gel
  - vitamin E oil

Other

❏ Try to exercise a little every day, avoiding over-stretching or exerting muscles nearby the area being treated—for example, no chest presses if you are receiving radiation for breast cancer.

❏ Meditate and reduce stress.

AT A GLANCE

DIET

⇒ Eat as nutritious a diet as you can. Fresh vegetables, fruit, legumes, and whole grains.

⇒ Although you may feel like "treating" yourself with cakes and sweets, they really are not helping your body to recover. Buy instead some delicious fruit or treat yourself with some flowers instead.

⇒ Avoid sugar.

⇒ If you feel too ill to eat a meal, try instead a small bowl of soup or perhaps a vegetable juice.

REMEDIES

⇒ If you are having chemotherapy always ask your team at the hospital what supplements if any are allowed.

⇒ Garlic helps immune system and protects healthy cells against the effects of radiation.

⇒ Vitamin C, zinc, echinacea, and andrographis will help boost your immune system. Vitamin C and zinc lozenges are good for mouth ulcers.

⇒ Probiotics are recommended, particularly after antibiotics have been administered postsurgery and especially if you are on chemotherapy.

⇒ Psyllium husks may help with both diarrhea and constipation.

⇒ The adaptogen herbs such as withania, Siberian ginseng, rhodiola, and Panax ginseng will help you get through this time and to convalesce safterward

OTHER

⇒ Now is the time to nurture yourself. Say no to any extra demands.

⇒ Meditate, or at the very least engage in activities that calm you.

⇒ The entire process from being diagnosed with cancer and throughout treatment is inherently stressful. Regular counseling can be beneficial. Talking things through with a non family member or friend can be liberating.

CANDIDA

WHAT IS IT?

Candida albicans is a yeast/fungus that lives within all humans. Known as a commensal microorganism, in good times, candida happily goes about its yeasty little life causing us no trouble at all. It's when candida gets too big for its own boots, expanding its fungal empire, that symptoms appear.

Yeasts, related to molds and fungi, prefer to live in a warm, dark, and moist environment, so the intestines, vagina, and even between soggy toes make ideal fungal hideaways. The trouble is when the community expands, *Candida albicans* is able to penetrate the lining of the bowel with thin thready roots. This has a twofold effect of creating a "leaky gut," where toxins found within the intestine are given access to the bloodstream, and the byproducts of candida (methane and acetaldehyde) enter the bloodstream. It is these substances that explain the diverse symptoms of candida ranging from bloating to dizziness.

SYMPTOMS

☑ Skin problems. These include pimples, eczema, psoriasis, tinea, jock itch and other fungal infections, swimmer's ear, itchy nose, and body odor.

☑ All in the mind. These are symptoms where you feel slightly off-color and may feel that you are imagining it or it is down to feeling flat. These include feeling drained, craving sugar, unable to concentrate, poor memory, frequent mood swings, headache, feeling "spacy" or "unreal," depression, and lethargy.

☑ Immune system. Signs of a faulty immune system include allergies and sensitivities and/or depleted immune system.

☑ Respiratory tract. These include wheezing or shortness of breath, sinus, and hay fever.

☑ Gastrointestinal tract. These include bad breath, constipation, diarrhea, abdominal pain, bloating, oral thrush, and itching around anus.

☑ Nerves and muscles. Sometimes there might be sensations such as numbness, tingling, muscular aches, muscular weakness, and fatigue.

☑ Reproductive and urinary system. Symptoms can include vaginal thrush, including itching and burning sensations or discharge, prostatitis, impotence, loss of sexual desire, menstrual problems, premenstrual syndrome (PMS), and recurrent cystitis.

WHAT CAUSES IT?

❑ Most people have had a course (or twelve) of antibiotics in their lives. As candida is not a bacterium but a yeast, it survives a dose of antibiotics. Antibiotics destroy the intended harmful bacteria as well as taking out some good bacteria as collateral damage. Certain species of good bacteria usually keep hoodlums like candida in-line. Once these guardians are out of the way, candida can party on, taking over. Antibiotics predispose you to candida because of this change to microflora populations in the digestive tract and elsewhere. Of particular concern are those of who have taken weeks and months of antibiotic treatment for conditions such as acne. Even if you studiously avoid taking antibiotics, watch for antibiotics in the food chain—for example, chickens and dairy cows are routinely given antibiotics, so buy organic chicken and eggs rather than their poor cousins. Organically produced cow's milk is also available or try sheep's or goat's milk products as these animals are rarely given antibiotics.

❏ Chlorine is added to our drinking water supply to prevent outbreaks of water-borne bacterial disease such as cholera and typhoid. Naturally enough, chlorine will also have an antibacterial effect on our internal microflora population, disturbing it day after day.

❏ The oral contraceptive pill and hormone replacement therapy can subtly change vaginal pH, making some women more susceptible to thrush (vaginal Candida albicans).

❏ Stress affects the immune system, allowing an infection such as candida to spread.

❏ Cortisone, the anti-inflammatory drug often given for aches, pains, and skin eruptions, suppresses the immune system's ability to fight bacteria, viruses, and yeasts such as candida.

❏ Diabetes is a condition that raises blood sugar levels. As candida thrives on sugar, diabetics are predisposed to candida. Insulin-dependent and noninsulin-dependent diabetics do well on the candida diet. Of course, close supervision from a doctor is necessary for those dependent on prescribed insulin.

❏ A diet containing white bread and pastries, sugar, alcohol, and pizza is more likely to promote candida than a healthy diet that encourages the growth of beneficial microflora.

WHAT TO DO

Treating candida requires a three-pronged approach. First, you need to reduce the candida population; this is done by starving them to death (the candida diet) in addition to killing them with antifungal agents. Next, you need to reintroduce friendlier probiotic bugs, and the final step is to improve and maintain the internal environment and immune system to prevent candida from recurring. All three "prongs" happen simultaneously, that is, the candida diet AND antifungal supplements AND probiotics. The diet is central to treating the problem.

In all except the most persistent cases the candida treatment will take four weeks. After the program has finished, reinstate "banned" foods slowly. People often find they no longer hanker after sugar as much, and choose to maintain many of the healthy choices of the candida diet.

Diet

❏ Foods to avoid

For four weeks avoid the following foods:

- Sugar, including sugar added to foods—for example, cakes, soft drinks, biscuits, most breakfast cereals, malt, molasses, honey, and golden syrup.

- Fruit juice, grapes, dried fruit, melons (papaya, watermelon, and rock melon).

- Yeasted bread, sour dough bread, and pizzas.

- Yeast spreads, such as Marmite and Vegemite.

"HANGOVER" SYMPTOMS

Occasionally some people can feel unwell for a few days due to "die-off," the reaction to a large percentage of the candida colony dying simultaneously. In their dying moments they release toxic substances such as acetaldehyde. The same chemical is released in the metabolism of alcohol. For this reason, you may experience "hangover" symptoms including fatigue, headaches, and nausea. Your existing symptoms may also worsen, but this is temporary. Take headache tablets, drink plenty of water, and symptoms will resolve in a few days.

- Beer, wine, fortified wine, liqueurs, sparkling wine, and champagne.
- Yellow cheese, soft cheeses such as camembert, brie, and so forth, and blue cheese.

❏ Foods to eat

- All vegetables and legumes/pulses.
- All fruit except grapes, dried fruit, and melons or fruit juice (limit other fruit to two pieces per day).
- All grains such as rice, corn, quinoa, and millet. Wheat products are fine except those with yeast added. For instance, wheat crackers and mountain bread are okay.
- All meat, chicken, fish, and eggs.
- All oils, especially coconut oil, as it contains acrylic acid, which is antifungal.
- White cheese, including ricotta, cottage, and feta.
- Probiotic foods miso, yogurt, kimchi, sauerkraut, and leben.
- Alcohol (vodka, gin, whiskey)—spirits are okay with soda or water, not soft drinks or juice.

Remedies

❏ Natural antifungals include garlic, acrylic acid (from coconut), pau d'arco, thyme, turmeric, calendula, goldenseal, and echinacea. Unless you are consulting a herbalist, the easiest supplement is garlic. Garlic is not only antifungal, it is also very good for the immune system. Take six cloves of raw garlic daily with food or the equivalent in freeze-dried supplement form, or two to three one-gram garlic tablets.

❏ Before breakfast take a good probiotic supplement. Invest in a good quality probiotic, one containing acidophilus, bifidus, and *saccharomyces boulardii* at a dosage of one teaspoon of powder or three capsules.

Other

❏ If thrush was one of the symptoms that alerted you to the fact that you have a candida overgrowth, it may be necessary to use a douche for the first three days of the program. Make a douche up by filling a squeezable plastic sauce bottle or rubber enema bulb three-quarters full with warm water. Add 30 ml white vinegar (to correct the pH), one teaspoon acidophilus powder (or the contents of three capsules) and two drops tea tree oil. Lie in a bathtub and squeeze the contents into the vagina. Don't worry that the water rushes out. Do this every night (or morning) before your shower or bath. Avoid douching during your period. It shouldn't sting; if it does, add more water; if still stinging don't use the tea tree oil. Men on the program can use this douche recipe as a wash for their dangly bits.

❏ On occasion, for severe cases, a pharmaceutical antifungal tablet could be taken in conjunction with above. These are available over the counter. One course should suffice.

❏ If your water supply is heavily chlorinated, boil your drinking water or leave it standing for a day or so to allow time for the chlorine to evaporate.

AROMATHERAPY

Tea tree oil has broad spectrum antimicrobial activity against bacteria, viruses, and fungi, making it a great choice to use in this instance, and combining it with lavender boosts these therapeutic properties.

Combine 4 drops of tea tree oil with 3 drops of lavender oil and mix thoroughly in 30 grams of unscented cream base or pure aloe vera gel and apply three to four times daily. This essential oil blend can also be used in a bath.

Diet

➠ Avoid sugar and all food that contains sugar, melons, grapes, dried fruit, yellow and creamy cheeses, yeasted and sour dough bread, pizza, wine, and beer.

➠ Include fruits (but see list of fruit to avoid above) and vegetables, crackers, spirits, white cheese such as cottage, oil, nuts, seeds, fish, meat, and legumes/pulses.

Remedies

➠ Garlic as an antifungal and/or antifungal supplements and herbs such as acrylic acid, pau d'arco, goldenseal, and calendula.

➠ Take a good quality probiotic supplement.

Other

➠ If you have thrush, use a douche for the first few days of the program.

CATARACTS

WHAT IS IT?

A cataract is a painless degenerative cloudiness of the lens of the eye. It is easily treated in the industrialized West, but cataracts are the leading cause of blindness in undeveloped countries. The lens, located just behind the pupil, should be clear and flexible. After we reach the age of forty-five years or so, proteins start to cloud the lens, and the lens itself becomes less flexible, and 20/20 vision is a thing of the past. By sixty years old, most people have cloudy vision, and it is the rare bird that does not have a cataract by age eighty.

SYMPTOMS

☑ Double vision

☑ Seeing a colored halo around lights

☑ Becoming sensitive to glare

☑ Poor night vision

☑ Loss of color intensity

☑ Eye glass prescriptions need changing more frequently.

WHAT CAUSES IT?

The jury is still out on the absolute cause of cataracts; certainly there appears to be oxidative damage, same as behind many of the aging symptoms. Below is a list of factors that hasten the progression of cataracts.

❏ Getting long in the tooth.

❏ Diabetes.

❏ Smoking.

❏ Strong sunlight and radiation. Pilots have a greater risk of cataracts.

❏ Cortisone medication.

❏ Injury or inflammation to the eye.

WHAT TO DO?

Once cataracts have formed and are affecting your quality of life, such as no longer being able to read or drive, then it's time for a cataract operation. The relatively painless procedure takes a little over ten minutes, where the faulty lens is replaced by an artificial, clear plastic version. Good as new. Natural therapies cannot replace the lens, but can go far in reducing the pace of progression of the condition.

Diet

❑ Control blood sugars. There is a connection between high blood sugar and the formation of cataracts. Avoid added sugar in your diet and eat low-glycemic carbohydrates.

❑ Antioxidant nutrients found in food reduce free radical damage and oxidation of tissue. Fruits and vegetables that are multihued have the largest percentage of antioxidants. These include blueberries, turmeric, and carrots.

❑ Trans-fatty acids increase oxidative damage. Avoid deep-fried foods, margarine, and packaged biscuits, pastries, and cakes.

❑ Drink more fluids, especially water; the lens is made up of water and protein.

❑ Eat more fruit and veggies. This time-honored piece of advice from grannies around the world proves right yet again. The following nutrients have been found to reduce the prevalence of cataracts: vitamin E, selenium, beta-carotene, lycopene, vitamin C, lutein, and zeaxanthin—and guess what? They are found in vegetables and fruit.

❑ Lutein—dark green leafy vegetables, Asian greens, kale, spinach; sweet corn, and egg yolk.

❑ Zeaxanthin—sweet corn, egg yolk, mandarins, tangerines, oranges, persimmons, and orange capsicum.

❑ Vitamin E—cold-pressed vegetable oils, especially wheat germ oil, nuts, seeds, spinach, kale, sweet potatoes, egg yolk, liver, soya beans, butter, and asparagus.

❑ Selenium—wheat germ, meat, fish, seafood, Brazil nuts, garlic, and brewer's yeast.

❑ Beta-carotene—Carrots, rock melon, broccoli, spinach, and the marine algae *Dunaliella salina.*

❑ Lycopene—Tomatoes and processed tomato products such as tomato sauce and dried tomatoes, watermelon, pink grapefruit, papaya, andguava.

❑ Vitamin C—berries, especially blackcurrants, chilies, capsicums, oranges, papaya, citrus fruits, mango, cabbage, cauliflower, broccoli, and tomato.

Remedies

❑ Herbally, a combination of bilberry and ginkgo biloba are a marriage made in heaven for cataract prevention. Bilberry is high in carotenoids beloved by eyes, and both herbs are excellent at improving microcirculation, improving blood flow to hard to reach places in the body, like the eyes.

❑ Vitamin E is an excellent antioxidant and improves circulation. No more than 500 IU daily.

❑ A buildup of a sugar-like substance, sorbitol, is thought to be behind the development of cataracts, particularly those in diabetics. The bioflavonoid quercetin helps to break sorbitol down into harmless compounds.

❑ Take an antioxidant supplement that contains vitamin E, selenium, vitamin C, and beta-carotene.

Other

❑ Cataract surgery today is a common procedure and is generally very safe and effective. If you need it, you need it.

❑ Wear a wide-brimmed hat to reduce glare and wear good quality sunglasses that cut out UVA and UVB sunlight.

□ Give up cigarettes. There is a very strong link between smoking (and the free radicals it generates) and cataract formation.

□ The eyes are how we view our lives and future; metaphorically, is there some fear about looking forward or into your future?

DIET

➧ Drink more water.

➧ Increase fruit and vegetables. Here are some to get you started: berries, citrus, tomatoes, green leafy vegetables, capsicum, and sweet corn.

REMEDIES

➧ The herbs bilberry and ginkgo biloba help circulation and are antioxidant rich.

➧ Take an antioxidant containing vitamin E, vitamin C, and beta-carotene. If it also contains selenium, all the better.

OTHER

➧ Protect your eyes from harsh sunlight and glare, wear good quality sunglasses and a hat.

➧ If your quality of life is becoming compromised, put yourself on a list for cataract surgery.

➧ Is the future scary to look at?

CELLULITE

WHAT IS IT?

Medically known as gynoid lipodystrophy, on the street cellulite goes by the less scary (but no less flattering) description of "the mattress phenomenon," "cottage cheese thighs," or "peu d'orange" (translated as the "orange peel" effect). It is merely a collection of fat deposits lurking below the skin. Although found within fatty tissue, cellulite affects women who are slim as well as the more voluptuous. Unlike cellulitis, a bacterial infection of connective tissue, cellulite is not a health problem, just a cause for aesthetic angst.

SYMPTOMS

☑ Cellulite generally strikes from the waist down, creating lumpy bits on thighs, buttocks, and hips.

☑ There are four distinct stages of cellulite. You can determine just how far down the path of orange peel you are by the good old pinch test. Between forefinger and thumb, gently grab a couple of centimeters of flesh, and assess:

1. The flesh on your thighs and buttocks is smooth; when pinched, it folds and furrows but does not pit or bulge. Good news.

2. Your skin looks okay, except when pinched the first signs of dimpling appear.

3. Your skin is smooth when you are lying down, but when you stand, it shows signs of pitting and bulging.

4. The "there can be no denying it" stage. Cellulite is apparent whether you stand up, lie down, and even wearing a caftan.

WHAT CAUSES IT?

- You are a woman. Cellulite is almost always a female complaint. Estrogen, the female hormone, is responsible for the way women's skin differs from that of men.

- Age. As women age, their skin gets progressively looser and thinner, and connective tissue becomes weaker. Elastin and collagen, two substances responsible for the tight, sleek lines of youth, become lax and loose.

- Poor blood and lymphatic circulation. The lymphatic system is largely responsible for clearing tissues of cellular waste, another possible contributor to cellulite.

WHAT TO DO

As cellulite is predominantly an aesthetic rather than a health-threatening complaint, it rather depends on how much effort you wish to expend to fix the problem.

Diet

- Drink 2 to 3 liters of fluid daily, including the herbal teas mentioned below.

- Eat fresh and predominantly raw food. Enjoy copious quantities of raw vegetables, salads, and fruit.

- Reduce salt. Avoid processed and fast foods, which tend to be high in salt.

- Increase foods that increase circulation. These include garlic, chilies, and ginger.

- Avoid fried foods, white flour products, high-fat dairy (e.g., cream), sugar, alcohol, artificial colorings, and preservatives.

Remedies

- Traditional lymphatic herbs are called for here. Best taken in tea form. Choose from one or a combination of burdock, clivers, nettle, calendula, and blue flag.

- The mineral silica strengthens skin, nails, hair, and connective tissue. Slack collagen fibers allow tissue fluids to leak, and silicon helps to check this process. Available in liquid or tablet form.

- The herb gotu kola is excellent for improving connective tissue, just the thing for cellulite control.

- Fluid retention only makes cellulite worse; if you are bothered by fluid retention then take vitamin B_6, 250 mg two times a day; the diuretic herb dandelion leaf (not root) will help. Drink a cup or two daily, or add to the detoxifying herbs mentioned above. Also good for fluid retention are juniper and celery tablets.

- If hormonal imbalance is part of your health picture, take some balancing herbs such as vitex and dong quai.

Other

- Massage. Although you can't break up cellulite, massage helps to boost general and lymphatic circulation. Enjoy a weekly or fortnightly massage if you can. Take along the essential oil combination mentioned below and ask your masseuse to use this on your floppy bits.

- Before showering, use a skin brush to improve circulation and encourage lymphatic circulation and drainage. Dry skin brushing sloughs dead cells from the skin's surface and encourages better elimination from the skin. Be a masochist: finish off your shower with a cold burst of water to further boost circulation.

- Take up walking, swimming, dancing, or gym classes. Aerobic exercise helps you to decrease body fat, tone muscles, increase circulation, and improve the elimination of body wastes via sweat. Three to five twenty-minute sessions is good, gradually building up to an optimum forty-five minutes each exercise session to keep you cellulite-free.

❑ Smoking inhibits circulation. Stop it.

❑ Avoid tight-fitting clothes that inhibit circulation.

AROMATHERAPY

Juniper and cypress are the two essential oils most effective in cellulite treatment. Juniper is well known for its diuretic (water-removing) qualities; cypress is also a diuretic and strengthens connective tissue. Mandarin and lavender complete the mixture, turning it into a delicious-scented and effective anticellulite treatment. Combine 5 drops of each into a base of 100 ml of almond or other base oil or body lotion. Apply after shower. Ingesting essential oils is toxic, so use this only externally on the body.

AT A GLANCE

DIET

➡ Drink 2 to 3 liters of fluid.

➡ Eat predominantly raw food.

➡ Avoid salt and highly processed foods.

REMEDIES

➡ Take silica in liquid or tablet form.

➡ Drink lymphatic cleansing teas including clivers, nettle, and burdock.

➡ If fluid retention is also a problem, drink dandelion leaf tea and take B_6 supplements.

OTHER

➡ Before your shower, use a dry skin brush, in circular movements from toes to tummy, and fingers to chest.

➡ After your shower massage in some almond or other oil, with a combination of the following essential oils: juniper, cypress, mandarin, and lavender.

CHICKENPOX

WHAT IS IT?

Chickenpox is caused by a varicella-zoster virus, a member of the herpes family. People rarely catch chickenpox twice; however, the virus hangs around in nerve endings and may become reactivated later in life as shingles, a painful rash, usually after a stressful event. Chickenpox is very contagious, spread by sneezing or coughing (at the onset of the infection) or contact with blisters (after the rash appears). After blisters heal the patient can no longer transmit the disease. From go to whoa, a bout of chickenpox lasts around ten days. Chickenpox is a self-limiting condition. It will resolve given time; however, symptoms such as fever and the itchy rash can be eased by natural remedies.

Chickenpox was a relatively mild childhood illness that is much less common since routine vaccinations were started in the United States around 1995.

WHAT CAUSES IT?

Chickenpox is a viral infection—one easily transmitted.

SYMPTOMS

☑ Chickenpox starts with a sudden onset of cold-like symptoms, a runny nose, and fever.

☑ The fever coincides with a rash that affects both skin and mucous membranes, such as inside the mouth.

☑ Within thirty-six hours the telltale poxy spots appear, looking a little like watery blisters. These spread from the trunk to the face, scalp, and limbs. These pox are intensely itchy.

☑ Headache, loss of appetite, and fatigue are also common symptoms.

WHAT TO DO

The following suggestions are appropriate for children as well as adults. If fever is severe, particularly for children, seek medical help.

Diet

❑ A light diet is best: soups and broths, steamed vegetables, white fish or chicken breasts, and boiled or poached eggs.

❑ Keep fluids up as the fever of chickenpox can be dehydrating.

❑ Fruit and vegetable juice.

❑ Barley water, lemon, and honey

❑ Avoid coffee, sugar, alcohol, and hot spicy foods.

INFORMATION ON THE SIDE

An old and persistent theory in traditional medicine is that early childhood conditions such as the measles, chickenpox, and mumps are transition processes, important to the child's physical, psychological, and psychic development and should not be "suppressed" by immunization. One explanation says that the fever and rash of chickenpox, for example, are eliminations of "toxins." Further, it is also said that if these run-of-the-mill childhood illnesses are suppressed via vaccination, the elimination of toxins is also suppressed, and may return many years later in a more insidious guise. I'll admit this sounds like eye-of-newt mumbo jumbo, but it would be nearly impossible to scientifically measure the effects of vaccination thirty, forty, and even seventy years after the event. No doubt the immunization controversy will continue, and there are arguments for both sides of the debate.

Remedies

❏ Traditional herbal teas to manage fever include lime flowers, yarrow, elder, and peppermint.

❏ Take the tissue salts ferrum. phos. and kali. mur., one of each every hour during the fever.

❏ Vitamins C and A, zinc, echinacea, cat's claw, and andrographis will help the immune system recover and prevent a secondary bacterial infection. Take these for one month after the illness.

❏ Take some antiviral herbs throughout and for a week or so after, to assist in recovery, such as echinacea, astragalus, cat's claw, and St. John's wort.

Other

❏ Avoid overly hot showers and baths.

❏ A cool bath or cool sponge with several drops of peppermint oil will reduce fever.

❏ The following things can be added to a cool bath or sponge bath (half the amounts for a sponge bath) to ease the insane itching—a cup of apple cider vinegar, a cup of bicarbonate of soda, 8 drops each of lavender and chamomile essential oil.

❏ An oat sock: place one cup of oats into a sock, tie off the end, add to the water, and use the creamy and calming liquid instead of soap.

❏ Wear loose-fitting cotton clothes.

❏ Rest as much as possible.

❏ Make sure fingernails are cut short, and resist scratching as much as possible to reduce infection and scarring. Wear cotton mittens or gloves to bed to reduce scratching overnight.

❏ Earl Grey tea bags, used and cold, placed on the spots, will soothe and heal.

❏ Witch hazel lotion (available from pharmacies) dabbed on the spots will help relieve the itch and dry the spots.

❏ Calendula, chickweed, tea tree, aloe vera gel, and lavender are all helpful for itching and healing. Use as cream or lotion.

❏ Vitamin E oil (pierce a capsule), applied after the spots have dried up, will help prevent scarring. Don't apply the oil onto open sores.

AROMATHERAPY

❏ 5 drops of lavender—analgesic, sedative, soothing, calming.

❏ 4 drops of roman chamomile—comforting, analgesic, sedative, temperature reducing.

❏ 3 drops of cajeput—analgesic, antimicrobial, antiseptic, fever reducing.

❏ 2 drops of tea tree—antiviral, immunostimulant.

❏ 2 drops of peppermint—analgesic, anti-itch, antiviral, cooling.

Add to the bath water for relief and a soothing soak. This mix can also aid in reducing temperature. Use 5 drops of lavender with 2 drops of tea tree in 10 ml witch hazel and use as a spot treatment.

Diet

- Keep hydrated with barley water and fruit and vegetable juices.

- Eat lightly: steamed vegetables, and for protein—chicken breast, white fish, or eggs.

- Avoid coffee, sugar, alcohol, and hot spicy foods.

Remedies

- Herbal teas to help manage a fever include lime flowers, yarrow, elder, and peppermint.

- Herbs to help you over the virus include echinacea, astragalus, cat's claw, and St. John's wort.

Other

- Rest as much as possible.

- Keep cool by sponging with water and a few drops of peppermint oil.

- To ease the itching add to a bath one of the following: a cup of apple cider vinegar or a cup of bicarbonate of soda.

- Calendula, chickweed, tea tree, aloe vera gel, and lavender are all helpful for itching and healing. Use as cream or lotion.

CHILBLAIN (PERNIOSIS)

WHAT IS IT?

Chilblain is a mild form of frostbite. When exposed to severe cold for long periods, the body hoards heat to keep the vital organs functioning by reducing blood circulation to the extremities. This leaves the nose, ear lobes, fingers, toes, and even the penis vulnerable to chilblain.

SYMPTOMS

- Affected parts initially redden, tingle, or ache.
- Swelling and inflammation occurs.
- Chilblain is intensely itchy.
- Sores and blisters occur when things are bad.
- Severe chilblain can cause permanent damage to blood vessels, nerves, and skin.

WHAT CAUSES IT?

- Icy-cold and blizzard-like weather conditions.
- Genetics play a role—poor circulation runs in families.
- Raynaud's syndrome is a condition where circulation is reduced in fingers, toes, and sometimes in nipples.
- Whenever there is limited blood flow, chilblain is more likely to occur.
- Thin people suffer more than more comfortably padded individuals.
- Sudden changes or extremes of temperature, from cold outside to very warm inside.

WHAT TO DO

The treatments given below are also recommended if you are generally prone to poor circulation. If you have suffered from chilblain in the past, don't wait for them to happen before beginning treatment. Start early, a month before the first cold snap.

Diet

❏ Be generous with circulation-enhancing spices and herbs in your meals, including chili, ginger, garlic, onion, horseradish, thyme, and turmeric.

❏ Legumes, such as kidney and lima beans, and the root vegetables are warming and good for the circulation.

❏ Eat more baked, stewed, and slow-cooked meals rather than raw food and salads. Energetically, baking and cooking food for hours has a grounding and warming effect. Salads and cold foods are lighter and cooler, better for summer and an overactive circulation.

❏ Avoid cold drinks; drink fluids at room temperature or warmer.

❏ Avoid alcohol; you may feel warmed up, but it is a dangerous illusion. Peripheral circulation diminishes, leaving your fingers and toes at risk.

Remedies

❏ Bayberry, ginkgo biloba, bilberry, horse chestnut, prickly ash, nettle, ginger, garlic, and chili are all herbs (and foods) that improve circulation. Take a combination in tablet, tincture, or tea form twice daily for a month before and during the cold season.

❏ Rutin, quercetin, and resveratrol as well as good old vitamin C are important for maintaining the strength of blood vessel walls and improving circulation. If you are a cold fish, take these all year long.

❏ Vitamin E improves circulation, take 500 IU daily.

❏ If chilblain has broken into open sores, apply some calendula cream.

Other

❏ Curtail your smoking as nicotine causes constriction to small blood vessels, further decreasing circulation.

❏ Avoid extremes of temperature, and bundle up before you go outside. When coming inside from the cold, don't toast your hands in front of the fire or heater immediately; wait until you have warmed up a little.

❏ Wear a hat or beanie; one-third of our body heat is lost from the head.

❏ Avoid wearing tight shoes, no matter how fashionable, as they restrict circulation.

❏ If you live near the beach, take a dip in the ocean every day, winter and summer. Be brave. Long term this will improve your circulation.

❏ Take warm footbaths and hand baths with ginger or thyme. Put six to seven sprigs of fresh thyme and a few drops of thyme oil, or a handful of grated ginger tied in a sock or stocking, into a basin or foot-sized bucket. Don't put frozen hands or feet straight into hot water; shake them around first, to get the blood flowing.

❏ The color red is warming, and is always in fashion.

❏ For fans of exploring the mind/body connection of ailments, the blood represents emotions. As chilblain is a condition where the blood flow is inhibited, the questions to pose are: "Are your emotions in danger of shutting down? Would it be helpful to speak and reveal more of your inner world?"

Belly breathing switches on the parasympathetic nervous system (PNS). The PNS governs the peripheral circulation. Belly (abdominal or diaphragmatic) breathing is the way we were meant to breathe. Initially, lie on your bed with a pillow beneath your head and knees. Place your hands palm down on your lower belly. Breathe in through your nose, counting slowly to three or four. Feel your tummy rise with the breath. Breathe out just as slowly, allowing the belly to drop. Once you feel comfortable with this, progress to doing this seated, and eventually you will be able to belly breathe all the time. The way nature intended.

Exercise is an excellent way to improve circulation. However, male cyclists and runners should wear an extra pair of shorts or thermal underpants to prevent penile chilblains or frostbite—a condition seldom talked about.

AROMATHERAPY

3 drops of marjoram sweet—has warming properties, making it an excellent choice in treating chilblains.

4 drops of kunzea—analgesic, anti-inflammatory.

3 drops of black pepper—stimulates circulation, detoxifies.

4 drops of lemon—stimulates circulation, diuretic, detoxifying, and tonifying.

Stir 6 to 8 drops of a combination of these essential oils into a foot/hand bath with 125 grams Epsom salts, or blend 6 to 8 drops of a combination of these essential oils into a bowl of warm water and use as a warm compress. Blend a combination of these essential oils into 20 grams unscented vitamin E cream with calendula or arnica and rub into the affected area. Use as a general body massage to improve circulation

At a Glance

Diet

Foods that improve circulation and warm the body include chili, ginger, thyme, garlic, turmeric, and horseradish

Steer clear of salads and raw cold foods; favor casseroles and baked meals, which are more warming.

Remedies

Herbs that improve circulation include prickly ash, ginkgo biloba, chili, garlic, bayberry, bilberry, and horse chestnut. Take in tincture, tablet, or tea form. Start taking a month before and during the cold season.

Vitamin C and the bioflavonoids rutin and quercetin.

Vitamin E, 500 IU daily.

Other

Avoid tight-fitting clothes and shoes that inhibit circulation.

Wear a warm hat as cold escapes from the head.

Belly (diaphragmatic) breathing switches on the parasympathetic nervous system, which governs the peripheral circulation, keeping nose, fingers, and toes supplied with warm blood.

Exercise keeps the blood pumping.

CHOLESTEROL, HIGH

WHAT IS IT?

High cholesterol increases your risk of having a stroke or heart attack. It's not the only risk factor; a blood test reading of high cholesterol is considered alongside a raft of other things including a family history of heart disease, high blood pressure, being male, getting older, being overweight, having diabetes, and smoking.

SYMPTOMS

There are no symptoms when your cholesterol is high. The first time you know about it is via a blood test. High blood pressure, another risk factor for heart disease, is also sneakily silent when it comes to symptoms. Therefore, regular checkups are key to knowing your heart disease risk status.

WHAT CAUSES IT?

❏ It used to be thought that if you ate a lot of high-cholesterol food such as eggs and shrimp, you would end up with high cholesterol in your bloodstream, but we now know this is not the case. Shellfish are off the hook, so to speak.

❏ What does appear to increase cholesterol levels is a diet high in sugar and refined carbohydrates (bread, sweets, pastries, biscuits, etc.). Trans-fatty acids are also to blame; these are found in fatty takeout foods and baked goods including pastries and cakes (again, there is a theme here). Steer clear of too much saturated fats such as the fattier cuts of meat and brie, camembert, and blue cheese. Favor the leaner meats such as chicken without the skin, and choose feta, ricotta, and cottage cheese rather than the creamier varieties.

❏ Stress is a major factor. Cortisol, the stress hormone, is manufactured from cholesterol. You need to make more cholesterol to make cortisol when you are stressed.

❏ Genetics. There is a hereditary condition known as familial hypercholesterolemia. No amount of dieting or exercise will significantly lower your cholesterol levels if you have this condition.

❏ Being overweight increases your risk of having high cholesterol.

❏ Being inactive is another causative factor.

WHAT TO DO

As there are no obvious symptoms to high cholesterol, it is wise to have regular blood tests just to keep an eye that everything is healthy in the heart department.

Diet

❏ Avoid or reduce sugar. A few pieces of fruit daily are fine, but avoid added sugar. Any sugar over 5 grams/100 grams on a packaged food is "added" sugar.

❏ Reduce saturated fats, especially animal fats, and in particular butter, yellow and decadent creamy cheese, cream, ice cream, lard, fattier cuts of beef, pork, and lamb, bacon, and deli meats.

❏ Avoid trans-fatty acids. Trans-fatty acids now need to be declared on food labels.

❏ Increase fish, especially the omega-3–rich fish such salmon, sardines, and mackerel.

❏ Use cold-pressed olive oil, coconut oil, and any nut oil.

❏ Increase fiber-rich whole grains, nuts, legumes, seeds, fruit, and vegetables, particularly those high in soluble fiber. (See Appendix D for food sources.)

❏ Foods with particular cholesterol-lowering effects include artichokes, ginger, cucumber, seaweed, banana, quince, onion, garlic, oatmeal, legumes, bitter melon, grapefruit, oranges, apples, yogurt, carrots, barley, eggplant, and shiitake mushrooms.

❏ Add foods high in antioxidants that contain beta-carotene, vitamin C, oligomeric proanthocyanidins, bioflavonoids, quercetin, resveratrol, vitamin E and zinc. (See Appendix D for food sources.) Add antioxidant foods to the diet. Broccoli and the brassica family reduce the risk of "bad" cholesterol becoming oxidized and causing damage to artery walls and atherosclerosis.

❏ Margarines that include plant sterols act to reduce absorption of cholesterol from the intestine. Studies have shown they have a small effect on lowering blood cholesterol levels. They are a highly processed food and choosing a spread of avocado or olive oil would be a naturopathic preference.

Remedies

❏ Soluble fiber reduces cholesterol by preventing it from being absorbed or reabsorbed from the intestines. The soluble fiber "chelates" or holds on to the cholesterol, and eliminates it via the bowel. In addition to dietary fiber, the following fiber supplements help lower cholesterol levels: one to two tablespoons of psyllium, pectin, chia seeds, oat bran, rice bran, or barley bran.

GOOD AND BAD CHOLESTEROL

Even more important than a blood test reading of high cholesterol is the ratio between "good" and "bad" cholesterol. Good cholesterol is high density lipoprotein (HDL) and bad cholesterol is low density lipoprotein (LDL). A lipoprotein is a vehicle that transports fats, including cholesterol, around the body in the bloodstream. Blood is predominantly water. Water and fat don't mix. So these transporters of fat are covered in a thin coat of protein, which *is* water soluble. Hence the name *lipo* (fat)—protein. Lipoproteins come in several shapes and sizes, and are named according to their proportions of fat to protein. The LDLs, containing more fat, are less dense than the HDLs, and have the job of distributing cholesterol (and fats) around the body. The HDLs return cholesterol back to the liver to be excreted as bile. Both lipoproteins are important, but as LDLs are responsible for depositing the cholesterol, they have been dubbed "bad cholesterol."

The story doesn't end here. Cholesterol in the LDLs can become oxidized by free radicals. When this oxidized cholesterol ends up in artery walls it creates a small wound, which recruits cholesterol, calcium, and various cells as a Band-Aid. This creates what is known as an atheroma or plaque, and not only narrows the artery, thereby increasing blood pressure, but has the potential to peel away, blocking arteries to the heart and brain, causing heart attacks and strokes.

The take-home message is to focus on the ratio between the lipoproteins; the higher the ratio of HDLs to LDLs, the lower the risk of heart disease. If you happen to have high LDL levels, and you are at a higher risk of heart disease, your doctor might also ask for further blood tests including high-sensitivity C-reactive protein (hsCRP) and Lipoprotein(a) [Lp(a)] levels. These are other blood markers of increased likelihood of heart disease.

- Take 10 ml of fish oil daily. This is a very effective way to reduce your cholesterol levels; 10 ml equates to 10 grams and it is much more economical and easy to buy a liquid fish oil product. Fear not, most varieties nowadays are relatively palatable.

- Krill oil has been found to be effective in reducing cholesterol levels, and you need to take a smaller dose than fish oil, but then again it is more expensive.

- Garlic helps lower cholesterol levels. Go for capsules or tablets that contain whole freeze-dried garlic.

- Herbs that help the liver excrete excess cholesterol include St. Mary's thistle, celery seed, dandelion root, globe artichoke, tribulus, and chelidonium.

- Polycosanol is a compound isolated from sugar cane (something useful coming from sugar!) that has been found in several studies to help lower cholesterol levels.

- Another supplement with some impressive results is red yeast rice, a traditional Chinese food and remedy.

- Vitamin B_3 (niacin) does lower cholesterol. However, it is required in fairly large amounts and has an unpleasant side effect of hot flashes.

- If you are taking statin drugs to lower cholesterol and experience muscle pain as a side effect, coenzyme Q_{10} and magnesium may be helpful.

Other

- Stress may be behind increased cholesterol levels. Endeavour to find ways to reduce your stress, and hopefully your cholesterol. Meditation, yoga, a pussycat perhaps?

- Aerobic exercise, anything that gets you huffing and puffing and your heart rate raised, lowers cholesterol levels and improves the HDL/LDL ratios.

- Being overweight raises cholesterol levels and losing weight lowers cholesterol levels.

BEHIND THE SCENES

Cholesterol is a type of fat manufactured by the liver of animals and man. Naturally occurring in animal foods such as chicken, eggs, lamb, beef, dairy, shellfish, and pork, you will not find cholesterol in plant foods—even those high in fat such as avocadoes and coconuts. Avocadoes and coconuts do not have livers and therefore cannot produce cholesterol.

Cholesterol is a vital molecule in the body, being the precursor to important substances including the digestive fluid bile, the sex hormones estrogen, progesterone, and testosterone, the stress hormone, cortisol, and vitamin D. Cholesterol is also an integral component of every cell membrane and forms part of the myelin sheath that surrounds nerve fibers. The alarm about cholesterol was raised several decades ago when it was found in the arteries of people with atherosclerosis. However, cholesterol in the arteries is just a sign, not the cause of atherosclerosis. Blaming cholesterol for heart disease is akin to shooting the messenger.

AT A GLANCE

DIET

⟹ Eat plenty of high-fiber foods; these help take cholesterol out of the body. Increase all vegetables, oats, brown rice, pears.

⟹ Eat at least three servings of omega-3 fish weekly such as sardines, salmon, and mackerel. Omega-3 fatty acids help to lower cholesterol.

⟹ Avoid or reduce sugar.

⟹ Steer clear of the fattier cuts of meat. Choose ricotta and feta over camembert and the high-fat cheeses.

⟹ Avoid trans-fatty acids; they are in takeout and commercial baked foods.

⟹ Include foods with particular cholesterol-lowering effects such as artichokes, ginger, cucumber, seaweed, banana, quince, onion, garlic, oatmeal, legumes, bitter melon, grapefruit, oranges, apples, yogurt, carrots, barley, eggplant, and shiitake mushrooms.

REMEDIES

⟹ Take 10 ml of fish oil daily. More economical to take as an oil rather than the equivalent 10 capsules. Citrus-flavored fish oils are available and can be more palatable.

⟹ Take a tablespoon of a soluble fiber supplement daily such as psyllium or chia seeds. Soluble fiber stops cholesterol from being reabsorbed back into the bloodstream.

⟹ Garlic helps lower cholesterol levels. Try capsules or tablets of whole freeze-dried garlic.

OTHER

⟹ Stress may be behind increased cholesterol levels. Endeavor to find ways to reduce your stress, and hopefully your cholesterol along with it. Try meditation, yoga, a pussycat.

⟹ Aerobic exercise, anything that gets you huffing and puffing and your heart rate raised, lowers cholesterol levels and improves the HDL/LDL ratios.

⟹ Being overweight raises cholesterol levels and losing weight lowers cholesterol levels. Do you need to lose weight?

CHRONIC FATIGUE SYNDROME

WHAT IS IT?

Chronic fatigue syndrome (CFS), dismissively named the "yuppie flu" in the 1980s, is now recognized as a seriously debilitating disease. Kerry Bone, a leading Australian herbalist, believes that chronic fatigue syndrome is not a new disorder, but one that was called "neurasthenia" in Victorian times.

SYMPTOMS

- Unfortunately, as yet there is no definitive diagnostic test for CFS.

- To be diagnosed as suffering with CFS, you must have tiredness in mind, body, and muscles for at least six months with all other possible disorders ruled out.

- People who have CFS are indeed fatigued, some to the extent of being bedridden, and most find it a strain to achieve their normal day-to-day activities.

- The syndrome is often initiated by flu-like symptoms that never really go away or return intermittently.

- Low-grade fever

- Heightened allergies

- Oversensitivities to food, chemicals, or other substances

- Frequent infections

- Weight gain or loss

- Sleep disturbances including night sweats

- Nonrestorative sleep and nightmares

- Sore throat; painful lymph nodes

- Muscle aches and pains without signs of inflammation

- Headaches

- Depression

- Brain fog

- Forgetfulness

- As the immune system is depressed, opportunistic infections such as the yeast organism *Candida albicans* (see also page 73), take advantage and often contribute to the symptom lineup.

WHAT CAUSES IT?

- There is a frustrating lack of information about what causes this condition. Even more than for other conditions, CFS differs case by case, in possible causes and symptoms.

- One common causative theme is stress, whether from relationship fractures, death of someone you love, overwork or overexacting personal standards.

- More women than men seem to be affected. A surprising number of sufferers are young, achievement-oriented go-getters who juggle

---

INTERESTING FACTS

It is thought that lead toxicity was partly to blame for the fall of the Roman Empire. Roman aqueducts and pipes were lined with lead along as were eating utensils and the ubiquitous goblets that were made from it. Metals such as mercury, lead, aluminum, arsenic, and copper can be present in our environment at relatively high levels. The early signs of lead and mercury poisoning include fatigue, muscle pain, and impaired attention span—all symptoms of CFS.

careers, families, and studies, and are used to being "on" all the time. Adjusting to the torpor of CFS is all the more difficult for them.

❏ Athletes also succumb to CFS, overdoing anything, including overtraining, will contribute to this syndrome.

❏ One theory is that a virus initiates CFS. Likely candidates include Ross River fever (a mosquito-borne infectious disease), glandular fever (Epstein-Barr virus), and even the ubiquitous herpes virus.

❏ Another theory is that CFS is caused by heavy metal toxicity.

■ WHAT TO DO

Chronic fatigue syndrome affects the adrenal glands, nervous, and immune systems, and CFS patients are often very sensitive, emotionally and physically. Sensitivity is always the sign to start slowly with treatment. Pushing too hard will be counterproductive. Patience is necessary with this condition, for the patient and the practitioner.

Diet

❏ Eat food that is close to nature; the less chemicals in your system the better.

❏ Avoid sugar as sugar suppresses the immune system.

❏ Avoid alcohol, which is a nervous system suppressant.

❏ Avoid caffeine completely. Although you might feel you need a "pick-me-up," stimulants such as coffee will only serve to flog an already tired horse. The same goes for nicotine.

❏ Food allergies are common in people with CFS. Treat accordingly. (See Food Allergies on page 152.)

❏ Eat plenty of fresh fruit and vegetables, as well as freshly made juices. It would do you well to invest in a juicer.

❏ Eat protein every day including organic eggs and fish. If you are a vegetarian, ensure that you have plenty of vegetable protein, namely legumes, nuts, and seeds.

❏ If there are signs of candida overgrowth (see page 73) go on the candida diet and program.

Remedies

❏ Herbs are excellent for CFS. Combine at least one from each of the following three groups:

• Immune-system-enhancing herbs such as astragalus, withania, echinacea, andrographis, goldenseal, and poke root (if glands are swollen).

• Adaptogens such as licorice, rehmannia, Siberian and Korean ginseng, rhodiola, and tulsi.

• Nervous system agents such as St. John's wort, oats, zizyphus, kava, passionflower, and valerian.

❏ Magnesium helps tired muscles and calms an overactive nervous system.

❏ Vitamin C and zinc are needed for the immune system.

❏ Coenzyme Q_{10} may help with energy levels.

❏ Take a good vitamin B complex each morning.

❏ The Bach flower remedy Olive is tailor-made for exhaustion.

Other

❏ Rest is the most important remedy of all. Rest means *rest,* so rest when you are lying in bed—that means no TV, no Internet, no reading. Restorative rest is not about lying in bed all day, it is about returning to bed after being active to restore and replenish energy levels.

- An excellent piece of advice, by Australian Kerry Bone, a world-leading herbalist for the treatment of CFS (and other illnesses where fatigue is an issue) is that as soon as you have got some extra energy, GO TO BED. This is the opposite of what you would like to do; after weeks and months of listlessness all you want to do is run around with excitement. Wrong! You need to build up your strength until there is a deep reservoir of energy.

- Reduce stress. The less you have to do the better. If you can, work fewer hours. Now is the time to call in all favors . . . babysitting, dog walking, cleaning the house.

- Learn some form of meditation and practice it at least twenty minutes daily. Transcendental meditation, tapes, guided visualization, or if you are strong enough, you might like to go on a retreat that focuses on meditation such as Vipassana to kick-start your practice.

- Warm baths with a handful of Epsom salts.

- Some gentle exercise every day is important to prevent your muscles from shrinking due to underuse. Don't exert yourself. Qi gong and tai chi are gentle Asian exercises that stimulate energy meridians.

- If you are not getting anywhere with treatment, it may be worthwhile checking for heavy metal toxicity. This is usually done with hair analysis testing.

- Do restorative yoga poses such as balasana (child's pose), and supta baddha konasana (goddess pose). For balasana, kneel on the floor and then sit back on your heels. Fold your body forward so that your chest rests on your knees and your forehead rests either on the floor or on a folded blanket. Either stretch your arms forward along the ground or rest them alongside your legs, facing your feet. For supta baddha konasana, lie on the ground, with your head resting comfortably on a pillow or folded blanket. Bring the soles of your feet together, with your knees out sideways, as close to your body as you can. Take your arms out to the side, at a 45-degree angle away from the body. Stay in these positions as long as comfortable—five to ten minutes would be ideal.

Another relaxing and restorative pose is savasana (corpse pose), and it is the ultimate letting go pose. Lie down on your back with your neck and head resting on a pillow or folded blanket. If your back hurts, place another pillow under both knees. Have your arms

---

INTERESTING FACTS

The term "adaptogen" was first coined in the late 1940s, when it was used to describe a medicine that can improve the body's response to stress. At that time, Russian scientists Professor N.V. Lazarev and his student Dr. Israel Breckman carried out research into the effect on the body of stressors, such as extreme physical and mental training, air and space travel, extremes of temperature, and chronic illness. Their findings? Basically not good. Herbs were then researched that reduced the effects of stress and increased physical and mental endurance and performance. These herbs were called adaptogens and include Siberian ginseng, licorice, Korean ginseng, schizandra, astragalus, gotu kola, tulsi, rhodiola, and withania. Adaptogens are indicated whenever there is stress on the body or fatigue, making them the perfect choice for those with CFS.

15 cm away from your body, palms facing toward the ceiling. Let your legs fall to the side with feet slightly apart. Mentally scan your body for areas of tension and allow them to relax: buttocks, jaw, forehead, and chest. Keep your mouth closed and place tongue at the roof of mouth, just behind your front teeth. Belly breathe. Chillax for twenty minutes.

At a Glance

Diet

⟹ Avoid sugar as sugar depletes the immune system and adrenal glands.

⟹ Avoid caffeine; the last thing you need is a nervous system stimulant when your nerves are exhausted.

⟹ Avoid any known food allergy, for example, wheat, dairy, soy.

⟹ Include protein with each meal such as lean meat, chicken, fish, eggs, nuts, seeds, and legumes.

⟹ If you have a candida overgrowth, see page 74 for information on the candida diet.

Remedies

⟹ Adaptogen herbs are well indicated for CFS; these include withania, Siberian ginseng, rhodiola, and licorice. Keep taking them. In addition, taking herbs for the immune and nervous system are helpful.

⟹ Coenzyme Q_{10} will increase energy production within muscles.

Other

⟹ It is very likely you got into this predicament by overdoing things. If this is the case, there is no time like the present to learn how to relax. This won't come easily to you. Do it anyway.

⟹ When you have more energy, go back to bed and rest.

COLD SORES, HERPES, AND SHINGLES

WHAT IS IT?

Cold sores are little blisters that erupt on the surface of the skin and mucous membranes, mainly on and around the lips. The virus responsible for cold sores is known as herpes simplex virus type 1 (HSV-1). Other members of the herpes family include HSV-2 (genital herpes), chickenpox, and shingles. Although appearing on the skin, the herpes virus lives within the roots of nerves, only manifesting when the nerves are activated by stress or other triggers.

SYMPTOMS

☑ Tingling on the skin before an outbreak

☑ Blisters or small ulcers erupt on the lips, gums, other parts of the face, and even the genitals. Genital herpes (HSV-2) also (obviously) appear on the genitals, but do not generally appear on the face. Both viruses are treated in a similar way.

☑ Fever

☑ Feeling of malaise

☑ Enlarged glands in the neck and/or groin

WHAT CAUSES IT?

❑ You caught it from someone, which is something that is outstandingly easy to do as the herpes virus is highly infectious. Also through direct contact with someone's saliva via a herpes blister, kissing, using the toothbrush of someone who has the infection, or sharing cutlery.

❑ There are triggers for herpes, and these include stress, infection, sun or wind exposure, before the menstrual period when the body's immune system is low, before a first date, or any potentially stressful situation.

WHAT TO DO

The most any treatment can offer is to lull the herpes virus into a long and dormant sleep. This is best done by supporting both immune and nervous systems. Many of the following suggestions can be taken as preventative measures, just increase the dose if an outbreak occurs. These suggestions are equally helpful for shingles and genital herpes.

Diet

❑ The two amino acids arginine and lysine are often trotted out in articles on herpes and natural remedies. While it is true that the herpes virus prefers arginine to lysine, and lysine taken in large amounts can help an outbreak, to eliminate arginine from the diet would be virtually impossible and mean cutting out some pretty good foods, including nuts and legumes. An outbreak of herpes is hardly likely to occur if you have been enjoying a lentil soup too many. It is much more likely to happen if you are stressed to the max, you've been drinking excess coffee, and you're living on takeout. However, if an attack is underway, by all means reduce foods high in arginine. These include chocolate, peanuts, soya beans, and other legumes, nuts, seeds, and carob. To improve the "lysine-to-arginine ratio" in the body, include more of the following foods in the diet—eggs, fish, chicken, milk, cheese, brewer's yeast, fruits, and vegetables.

❑ Avoid coffee, alcohol, and sugar, none of which are beneficial for the nervous or immune system.

Remedies

❑ Herbs to support the immune system include echinacea, cat's claw, and andrographis. At a low dose these can be taken long term. At the first sign of an outbreak increase one or more to larger doses.

❏ Herbs to support the nervous system include St. John's wort, lemon balm, chamomile, and green oats. St. John's wort deserves special mention as it is not only restorative for the nervous system, but it also has antiviral properties specifically against the herpes virus.

❏ Vitamin C, 500 grams daily, and zinc, 22 mg daily, as preventatives; increase to three times a day. (A smaller dose for children.)

❏ Take a lysine tablet three times a day between meals. Generally, the dose when an attack has hit should be up to 1,000 mg per day. You could also take lysine at a lower dose (around 50 to 100 mg a day) as a preventative, particularly when you are run down or feel vulnerable to an episode of herpes. (Note: lysine doesn't work for everyone; if there is no improvement for you, stop taking it.)

❏ Take a vitamin B complex daily for the nerves as a preventative measure; take one at breakfast and at lunch during stressful times.

Topical Remedies

❏ Dab a small amount of zinc sulfate solution to heal.

❏ Aloe vera gel helps to heal and dry blisters.

❏ Licorice root extract is particularly good applied straight onto the blister.

❏ To help blisters dry out, wash with a diluted mixture of apple cider vinegar and water, about one teaspoon per cup of water.

❏ After the blisters have dried, apply some vitamin E straight from a capsule to prevent scarring.

❏ A good and inexpensive remedy to ease the pain is a used Earl Grey tea bag. Apply the cool tea bag to the blisters for ten minutes, two or three times daily.

❏ Ice is nice. From the moment you notice any warning tingle or pain, place ice wrapped in a tea towel or even a bag of frozen peas on the area affected. If you are lucky, this could stop an attack in its tracks.

❏ If the blisters occur around the genitals, urination can be painful. Spray them with cold water from a spray bottle when you are urinating. Or urinate in the shower.

Other

❏ Stress is the most common cause of herpes outbreaks. Do what you can to keep the nervous system calm to prevent flare-ups; this could involve yoga, meditation, whatever takes your fancy.

❏ Wear a wide-brimmed hat and avoid direct sunlight as this can trigger an outbreak.

❏ Avoid kissing or hugging anyone with an outbreak of herpes on their lips.

BEHIND THE SCENES

The incubation period for herpes is two to twelve days, so you could have the virus for nearly two weeks before there is any sign of a cold sore, although herpes is at its most contagious when the blisters are visible. An outbreak of blisters can last from a couple of days to a couple of weeks, but usually resolves within two or three weeks. You can feel rundown in the days before the blisters appear, and a warning tingling on the skin may precede an outbreak. The bad news is that once caught, the herpes virus resides permanently in nerve endings, willing and able to break out at any time. The good news is that the first attack is generally the worst, and subsequent bouts are less and less severe. The virus may eventually burn itself out.

AROMATHERAPY

❑ 5 drops of tea tree—anti-inflammatory, antiseptic, antiviral, immune-stimulant.

❑ 3 drops of geranium—astringent, antiseptic, anti-inflammatory, styptic.

❑ 2 drops of ravensara—antiseptic, antimicrobial, antiviral, immunomodulator. (See Appendix A: Essential Oil Therapeutic Properties.)

❑ 2 drops of lemon myrtle—anesthetic, antimicrobial.

Make into a balm by melting 15 to 20 grams beeswax or cocoa butter with 80 to 85 ml vegetable oil. Once the mixture starts to cool, add the essential oils and stir thoroughly. Pour into a sterilized container and seal once balm is cooled completely. Label and date your balm. Apply as needed. Wash your hands thoroughly before use.

Or . . .

❑ 6 drops of true lavender—analgesic, antiseptic, antiphlogistic, cytophylactic. (See Appendix A: Essential Oil Therapeutic Properties.)

❑ 4 drops of blue cypress—anti-infectious, anti-inflammatory, antiseptic, antiviral, analgesic, antibacterial, antihistamine.

❑ 4 drops of German chamomile—analgesic, anti-inflammatory, antiphlogistic, vulnerary. (See Appendix A: Essential Oil Therapeutic Properties.)

❑ 1 drop of peppermint—analgesic, anesthetic, astringent, nervine.

This blend will help reduce the pain and discomfort associated with shingles. Add to a bath with some bicarbonate soda or add to 30 grams aloe vera gel that may be applied directly on the lesions.

AT A GLANCE

DIET

➡ Avoid caffeine, sugar, and alcohol. They do not support the immune or the nervous system, both of which you need in tip-top shape to prevent further outbreaks.

➡ Decrease arginine foods at the time of an outbreak. This is found in the following foods: chocolate, peanuts, soya beans and other legumes, nuts, seeds, and carob.

REMEDIES

➡ Take herbs that improve immune function such as echinacea, cat's claw, andrographis. Increase the dosage as soon as you are aware of an outbreak.

➡ Take the following herbs to calm the nervous system—St. John's wort, lemon balm, green oats, chamomile.

➡ Supplements for the immune system include zinc and vitamin C. Take regularly and increase with an outbreak of herpes.

➡ Topically apply tincture of licorice root or zinc sulphite.

➡ Dry the blisters with diluted apple cider vinegar.

OTHER

➡ Stay out of strong sunlight or at least wear a hat.

➡ Knowing that stress is a huge trigger for herpes, adopt some calming practices into your life such as meditation, yoga, gardening.

➡ Wave good-bye to your loved ones rather than kiss when cold sores are hanging around.

COLDS AND FLU

WHAT IS IT?

Colds and flu (influenza) are both viral infections. Head colds tend to be affairs of the upper respiratory tract (nose, throat, and sinuses) and chest colds affect the lungs. Influenza or flu is felt all over the body with muscular aches and pains and often fever. Influenza is a much more serious condition than the common cold, although treatment is similar for both conditions.

Naturopathic old-timers consider that having a cold once every couple of years is an effective way to eliminate toxins from the body, or at least a good excuse to spend a day cuddled up in bed. Certainly, there is a difference between a "good" cold, where symptoms progress rapidly from sore throat to drippy nose, all over in a few days, and the "bad" kind that persists for weeks and escalates to something nasty like bronchitis (see page 51) or pneumonia.

SYMPTOMS

Cold symptoms include:

☑ Stuffy nose.

☑ Sore throat.

☑ Sneezing.

☑ Cough.

☑ Sore chest.

Flu symptoms can be the same as for a cold as well as:

☑ Headache.

☑ Extreme exhaustion.

☑ Aches and pains in joints and muscles.

☑ Fever.

WHAT CAUSES IT?

❏ Viruses abound in the air we breathe. There are more than 200 varieties of virus that can cause a cold or flu.

❏ In many cases, a cold or flu is a signal from the body to let us know we need rest. Have you ever noticed that you tend to get a cold during or at the end of a stressful period? If we take heed of this eloquent request for a couple of days in bed, the cold is more likely to resolve itself easily and quickly. Unfortunately, many people battle on with an arsenal of nasal sprays, decongestants, cough syrups, and pills, refusing to take so much as an afternoon off. Even with the best intentions, there are a few malevolent viruses to which even the healthiest person will succumb.

❏ Cold and flu season is often in the middle of winter. It's due to the change of seasons when the weather is unpredictable that you are more likely to catch a cold.

WHAT TO DO

Diet

❏ "Feed a cold and starve a fever" is an old proverb that has been misinterpreted in the past to encourage eating voraciously during a cold and abstaining from food only during a fever. However, the saying originally meant: don't feed a cold and you won't get a fever.

❏ Fasting, or eating very little during any short-term illness, is old wisdom and is still valid. If we took our cue from the animal kingdom, we would fast through the days of fever and flu. Sadly we've lost this intuitive response to illness. Appetite will return as soon as your body is ready to digest more solid sustenance. However, it is important to consume plenty of fluids.

❏ "If you have a cold, build a fire in your stomach" is a wise Chinese saying. Ginger, cinnamon, chili, garlic, and horseradish are all traditional "warming" remedies, which will speed you through a cold or flu.

❏ Drink copious quantities of fluid, which means about 3 liters daily. Fluids, especially if they're hot and clear, help to mobilize the lymphatic system, which carries white blood cells, and to thin out mucus, which tends to become infected if it thickens up.

❏ Soup is a winner on several fronts. It provides warmth, fluid, and easily digestible nourishment. Make a broth from vegetable, fish, chicken, or beef stock, add vegetables, onions, beans, and garlic, and you have a couple of days' worth of nourishing and healing food. Maimonides, the twelfth-century Jewish physician, recommended chicken soup for a cold. He was probably passing on his bubbe's (*Bubbeh,* Yiddish for grandmother) favorite recipe. Chili hot soups, like the Thai favorite, tom yum, is also an excellent choice, and one you can order as takeout from your sick bed. Avoid soups based on cream, cheese, or milk.

❏ Avoid sugar. Studies have shown that within a few minutes of sugar consumption lymphocyte activity is reduced markedly. Lymphocytes (white blood cells) are major players in the immune system. Sugar also tends to increase mucus. A little raw honey is better and soothes a sore throat.

❏ Nasturtiums are very good for coughs. If you have nasturtiums growing in your garden, gather the leaves and a few flowers and add to a salad.

❏ Garlic helps the immune system and is excel-lent for clearing mucus from lungs, nose, and sinuses.

❏ Avoid alcohol. Alcohol swells the mucous lining of the nasal passages and bronchial tissue, exacerbating inflammation.

❏ Milk and milk products, especially milk and yellow cheese, may increase mucus during a cold, so avoid them during this time.

❏ Increase eating foods that are high in vitamin C, including citrus, papaya, kiwifruit, strawberries, pineapple, guava, rock melon, broccoli, cauliflower, Brussels sprouts, and capsicum.

Remedies

❏ The herb echinacea is one of the best herbs for stimulating immunity and treating the effects of a cold or flu. If you are prone to viral infections, start taking echinacea as a precaution before cold season begins.

❏ Other excellent herbs for times of infection include garlic, andrographis, cat's claw, goldenseal, olive leaf, and elder. Andrographis is "the" herb to use in an acute infection. Brilliant for reducing symptoms and if you get to it in time, may stop the progression of the virus.

❏ This following tea is guaranteed to prevent and treat even the most evil cold. In your favorite teapot, plunger, or thermos, combine the juice of one lemon and add half of the lemon rind, chopped up, half a stick of cinnamon, a handful of fresh thyme crushed or chopped, a half inch of fresh ginger root thinly sliced or grated, and a good dollop of honey. Add boiling water and let stand for five minutes (or hours in the thermos). Drink two to three cups daily.

❏ The change of seasons (depending on where you live in the world, this will occur two to four times a year) is when you are most vulnerable to catching a cold or flu, and is also the time to boost your immune system. You can't go wrong with a combination of garlic, echinacea, vitamin C, and zinc. Throw in a cod liver oil capsule if you are prone to lung infections.

❏ Increase body temperature and encourage perspiration. Increasing body temperature during infection is a treatment that goes back hundreds of years. The principle behind the "sweat it out" theory is that an increase in body temperature by a Celsius degree or two is thought to slow down the rate at which viruses replicate. Heat also revs up action in immune cells.

❏ Vitamin C not only reduces the signs and symptoms of the common cold, but helps you to avoid them in the first place. Take 500 mg to 1 gram of vitamin C every couple of waking hours. If you develop flatulence or diarrhea (the signs of overdoing vitamin C), reduce the dose accordingly.

❏ Vitamin A plays an essential role in maintaining all mucous membrane surfaces such as the lungs and throat areas, which become sore and inflamed during coughs and colds. Vitamin A also has been shown to stimulate and enhance numerous immune processes.

❏ Cod liver oil contains vitamin A and vitamin D, another important vitamin for the immune system; take one or two cod liver oil capsules daily as a preventative before the change of season.

❏ Zinc and vitamin C lozenges soothe an inflamed throat and boost immunity.

❏ Sucking on propolis lozenges will soothe the throat and helps if there is an infection of the tonsils or throat. Propolis is a resinous bee product that combines the soothing effect of honey with the potential to slow down the growth of the flu virus.

❏ The homoeopathic remedy Allium cepa is very good for colds where there is clear, runny mucus.

Other

❏ Don't attempt your normal exercise program when you have a cold or flu. A stroll in the sunshine or a couple of stretches is all that is necessary while you have a cold. Avoid strong winds or drafts. Some people go for a jog on the "sweat it out" theory already mentioned, but vigorous exercise is recommended only for the very early or very late stages. Remember

THE WINDOW OF OPPORTUNITY

There is a window of opportunity in which you can avoid getting a cold or flu. This window is literally hours long. Most of us know our own particular "uh oh . . . I'm getting a cold" set of symptoms. They may include feeling a wave of fatigue, sneezing, or tickling at the back of the throat. The moment you feel these signs is the time to act; wait a few hours and the virus will have taken hold. If you are able to catch it in time, take very large doses of natural remedies such as echinacea, andrographis, and vitamin C throughout the day, and if you are lucky you will escape the infection, or if not, you will minimize its duration and intensity.

The beauty of natural remedies as opposed to antibiotics is that they enhance the body's natural ability to fight the infection, building up your resistance to future infections.

your body is trying its hardest to get you to rest. Cancel the triathlon.

❏ A sauna or steam bath increases body temperature, thus invigorating the immune cells, but again is recommended only for the very early or fading stages of a cold as it can be very draining for your body. A few drops of eucalyptus oil in the steam bath or thrown with some water on hot sauna rocks will help clear nose and throat, and bring healing to the lungs. Have a sauna only if your body craves the heat, otherwise it will sap your strength. Wrap up warmly afterward and hop straight into bed.

❏ Vicks VapoRub is a decongestant that holds a place of honor in most cupboards, as it makes an excellent inhalation base. Place a blob of it in a basin of boiling hot water, inhale the vapors deeply, and feel how much more easily you can breathe. Rub Vicks on your chest, back, under your nose, and even the soles of the feet before bed.

❏ A hot foot bath takes congestion away from the head. Truly. Dissolve two teaspoons of hot mustard or chili powder in a little water, then add to a bucket or basin of tolerably hot water. Soak your feet in this for about fifteen minutes, rinse well, put some woolly socks on, then go back to bed.

❏ Inverted postures, to which the yogis are so partial, improve immunity probably by stimulating the thymus gland (located in the chest) and the lymphatic system. "Inverted" means a position where the legs are higher than the heart and is a very restorative posture. If you are in the throes of a cold, the only inverted posture you are likely to cope with is lying with your legs up the wall. To boost your immunity against colds and flu, practice the inverted postures regularly.

❏ Another old Chinese proverb tells of colds that enter the body at the back of the neck, via the wind. Good advice—wear a scarf in cold or windy weather.

❏ The fastest way to turn a "good" cold into a "bad" one is to refuse to rest. Learn to accept that a cold is your body's way of telling you to slow down and rest in bed. Give yourself time to regenerate and contemplate. If you cannot completely surrender to the cold because of unavoidable responsibilities, then try to minimize your workload and ask for support.

❏ Viruses spread easily via coughs and sneezes. Remember germ etiquette and keep your hands clean (soap and water or alcohol wipes), dispose of tissues after use, and if you have forgotten your hanky or tissue, cough into the crook of your elbow rather than your hands.

AROMATHERAPY

❏ 6 drops of sandalwood—anti-inflammatory, antiseptic, antispasmodic, reduces congestion.

❏ 4 drops of ravensara—antimicrobial, antiviral, antiseptic, immune stimulant, expectorant.

❏ 4 drops of cajeput—analgesic, febrifuge, antiseptic, expectorant.

This is a wonderful antiviral, antimicrobial, and soothing blend. The above blend may be used as a room spray by combining it with distilled water in an essential oil dispersant. For dry inhalation, put 6 to 8 drops of the essential oil blend onto a tissue or into a bowl of steaming water as a steam inhalation. Blend with unscented vitamin E cream and use as a chest rub.

At a Glance

Diet

⟹ Avoid sugar. Sucrose decreases immune capability. You need all the help you can get right now.

⟹ If dairy products increase mucus, avoid them too.

⟹ Drink plenty of clear hot fluids to allow the mucus to flow out. Soups are an excellent choice—anything that involves chicken, garlic, and is spicy.

⟹ Garlic is antimicrobial and mucolytic (decreases stickiness of mucus). Eat plenty of it while your cold is raging.

⟹ Ginger, cinnamon, chili, garlic, and horseradish are all traditional "warming" remedies, which will speed you through a cold or flu.

Remedies

⟹ Herbs to choose to ward off and cure a cold include echinacea, andrographis, astragalus, cat's claw, and propolis (the last one is a bee product, not a herb).

⟹ Vitamin C, zinc, and vitamin A are a winning combination. Take together to help get through your cold or flu quickly.

⟹ This winning tea tastes fabulous and contains herbs and foods that are guaranteed to reduce the symptoms if not send that cold into oblivion. In a teapot or plunger combine the juice of one lemon, half the lemon rind, chopped, half a stick of cinnamon, a handful of fresh thyme crushed or chopped, a half inch of fresh ginger root, thinly sliced or grated, and a tablespoon of honey. Add boiling water and let stand for five minutes. Drink two to three cups daily.

Other

⟹ You are bound to get a cold or flu just when you least want it, usually when you are tired, stressed, and rundown. Don't let it happen to you. Or at the very least, acknowledge you are not at your best and take some preventative herbs and supplements.

⟹ Keep out of the cold and drafts. If you are in them, wear a scarf.

⟹ Put a hold on your gym membership until you fully recover. You will only prolong the infection if you push yourself too early.

CONJUNCTIVITIS

WHAT IS IT?

Conjunctivitis, or pink eye, is an inflammation of the conjunctiva, the membrane lining the eyes.

SYMPTOMS

- ☑ Bloodshot eyes
- ☑ Blurred vision
- ☑ Crustiness around the eyelashes
- ☑ Sensitivity to light and glare
- ☑ Eyes feel gritty and itchy.
- ☑ Occasionally there is a pus discharge.

WHAT CAUSES IT?

- ❑ Conjunctivitis can be viral, bacterial, or allergic. The latter is not contagious.

- ❑ The allergic reaction can be to cosmetics (especially mascara), pollution, pets, dust mites, or pollen.

- ❑ Regular bouts of conjunctivitis may be a sign that your immune system is low.

Conjunctivitis can sometimes look like another condition called blepharitis, which is a bacterial infection of the eyelash follicles. In blepharitis, the eyelashes gum together and there is a noticeable crusty mucus. The natural treatment for blepharitis is the same as for conjunctivitis.

WHAT TO DO

Diet

- ❑ Avoid sugar and alcohol as they lower your immune system.

- ❑ Eat onions and garlic daily to improve your immunity.

- ❑ Drink a daily vegetable juice based on raw carrots with celery, beetroot, and/or parsley.

Remedies

- ❑ Make up a strong tea of a few of the following herbs: calendula, goldenseal, echinacea, goldenrod, chamomile, and/or eyebright. Wait until the tea has cooled then use it as an eyewash or saturate a cotton swab or gauze pad with the tea and rinse the eyes. Take care to clean in one direction only—from the nose to the outside of each eye—and make sure you use a new cotton swab with each application. Even if only one eye is affected, wash out both eyes as conjunctivitis has a habit of jumping ship. The tea will last a couple of days in the fridge before needing to be made afresh. Alternatively, add 2 ml of herbal tincture to 25 ml of purified water or saline solution and use in a similar fashion. The tea and tincture are also good taken orally. These herbs all have antibiotic properties and are immune boosters as well as being eye focused. Goldenseal is excellent for healing mucous membranes.

- ❑ Take vitamins C and A and zinc for immunity. Vitamin A is particularly important for the mucous membranes, such as the conjunctiva.

- ❑ If conjunctivitis is a regular part of your life, cod liver oil capsules, taken daily, can be helpful.

- ❑ If you are at work or away from your herbs, apply a cool teabag (green, black, or chamomile tea are all good) to ease the discomfort. Tea has anti-inflammatory and antimicrobial actions.

- ❑ If you don't have any tea or herbs on hand, rinse both eyes with a saline solution at the first sign of redness or soreness.

- If yours is allergic conjunctivitis, and it is an ongoing problem, it may be worthwhile being desensitized. Treatment involves first isolating the allergens (dust mites, and so on), then applying regular desensitization treatments in the form of drops or injections.

Other

- It's hard to resist, but don't scratch or rub your eyes—this will only spread the infection.
- A daily change of pillowcase, washcloth, and towel will minimize recontamination.

- If you usually wear contact lenses, swap to glasses for a while until your eyes are clear again.
- Wearing some sort of eye protection in windy weather will help guard against pollens and other irritants.
- Don't share your eye makeup and regularly replace items such as mascara.
- Swim in the ocean without goggles.

AT A GLANCE

Diet

- Drink a daily vegetable juice and increase your garlic and onion intake.
- Avoid sugar and alcohol due to their immune-lowering effects.

Remedies

- Use a herbal eyewash twice a day or rinse eyes with a saline solution or a cold teabag if you don't have any herbs handy.
- Take vitamins C and A and zinc for your immune system.

Other

- Change your pillowcase and towels often and wash in hot water with tea tree oil.
- Don't share eye makeup, especially mascara.
- Wear glasses for a while if you normally use contact lenses.

CONSTIPATION

Horace Fletcher (1849–1919), a self-taught American nutritionist, was known as "the great masticator" for his advice that one must chew each mouthful of food thirty-two times before swallowing. Horace had more on his mind than just mastication, however. He was also a bowel man. With firm ideas about what constituted the ideal bowel movement, Horace claimed it must be the "shape of a small banana and smell as sweet as a biscuit."

WHAT IS IT?

Normal bowel movements are defined as those that occur anywhere from three times a day to three times a week. Anything less is constipation. Most people feel better with one or two bowel movements a day. Not least because the act itself is satisfying (when we defecate, the brain waves change from alpha to beta, a more meditative and calming state of mind). While you can suffer from an isolated bout of constipation, more commonly it is a long-term condition. A little detective work to find the cause will hopefully cure constipation forever.

SYMPTOMS

☑ Having less than three bowel movements weekly.

☑ Straining when you go to the toilet.

☑ A feeling of incomplete evacuation

☑ Lumpy or hard bowel movements

☑ Accompanying signs may include bad breath, tiredness, headaches, loss of appetite, coated tongue, bloated tummy, body odor, flatulence, and skin problems.

WHAT CAUSES IT?

❏ Not drinking enough fluid is often the most simple and only cause of constipation. Without sufficient fluid, the contents of the bowel become dried out and difficult to pass.

❏ The fiber connection. When it comes to bowels, much depends on "transit time" (the time it takes for food to pass through your entire twenty-eight feet of digestive tubing). In countries where the diet is mostly fibrous grains and vegetables, the transit time is less than twenty-four hours and up to just over one pound a day can be eliminated from the bowel. In more highly industrialized countries like ours, transit time may take several days and stools weigh in at a paltry three and a half ounces. The obvious conclusion is that fiber speeds up the transit of body waste. For many people, therefore, fiber is the key to curing constipation.

❏ Stress tightens many muscles, including the muscles lining the digestive tract. For some people, a stressful situation can cause diarrhea. However, others react to stress by holding on internally. The tightness of the intestinal muscles causes the stressed stools to look like small pellets or animal droppings (variously described as looking like the droppings of a goat, or if extremely stressed, a rabbit).

❏ Gluten intolerance may cause constipation. Especially if there is bloating, it is well worth trialing a gluten-free diet for a month to see if things improve. (See Gluten Intolerance on page 168.)

❏ The wrong bugs. The more we find out about the bacteria living within our bowel, the more important they appear to be. For instance, some bacteria secrete substances that can paralyze the bowel wall, putting a stop to peristalsis in that section of the bowel, causing constipation.

❑ The truism "a change is as good as a holiday," doesn't work for many bowels. Changes in routine, travel, and work can cause constipation. The bowel is a creature of habit, preferring regular meal and sleep times. For this reason, many shift workers and constant travellers suffer from constipation.

❑ Some iron supplements can cause constipation, typically iron sulphate. Although well absorbed, which is a good thing, it may bind the bowel. Other iron supplements are available that do not constipate yet will still boost iron stores and blood levels. (See Iron Deficiency Anemia on page 10.)

❑ The female hormone progesterone slows down the peristaltic movement of the bowel. This is why many women become constipated at certain times of their menstrual cycle and early in pregnancy.

❑ Sufferers of irritable bowel syndrome usually experience an alternation between constipation and diarrhea. (See also Irritable Bowel Syndrome on page 211.)

❑ If taken daily for several years, laxatives that have a stimulant effect on the bowel can make the bowel lazy. This includes over-the-counter brands and Epsom salts as well as natural senna and cascara tablets and teas.

❑ Poor abdominal muscle tone may contribute to constipation.

WHAT TO DO

Diet

❑ A high-fiber diet is mandatory. "Fiber added" products are available—usually a refined-flour food with bran added. But why not eat food that has retained its original fiber? Eat bread made from 100 percent of the grain instead of white bread with a few flakes of added bran, fruit instead of fruit juice, brown instead of white rice, potatoes with their skins instead of chips, rolled or puffed whole grains for breakfast rather than highly processed cereals. High-fiber foods include dried fruits, nuts, legumes, seeds (especially chia and linseeds), pears, sprouts, apples, quince, passionfruit, oranges, and corn.

❑ Eat your meals at regular times during the day. Bowels work best with routine.

❑ Chew each mouthful well. The chug-a-lug downward movement of the bowel, peristalsis, starts when you begin to chew.

❑ Coffee rarely gets the thumbs up in any book about natural health. However, there are many people who cannot go to the toilet without first drinking a cup of strong coffee and/or smoking a cigarette. If this is true for you, it is a sign that the muscle of your bowel is tense. Caffeine (and nicotine) relax smooth muscle, and the bowel is predominantly smooth muscle. A cup of coffee a day is hardly a problem if this is all you need to have a healthy daily bowel movement.

❑ Avoid foods that may contribute to constipation, including sugar, white-flour products, carob, chocolate, tea, yellow cheese, and red meat.

❑ Try a gluten-free challenge for one month to see if this may be the cause of your constipation. (See Gluten Intolerance page 168.) Avoid any foods containing wheat, rye, triticale, spelt, barley, or oats. If you notice an improvement in your bowel movements, keep gluten to a minimum.

❑ Prunes are a tried-and-true constipation remedy. Place two to three prunes in hot water and leave overnight. Eat the prunes and drink the remaining fluid the following morning.

❑ Don't allow the contents of the bowel to dry out. Be sure to drink 2 liters of fluid every day.

- First thing every morning drink a large glass of warm water containing the juice of half a lemon. The warm water and lemon stimulate the bowel and the liver.

- Increase the amount of good oil in your diet (flaxseed oil, olive oil, any cold-pressed seed or nut oil, and coconut oil.) This can help to lubricate things.

- Probiotics and prebiotics. The human bowel contains around four pounds of bacteria, many of which are necessary for bowel health and function. Increasing probiotic foods such as yogurt, miso, sauerkraut, kefir, natto, tempeh, and the Korean delicacy kimchi often helps constipation. Prebiotics is food for probiotics. Prebiotics are found in certain vegetables (especially asparagus, Jerusalem artichokes, leeks, and onions), legumes (such as baked beans, chickpeas, and lentils), and supplementary fibers (including psyllium, pectin, guar gum, and slippery elm).

Remedies

- For a tense bowel, magnesium can reduce muscle spasm and tension. Take a large dose (over 400 mg) twice daily. Smaller doses for children, or perhaps the tissue salt mag. phos.

- The herbs valerian, passionflower, skullcap, chamomile, and kava can help when stress is a causative factor.

- Herbal bitters are a traditional herbal treatment for many digestive complaints. Bitter herbs include artichoke leaf, angelica, dandelion, yarrow, wormwood, and others. High-quality bitter tonics are available in liquid form and contain several varieties of herbs. Take one teaspoon of herbal bitters in water before dinner

LAXATIVES

Laxatives increase peristalsis, the rhythmic downward movement of the muscles lining the bowel. Peristalsis means that it's theoretically possible for you to eat a meal standing on your head and the food will still travel in a downward (or in this case, upward) direction.

There are several sorts of laxatives including stimulant, osmotic, and bulking. The stimulant kind (e.g., the herbs cascara and senna) irritates the bowel, causing it to contract and spasm, increasing the rate of peristalsis. This often causes diarrhea and tummy cramps. While they are okay to use from time to time, if stimulant laxatives are used daily, the bowel will become reliant on them, creating a "lazy bowel."

Osmotic laxatives (such as Epsom salts) cause body fluids to enter the bowel due to a difference in osmotic pressure. These are the laxatives of choice before a colonoscopy as they cause a complete and often urgent evacuation of the bowel contents. This is a concern for two reasons: diarrhea leaves you at risk of dehydration, and the bowel is not meant to be empty. You may not like to think of it, but the bowel should be full of bacteria, fiber, and poo.

Bulking laxatives work more slowly than stimulant or osmotic laxatives. The fibers soak up fluid causing the stool to increase in volume and weight. This allows the bowel wall to be stretched, in particular the rectum. There are nerve endings in the rectum that relay the information to the brain that a bowel movement is desirable and imminent. Additionally, the soluble fibers that create the bulking of the stool are utilized by resident bowel bacteria to create beneficial substances for the health of the bowel. The one thing to keep in mind with bulking laxatives is that you need to drink plenty of fluids, otherwise the stool will dry out and further increase constipation.

each night. The bitter taste stimulates the vagus nerve, which improves the functioning of all digestive organs including the liver. As the liver produces and excretes bile into the intestine, this promotes peristalsis. Just what the naturopath ordered. Bile is the body's own laxative.

❑ Herbs that can improve the healthy functioning of the bowel include licorice, yellow dock, dandelion root, and rhubarb. Take in tablet, tincture, or tea form daily.

❑ Several fibers have the capacity to swell considerably in the bowel making the stool softer and easier to pass. These are known as soluble fibers due to their capacity to dissolve in water. These include psyllium husks, chia seeds, linseeds, slippery elm, oats, and oat bran. Start with one teaspoon and build up to three after dinner each night. Ensure you are drinking at least 2 liters of water each day as these fibers soak up a lot of liquid.

❑ The right bugs. Just as there are malevolent bacteria in the bowel that can cause constipation by halting peristalsis, there are beneficial bacteria that improve functioning of the bowel. Take a good broad-based probiotic supplement that includes a bug called *lactobacillus plantarum* every morning.

❑ If your iron supplement is causing constipation, switch to another.

❑ If your routine is upset by holiday, work, or travel, try taking a cup of weak senna-pod tea (available in tea bags) after dinner the night before you travel, and once again on the first evening. The very occasional stimulant laxative will not cause a dependency.

Other

❑ The bowel is lined with smooth muscle. This type of muscle is not under your conscious control so when it is tense or holding stress, it may interfere with peristalsis, resulting in constipation. Belly (diaphragmatic) breathing, however, switches on the parasympathetic nervous system, which in turn relaxes smooth muscle, thereby assisting peristaltic movement of the bowel. To do this, breathe through your nose, inflating the lower abdomen with your breath on the inhalation and relaxing the abdomen on the exhalation. The downward movement of the diaphragm will also massage the bowel.

❑ Try to visit the toilet at the same time each day. Many people find that after breakfast works well. Make sure you allow enough time: no bowel likes to be rushed.

❑ There are lengthy naturopathic discourses on toilet technique. The Western style toilet—a contraption that is not well suited to its task—has transformed what should be a natural act of nature. Squatting has been the favored position for millennia. It activates the abdominal muscles and the rectum and anus to widen out, making a more efficient funnel shape. While I do not suggest crouching over the rim of porcelain in stilettos or ripping out your toilet in favor of a simple hole, there are some alternatives. Try putting a few old phone books or blocks on either side of the toilet so that your knees are slightly raised. (Or look for the commercially marketed plastic shapes that fit around the toilet).

❑ An invaluable tidbit of anatomical curiosity is that our sphincters—oral and anal—are said to copy one another. So instead of pursing your lips, relax them.

❑ Any exercise that uses the abdominals will help build muscle tone. Lack of tone in the pelvic floor muscles—common after pregnancy or abdominal surgery—also contributes to constipation. Try Pilates, yoga, or the martial arts—any of these emphasize switching on the internal muscles that can help move things along.

❏ A brisk walk—the old-fashioned constitutional—may be just the thing to bring those bowels into line.

AROMATHERAPY

Mix the following blend of aromatherapy oils with 30 grams of warm coconut oil and massage into the abdomen in a clockwise direction. Massage to the lower back can also be helpful. Alternatively, sprinkle 6 to 8 drops onto a washcloth rinsed in some cool or warm water and use as a compress on the abdomen.

❏ 3 drops of carrot seed oil—stimulating to the digestive system and smooth muscle relaxant

❏ 2 drops of cardamom oil—digestive, carminative, stomachic, and diuretic

❏ 4 drops of black pepper oil—laxative, diuretic, calming, stomachic, and tonifying

❏ 4 drops of grapefruit oil—digestive stimulant, purifying, and cleansing

❏ 2 drops of juniper oil—diuretic, calming, detoxifying, and stomachic

AT A GLANCE

DIET

➡ Eat high-fiber foods (whole grains, nuts, seeds, vegetables).

➡ Drink at least 2 liters of clear fluid daily.

➡ Try a glass of warm water with the juice of half a lemon every morning. This will stimulate the liver, which in turn stimulates the bowel.

➡ Avoid foods that may cause constipation (yellow cheese, tea, sugar, white-flour products, red meat).

➡ Prunes are a tried-and-true remedy for constipation. Soak them overnight before eating and drink the juice too.

➡ Avoid gluten for one month, especially if you are bloated, to see if gluten intolerance could be causing constipation.

REMEDIES

➡ Soluble fiber supplements, also known as bulking laxatives, allow the stool to increase in size and stimulate peristalsis. Choose from psyllium husks, chia seeds, linseeds.

➡ If you suffer from anxiety and stress, chances are your bowel does too. Take a large dose of magnesium morning and night to relax the bowel wall and try the following stress-beating herbs: valerian, passionflower, skullcap, chamomile, and/or kava.

➡ Herbal bitters are a group of herbs that improve bowel function. Take a teaspoon in water before each meal.

➡ Take a good probiotic supplement every morning.

OTHER

➡ Belly breathing switches on the parasympathetic nervous system, which helps to relax the smooth muscle lining of the bowel. Relaxed muscles equal relaxed bowel movements. Beautiful.

➡ The bowels are creatures of habit, preferring meals to be eaten at the same time. Same goes for the toilet. Try to move your bowels at the same time, preferably after breakfast.

COUGH

WHAT IS IT?

Coughing is an important bodily function. Normally the cilia, or the tiny hairs that line the airways, move in unison (like a stadium "wave") and transport mucus and particles up from the lungs and bronchi to be cleared from the throat, resulting in a little *humphing* sound. Coughing is a more forceful removal of unwanted matter, ejecting particles snared in mucus from the lungs at a velocity of up to almost 100 miles an hour.

Coughs are described as being either productive or unproductive, depending on the amount of phlegm or mucus brought up. It is preferable to get rid of the mucus rather than swallowing it, as this can lead to nausea. After a productive cough, examine the color of your mucus (in private). Clear mucus indicates an irritation, a virus, or an allergy, while yellow to green may be sign of a bacterial infection. The presence of blood means that you have been coughing very hard, or possibly something more serious. In either case, mention it to your doctor.

SYMPTOMS

☑ A cough may be a symptom of an underlying condition. But sometimes a cough is just a cough.

WHAT CAUSES IT?

❏ A single cough is usually about expelling dust or something caught in the throat.

❏ Bronchitis is an infection or irritation of the bronchial tree, the airways leading down to the lungs. Bouts of coughing can occur with or without mucus. You can also wheeze if you have bronchitis.

❏ Air conditioning can dry out the membranes of the nose, throat, and lungs. In susceptible people, this will cause irritation and may trigger coughing.

❏ Reflux is where there is a regurgitation of the acid contents of the stomach into the esophagus, irritating the mucous membranes and causing a cough. Silent reflux is when you are unaware that this is happening, so while the cough seems entirely random, it is in fact in response to the esophageal irritation. If more obvious reasons for your cough have been addressed, silent reflux is worth investigating with your doctor.

❏ Coughing can be a side effect of certain medications.

❏ Some people cough when they are nervous.

❏ Allergies may cause coughing. Common allergens include preservatives in food or wine, pets, certain plants, mold, and cleaning chemicals.

❏ Coughing can be the sign of a more serious condition such as tuberculosis or lung cancer. If you are concerned about an unexplained cough, ask your doctor to examine your chest, listen to your cough, and order whatever tests may be necessary to determine the cause.

WHAT TO DO

Coughing is a natural way of eliminating matter from the lungs. Unfortunately, many pharmaceutical cough mixtures contain substances that suppress the cough reflex. Therefore, the best cough treatments reduce the viscosity (stickiness) of the mucus and open up constricted airways so that the mucous can be more easily eliminated. Cough suppressants (antitussives) can be used at night to help with a good night's sleep. Persistent coughing irritates and inflames the membrane lining of throat and lungs so something soothing and healing needs to be included. Infection, which is more likely if mucus is green or yellow, must also be attended to.

Diet

❑ Fluid makes the mucus less sticky, and elimination therefore easier. It is very important to drink 2 to 3 liters of clear liquids daily such as water. Hot fluids are best—hot honey and lemon, herbal teas, broths, miso soup, spicy soups, or chicken soup.

❑ Try this fabulous cough-busting brew:

Juice of one lemon

Rind of half the lemon, chopped

1 stick of cinnamon (optional)

1 handful of fresh thyme, crushed

1 inch of fresh ginger root, grated

2–3 tablespoons of honey

Place all the ingredients into a teapot. Add boiling water and let stand for five minutes. Drink three cups daily.

❑ The old-fashioned hot toddy can also work a treat to help you get off to sleep. Pour a shot of whisky, brandy, or rum into a cup of hot water and add some lemon juice and honey.

❑ For some people, dairy products increase mucus. Avoid them if necessary.

❑ Eat fresh pineapples and drink pineapple juice—they contain bromelain, a substance that helps to break down mucus.

❑ Foods that are good for the lungs include onion, garlic, pepper, aniseed, and cinnamon.

Remedies

❑ Onion cough syrup. Sounds yuck, but tastes yum. Roughly chop an onion (red, brown, or white) and place into a bowl. Pour over some runny honey until covered. Leave in warm place for a few hours or overnight. Adults can take one tablespoon of onion syrup every hour, or one teaspoon for a child. Onions are part of the *Allium* family, as is garlic, and they both have bug-killing and mucus-thinning properties.

❑ Herbs can also help relieve coughing in several ways. Some have expectorant properties that can encourage mucus to move up and out of the airways, while some have antimicrobial properties that can help fight viral, bacterial, and fungal infections. Others have mucolytic properties that can reduce the viscosity or stickiness of mucus, allowing it to be more easily removed. Antispasmodic herbs can reduce excessive coughing, promoting a restful night's sleep. Many herbs combine several of these actions. The following herbs are traditional lung tonics: mullein, grindelia, licorice, thyme, marshmallow, euphorbia, elder, white horehound, garlic, and saffron. A mixture of several of these in a tincture or in tea form three times a day can relieve the most stubborn cough.

❑ Quercetin is known for its ability to reduce the inflammation often associated with allergies and respiratory complaints.

❑ Cod liver oil, which contains vitamin A for mucous membrane support and vitamin D for immunity, can be helpful in preventing coughs. It is good for children, too. Now available in capsule form, rather than the psychologically scarring spoonful of yesteryear.

❑ Vitamin C and zinc can help prevent and resolve an infection.

❑ Magnesium (200 mg) taken twice a day can ease the muscular strain of excessive coughing.

❑ Magnesium phosphate (mag. phos.) tissue salts can help remedy a chronic, hacking, unproductive cough.

❑ The homoeopathic remedies ipecac and antimonium tartaricum (ant. tart.) are also good for productive coughs, especially if there is gagging.

Other

❑ Humidifiers, available from pharmacists, can help moisten the airways and allow for a peaceful night's sleep. Add a dab of Vicks or a few drops of essential oil to the water in the humidifier (eucalyptus and/or thyme oil for an infection; lavender for a calming effect).

❑ Coughing can both cause and be caused by a spasm in the smooth muscles that line the airways. If your cough is driving you mad (and those around you), switching on the parasympathetic nervous system by a slight increase in carbon dioxide can relax the smooth muscle and stop the coughing. Sound simple? It is. Try this. Close your mouth. Take a small breath in, then out. With the thumb and forefinger of one hand, gently hold your nose closed for five seconds. Release and relax for ten seconds, breathing gently through your nose. Repeat ten times or until the coughing stops. (See Appendix F on Buteyko breathing.)

❑ Try a steam inhalation once or twice a day, and definitely before bed. Steam inhalations relax the airways and help the elimination of mucus. Simply bring a kettle of water to the boil. Pour the water into a large bowl or pot and add a teaspoon of Vicks or eucalyptus oil.

Place the bowl on a table and sit close by, draping a towel over your head and the bowl. Keeping a slight distance from the water, breathe the vapors in through your nose. Stay for as long as comfortable.

❑ Postural drainage uses gravity to help you cough. It is a very useful technique for loosening congestion, and is best done after a steam inhalation. First, lie face down across the bed, bending at the waist so that your hips and legs are on the bed and your trunk is hanging over the side. Place a bowl or towel within striking distance. Make yourself comfortable by resting on your forearms on the floor. In this position, your lungs are upside down. Very gently begin to cough. If you have a helper, ask them to thump rhythmically and lightly on your back, especially on the side and bottom ribs. This can be too rough for some, however. Children, babies, and older people can therefore lie on the bed fully and prop several pillows under their middle so that their head is lower than their chest. The helper should apply gentle percussion to the upper back to dislodge phlegm. This is very good for children who vomit up mucus in the night.

❑ For those with a chronic cough or lung congestion, place bricks or books under the base of your bed so you are lying slanting down towards the bedhead. This will help drain the lungs.

❑ Don't smoke.

DIET

→ Drink at least 2 liters of clear fluid to allow for the easy elimination of mucus.

→ Hot fluids are best, especially the fabulous lemon-honey cough-busting brew described earlier. Drink three cups daily.

→ Lung-friendly foods include pineapple, onion, garlic, pepper, aniseed, and cinnamon.

REMEDIES

→ Onion cough syrup (see earlier) is a powerful cough medicine for both the young and old alike.

→ Herbs that can be helpful for a cough include mullein, grindelia, licorice, thyme, marshmallow, euphorbia, elder, white horehound, garlic, and/or saffron. Take as a tablet, tincture, or in tea form.

→ For a chronic cough, take cod liver oil daily.

OTHER

→ A steam inhalation (see earlier), especially at night, will help clear the airways and allow for a restful, cough-free sleep.

CYSTITIS

WHAT IS IT?

Cystitis, also known as a urinary tract infection (UTI), is quite common in women and young girls and frankly, can be described as like "weeing razor blades." Caused by a bacterial infection, cystitis affects women most often because the journey from the outside world where bacteria lurk (near the anus), to the bladder, is much shorter than it is in men. The infection inflames the lining of the bladder and urethra (the tube that takes urine from the bladder to the outside world). It is therefore very important to treat cystitis before any infection travels to the kidney via the ureters (the pair of tubes that take urine from the kidneys down to the bladder). A kidney infection is a much more serious affair. If you begin to experience a fever, vomiting, or chills, this may be a sign that the kidneys have been affected, so contact your doctor straight away.

If men have symptoms similar to those of cystitis, it may be a sign of an enlarged prostate gland or a condition known as nonspecific urethritis (NSU), a sexually transmitted disease that must be treated by your general practitioner. Cystitis in women may occur after intercourse, but is not sexually transmitted.

SYMPTOMS

☑ Painful urination

☑ A frequent urge to urinate only to be disappointed by a tiny output, and/or feeling the urge to go again a few minutes later

☑ The need to urinate frequently during the night

☑ Pain in the lower abdomen

☑ Smelly urine or urine of an unusual color or cloudiness

WHAT CAUSES IT?

❑ Cystitis used to be called the "honeymooner's disease" because frequent sex, and the mechanical rubbing against the urethra during intercourse, increases the opportunity for bacteria to travel to the urinary tract.

❑ Women who use a diaphragm for contraception are more prone to cystitis because it must be physically inserted.

❑ After menopause, when there is less estrogen present, the lining of the urethra thins, increasing the chance of cystitis.

❑ The oral contraceptive pill and other medications can make women more susceptible to cystitis.

❑ *Candida albicans,* a yeast that commonly occurs in the vagina, can sometimes become troublesome and travel to the bladder, creating symptoms very similar to cystitis.

❑ Diabetics are more prone to cystitis, possibly due to an increase of sugar in the body. Bacteria just love sugar.

❑ Pregnancy is also a time when cystitis is more common. The change in hormones and pressure on the bladder are two likely triggers.

❑ Stress lowers your immunity and makes you more susceptible to infections like cystitis.

WHAT TO DO

Diet

❑ Even though you might be running to the toilet all the time, now is the time to keep drinking. Drink at least 3 liters of fluid daily to flush out the bugs from your bladder. At least 2 liters of your daily intake should consist of pure water.

❑ Barley water is a traditional remedy for cystitis. Boil 1 liter of water with a handful of pearl barley. Simmer to reduce it down to about 500 ml. Drink when the liquid has cooled. A little lemon juice can be added for taste.

❑ Corn silk. If you have access to fresh heads of corn, use the hair or silk that surrounds the cob and use in a similar way to pearl barley above, or add to the brew if you have both.

❑ Cranberry juice. Drink two glasses of unsweetened cranberry juice a day. Cranberries can inhibit the ability of bacteria to adhere to the lining of the bladder, as can blueberries. Add a handful to your fruit salad or smoothie.

❑ Avoid coffee. It is a bladder irritant. This goes for decaf as well.

❑ Garlic and onions are naturally antibiotic.

❑ Avoid sugar. It lowers the immune response.

Remedies

❑ Herbal teas are an excellent way to treat cystitis. They combine the therapeutic actions of the herbs with the very necessary extra fluid. Use crataeva, goldenrod, juniper, celery seed, corn silk, buchu, uva ursi, and/or shepherd's purse.

❑ If this is not your first bout of cystitis, it can be worthwhile upping the stakes and taking the herbs in tablet or tincture form as well as in a herbal tea.

❑ Cranberry tablets can be taken as part of a treatment as well as a preventative if you are prone to cystitis.

❑ The probiotic acidophilus can help to normalize bacteria. Try a tablespoon of acidophilus yogurt or take a teaspoon of powder in water each morning. If you are in a lot of pain, apply a handful of cool, plain yogurt to the area.

❑ A buffered form of vitamin C can help fight any infection without causing further acidity.

❑ Echinacea, vitamin A, and zinc can also fight infection. Vitamin A is particularly good for healing the inflamed bladder lining.

❑ Normally, urine should be slightly acid (around pH 5–6). During a bout of cystitis, however, alkalizing the urine will calm the inflamed bladder. This is why over-the-counter sachets for cystitis can work in the short term. A kitchen remedy that will also alkalize the urine is drinking a cup of water containing a teaspoon of bicarbonate of soda. Note that this merely helps relieve the symptoms and does not treat the infection.

❑ The homoeopathic remedy cantharis, or Spanish fly, can also be very good, particularly if there is a burning sensation, a nonstop urge to urinate, and an inability to empty your bladder completely.

❑ If you feel your cystitis has an emotional or psychological trigger (that is, you are pissed off) then the Bach flower Willow and/or Chicory for resentment may help.

Other

❑ Avoid bubble baths, bath salts, scented soaps, and deodorant sprays as they will irritate the area further. Use a low-allergy body wash or a sock or stocking filled with oats in the bath.

❑ Sandalwood oil is recommended for cystitis. Not to be taken internally, add a couple of drops to your bathwater.

❑ Adding a cup of bicarbonate of soda to your bathwater can also help relieve any burning.

❑ Wash before and after intercourse. A bidet or handheld shower is well suited to washing hard-to-reach places. Urinating after intercourse can also help flush away any bacteria.

❑ If urinating is painful, do so in a warm bath or spray on some warm water.

❑ Wipe from front to back with each visit to the toilet.

❑ Some women find tampons may aggravate chronic cystitis or can set off an infection.

❑ Change sanitary pads regularly (every three hours or so) to prevent bacterial growth.

❑ A hot, sweaty environment is what every bacterium likes. Swap synthetic underpants and tights for a pair of cotton underpants and knee-highs.

❑ For many women, cystitis is the body's eloquent way of saying, "I'm pissed off."

AROMATHERAPY

Try this soothing bath oil.

❑ 2 drops of sandalwood (Australian) oil—a known urinary antiseptic

❑ 1 drop of atlas cedarwood oil—anti-infectious, decongesting

❑ 1 drop of tea tree oil—antibacterial, antiviral, anti-infectious, analgesic

Use in a sitz (hip) bath or double the amount of drops and use in a full bath. Make sure the essential oils are mixed well through the water before sitting down in the bath.

DIET

➡ Drink at least 3 liters of fluid daily in order to flush the bacteria from your bladder.

➡ Avoid coffee and sugar. Coffee is a bladder irritant and sugar has a negative effect on the immune system.

➡ Drink unsweetened cranberry juice. Cranberries inhibit the bacteria from attaching to the bladder wall.

REMEDIES

➡ Drink herbal teas made from echinacea, crataeva, goldenrod, juniper, celery seed, corn silk, buchu, uva ursi, and/or shepherd's purse.

➡ Buffered (nonacidic) vitamin C, vitamin A, and zinc are all good for the immune system, which needs a boost right now.

➡ To ease the burning pain of cystitis, drink a cup of water to which a teaspoon of bicarbonate of soda has been added. This will only help relieve the symptoms, not treat the cause, which is a bacterial infection.

OTHER

➡ Avoid anything likely to irritate the area.

➡ Wash before and after intercourse.

➡ Wear cotton underwear and avoid pantyhose for a while.

➡ Consider if you are "pissed off" with something or someone.

DANDRUFF

WHAT IS IT?

Dandruff is a condition whereby the skin of the scalp sheds in white scales. Dandruff is not contagious, nor is it a sign of poor hygiene, but it can be a cause of sartorial concern for those who prefer dark-colored sweaters and coats.

Seborrheic dermatitis has a similar presentation to dandruff, but there is generally more redness and the scales are colored cream to yellow. This condition spreads to the hairline, behind the ears, eyebrows, bridge of the nose, around the nose, genitals, and anus. In addition to the remedies for eczema, seborrheic dermatitis can respond well to the treatment for dandruff. The same condition is called cradle cap in babies. Dandruff can also look similar to psoriasis, another condition that frequently affects the scalp.

WHAT CAUSES IT?

❏ No-one is quite sure of the cause of dandruff; however, a small fungal/yeast organism is always found at the scene. *Pityrosporum ovale* (also known by the more exotic name of *malassezia furfur*) is either attracted to the inflamed skin or is the cause of the problem. Either way, eliminating Monsieur FurFur can help to get rid of your dandruff problem.

❏ Overuse of hairsprays, gels, dyes, and other grooming products.

- Hormonal imbalance. Puberty is commonly a time when adolescents experience dandruff, acne, and unrequited love.

- Stress is nearly always a factor in skin conditions and dandruff is no exception.

- A diet low in essential fatty acids.

- Poor circulation.

- Genetics.

WHAT TO DO

The goal is to eliminate the fungal factor and generally improve skin quality.

Diet

- Drink 2 liters of water daily to keep the skin hydrated.

- As Monsieur FurFur is a major factor in terms of dandruff, the best advice is to follow the candida diet (see page 74). The basics of this month-long diet are to forgo sugar and yeasted foods.

- If you are not yet prepared to take the candida diet plunge, at the very least, eliminate all added sugar from your diet.

- Increase good oils including cold-pressed olive oil, cold-pressed nut oils, coconut oil, and foods with beneficial fatty acids, including fish, nuts, seeds, and avocadoes.

Remedies

- Make up a strong tea using dried or fresh thyme. Allow to cool and strain. Use as a rinse after you have finished washing your hair, leaving the tea in the hair without further rinsing.

- Use a shampoo containing the antifungal minerals selenium and zinc. Several antidandruff shampoos incorporate these minerals into their formulation.

- Rinse your hair with a solution of one-quarter cup of apple cider vinegar diluted in 1 liter of water. Another good rinse is the juice of one lemon added to 1 liter of warm water. Pour over your head and massage in. If possible, and if weather permits, dry in direct sunshine.

- Once or twice a week, before bed, massage your scalp with a mixture of olive oil with a few drops of antifungal tea tree oil added. You could also add lavender, rosemary, and/or sandalwood oils as they are also antifungal and smell a little sweeter. Cover your pillow with a towel to avoid staining and shampoo out in the morning.

- Give babies with cradle cap a gentle scalp massage with olive, sweet almond, or apricot kernel oil with a couple of drops of tea tree or rosemary oil every day.

- Add 2–3 drops of tea-tree oil to any shampoo you use. Tea-tree oil is antifungal.

- Take some fish oil and evening primrose oil daily (3 grams of each).

- Take a probiotic containing acidophilus, bifidus, and *lactobacillus rhamnosus* GG.

- Biotin, vitamin A, and zinc are all necessary for healthy skin.

- The tissue salt potassium sulphate (kali. sulph.) is recommended for dry, scaly skin.

Other

- Don't wear dark-colored shirts.

- If you live close to the beach, try to swim in the seawater, allowing the sun to dry your hair.

- Inverted postures—where the head is lower than your hips—improve circulation to the head and scalp. Try lying with your legs up the wall, bottom resting on a cushion. For the more adventurous (and strong of neck and back), yoga shoulder and headstands will also do the trick.

❏ Steer clear of hair products, gel, and dyes as they can be irritating to the scalp.

❏ Don't lend or borrow hairbrushes or combs.

❏ Invest in a shower filter that minimizes chlorine and other chemicals added to the water.

AROMATHERAPY

The following blend of essential oils can be blended with 30 ml of warmed coconut or jojoba oil and massaged into the scalp. Wrap the hair in a warm towel and leave for an hour then wash hair. Repeat weekly. Alternatively, the blend can be made into a neutral shampoo base and/or a neutral conditioner base and used as normal.

❏ 3 drops of tea tree oil—antiseptic

❏ 4 drops of lemongrass oil—antipyretic, bactericide, tonic

❏ 3 drops of clary sage oil—excellent for oily hair, antiseptic, astringent

❏ 5 drops of rosemary oil—antiseptic, restorative, stimulating

AT A GLANCE

DIET

➠ Avoid sugar and yeast. This will starve the yeast organism involved in dandruff.

➠ The best option is to go on the candida diet for one month (see page 74).

➠ Dandruff is a skin condition. Improving overall skin quality will help prevent and treat dandruff. Increasing foods high in essential fatty acids (such as fish, nuts, seeds, and avocadoes) as well as the good oils (olive oil, nut oils, and coconut oil) can be beneficial.

REMEDIES

➠ Add a few drops of tea tree, lavender, or sandalwood oil to your shampoo. After washing, apply a strong thyme tea preparation and don't rinse out.

➠ Take some probiotics.

➠ Biotin, vitamin A, and zinc are all recommended for healthy skin.

➠ Evening primrose oil and fish oil will help improve skin quality and prevent further outbreaks of dandruff.

OTHER

➠ Keep your favorite black clothing for when your dandruff has been treated.

➠ Swim in seawater, let your locks flow freely, and allow the sunshine to dry your hair naturally.

➠ Avoid using chemicals such as hair dye, gels, and other hair products.

DEPRESSION

WHAT IS IT?

For a rainbow to be a rainbow, all the colors must be there—from bright yellow to somber indigo. A depressed mood is part of being human, but depression is more than just a mood. Depression is as much physiological as psychological: neurotransmitters produced by the body (including serotonin and dopamine) affect our thoughts and mood. Regarded as the common cold of psychiatry, depression is unfortunately for many, a lifelong companion.

SYMPTOMS

Some signs that you might be depressed are given by the Depression and Bipolar Support Alliance (http://www.dbsalliance.org/site/PageServer?pagename=education_depression), one of the top U.S. organizations that deals with depression and other mood disorder. They include:

- ☑ Prolonged sadness or unexplained crying spells
- ☑ Significant changes in appetite and sleep patterns
- ☑ Irritability, anger, worry, agitation, anxiety
- ☑ Pessimism, indifference
- ☑ Loss of energy, persistent lethargy
- ☑ Feelings of guilt, worthlessness
- ☑ Inability to concentrate, indecisiveness
- ☑ Inability to take pleasure in former interests, social withdrawal

A spell of depression is normal when grieving, after a separation, and so on. However, if your depression doesn't have an obvious cause, or has not lifted after six months, seek help. Depression is a condition that must be taken seriously.

WHAT CAUSES IT?

- ❏ Negative life events (including abuse, poverty, or illness and particularly events or situations stemming from childhood where we learn much of our behavior), may contribute to later depression.

- ❏ If depression or anxiety taints your family tree, you have a higher risk of suffering this condition.

- ❏ Depression is not caused by a virus or bacteria, although occasionally infection may trigger a bout of depression.

- ❏ Other physical causes may include hormonal imbalance, low thyroid function, and low iron levels. Get these checked also.

- ❏ Chronic illness or pain is a frequent cause of depression. In fact, if you suffer from a long-term health condition, it's likely that you will also become depressed. Cortisol, the stress hormone that increases with any stressor (including illness) decreases serotonin, the "happy" neurotransmitter. Low serotonin equals low happiness.

- ❏ Long-term stress. Relationship, financial, and job stress or being a caretaker will increase cortisol.

- ❏ People who are at a life crossroads, or those who have recently experienced a high such as having a baby, getting married, or graduating from studies can become depressed when the good times are over, with seemingly nothing to look forward to after months or years of expectation.

WHAT TO DO

Any treatment for depression needs to work on both levels, psychological and physically. After all, mind and body are intimately connected. Regardless of the cause of depression, there are natural remedies as well as dietary and lifestyle changes that may help.

Diet

❏ When depressed, cooking and eating well might be difficult to do, but a poor diet will only contribute to the problem. If you live alone, perhaps invite a friend over once a week and make a point of cooking a nutritious and delicious meal. Freeze leftovers for later in the week.

❏ Erratic blood sugar levels can influence mood. Keep blood sugar levels steady by eating small meals containing protein every two to three hours. Avoid sugar.

❏ Reduce caffeine. Depression is associated with levels of caffeine above 700 mg daily (4 to 5 cups of coffee).

❏ Alcohol is a nervous-system depressant. In particular, beer should be avoided—it contains hops that may have a depressive effect on the body. You be the judge. If a glass or two of alcohol a day helps you to relax and your sleep and mood are not affected, then enjoy. If this is not the case, resist.

❏ Eat plenty of whole grains, legumes, fresh fruit, and vegetables to supply sufficient B vitamins, zinc, and chromium—all nutrients important for optimum nervous-system function.

❏ People who enjoy the Mediterranean diet— where the emphasis is on vegetables, legumes, fish, olive oil, and a splash of red wine—have lower levels of depression. This diet also offers other health benefits, such as lower heart disease, diabetes, and osteoporosis.

❏ Oats are good for depression. Eat them in muesli or as oatmeal.

❏ Food allergies or sensitivities may also affect mood. If you notice your mood is changeable and can't pick an obvious trigger, make a food diary for a couple of weeks and see if you can track a pattern.

❏ Avoid processed foods such as soft drinks, cordials, packaged food, and takeout.

❏ Certain foods can interact if you are taking a particular (older) class of antidepressants known as monoamine oxidase inhibitors (MAOIs). Avoid all food sources of tyramine including aged cheeses, avocado, ripe bananas, broad beans, chicken liver, pickled herrings, wine, beer, yeast extract (e.g., Vegemite), or an excess of licorice.

Remedies

❏ St. John's wort is famous for banishing the blues. It is also the most frequently prescribed medication (herbal or pharmaceutical) for depression in Germany and is the most studied herb for depression. However, it is not the only effective herb. Others that have traditionally been used for melancholy include panax ginseng, damiana, tribulus, rhodiola, lemon balm, and verbena. If you are considering taking St. John's wort, let your doctor know as it may interact with certain medications.

❏ All the B vitamins are good for depression in one way or another. Take a fulsome B complex daily.

❏ The fatty acids EPA and especially DHA are needed for nervous system and brain function. They can also help prevent and treat depression. Take 6 capsules or 5 ml of a strong supplement daily.

❑ SAM-e (or S-adenosylmethionine) is a natural compound that is made in the body, although production diminishes with age. It can help depression and is thought to be involved in the creation and transport of the neurotransmitters serotonin and dopamine, both important for mood stabilization.

❑ L-tryptophan is an amino acid that can convert to serotonin in the body. Vitamins B_3 and B_6 and magnesium are also necessary for the conversion.

❑ Royal jelly is an excellent tonic for the nervous system. It is particularly high in B_5, which assists the adrenal glands. Take one vial or capsule each morning. (Important: do not take royal jelly if you are allergic to bees.)

❑ The Bach flower Mustard is good if your depression is like a dark cloud above you, coming on without apparent reason, whereas Gorse is the remedy for despondency.

Other

❑ Exercise alone has a tremendous impact on improving mood. By the 1970s, scientists discovered that endorphins (chemicals produced in the brain) function to deaden pain, improve mood, and have a tranquilizing effect. Endorphins, our natural opiates, are released during vigorous exercise, and are thought to be behind the phenomenon of "runner's high." When you are depressed, you probably won't feel like exercising. Too bad. Make a pact with yourself that you will do some exercise every day for ten days. Guaranteed you will feel brighter.

❑ Low thyroid activity and low iron levels can be the cause of depression. Get some blood tests to at least disqualify these variables.

❑ The pineal gland is a tiny pea-shaped organ sitting neatly near the base of the brain. It was described by Descartes as the "seat of the soul." The pineal behaves as a biological clock, keeping our bodies in sync with the rhythms of nature, the seasons, and day and night, adjusting our physiology to the environment. It translates light signals into nerve impulses, which in turn stimulate the endocrine glands to produce hormones such as melatonin. It is due to this mechanism that lack of sunlight may contribute to depression. Although we live in a sunlit land, many of us work inside for much of the day or cover up from the sun. Artificial lights do not seem to have the same beneficial effect as daylight. Sunlight contains the full spectrum of colors including ultraviolet and infrared. Walking in the sunlight for twenty minutes a day is enough to activate the pineal gland. Early morning sunlight is said to have a particularly beneficial effect.

❑ Seasonal affective disorder (SAD) is a particular variety of depression that starts in the autumn and disappears in the spring. Colder, darker nations are particularly susceptible. The treatment for SAD is simply sunlight.

❑ The Greek philosopher, Epictetus, who lived in the first century AD wrote that "men feel disturbed not by things, but by the view which they take of them." There is nothing to be lost and much to be gained by seeking professional psychological guidance. A good psychiatrist or psychologist will gently help you to unravel and heal the hurt inside. Even if you have to kiss a few frogs before finding the right therapist, be courageous.

❑ Notice your internal dialogue—or monologue, depending on how bad things are in there! Negative self-talk such as, "You are no good at blah" or "No wonder your life is s&$!" isn't going to help you.

❏ Wear bright colors. Red, orange, yellow. Bring a smile to your dial. Bypass black.

❏ Drinking morning urine (amaroli) has been used in certain cultures for depression and insomnia. Interestingly, melatonin is present in morning urine in significant quantities. Urine straight from the healthy bladder is free from germs. Best to drink your own, not a friend's!

❏ Gather things of beauty. Florence Nightingale wrote in 1859 in her *Notes on Nursing* that "The effect in sickness of beautiful objects is hardly at all appreciated. [They are an] actual means of recovery." Way to go, Flo. Keep beautiful objects around you and witness natural things of beauty—trees, flowers, animals.

AROMATHERAPY

The sense of smell bypasses the cognitive part of the brain and stimulates the limbic system (the primitive emotional brain). Aromatherapy oils are a wonderful way of calming and lifting mood. Use as a perfume, an aromatherapy candle in the bathroom, some drops in your bath, or as a vaporizer in your work space or bedroom. Aromatherapy oils used for depression include basil, lavender, neroli, Roman chamomile, frankincense, and bergamot.

Blend the following oils with jojoba oil for a personal perfume. Or omit the basil and use in a spray bottle with some essential oil dispersant (use orange flower or rose water as the base) and spray onto your pillow or bed linen before retiring. Use this blend in 30 ml of sweet almond oil for a relaxing full body massage or sprinkle 10 drops into 125 grams of Epsom salts and mix into the bath water. Lie back and relax.

❏ 1 drop of ylang ylang oil—sedative, antidepressant, nervine, aphrodisiac, euphoric

❏ 2 drops of basil oil—uplifting and clearing to the mind, nervine, antidepressant

❏ 3 drops of neroli oil—antidepressant, nervine, antistress

❏ 4 drops of lavender oil—hypotensive, antidepressant, nervine, sedative

❏ 5 drops of bergamot oil—uplifting, antidepressant, tonifying

At a Glance

Diet

➠ Avoid or reduce alcohol. It is a nervous-system depressant.

➠ Keep blood sugar levels steady to steady your mood. Avoid sugar and coffee and eat small meals frequently, making sure each meal contains some protein.

➠ The Mediterranean diet—with lots of vegetables, legumes, fish, and olive oil—is associated with lower levels of depression.

➠ Horses are given oats to pep them up. Why don't you give them a go? Eat them every morning as muesli or oatmeal.

Remedies

➠ St. John's wort is a proven herb for treating depression. Other herbs for the blues include panax ginseng, damiana, tribulus, rhodiola, lemon balm, and verbena.

➠ The nervous system relies on the B group of vitamins. Make sure you have plenty by taking a multi-B vitamin each day.

➠ EPA and DHA are the omega-3 fatty acids that have been extensively studied for their mood-enhancing activities. Take as a supplement daily.

Other

➠ Even though it might feel like the last thing you want to do, exercise increases endorphins and serotonin levels—both important for tackling depression.

➠ Sunshine is an excellent medicine for both mind and mood. Acting via the pineal gland in the brain, sunlight activates mood-enhancing hormones. Get outside now.

➠ Get checked for low thyroid hormones and iron levels. Sometimes depression is purely physical.

➠ Watch your self-talk. If you catch yourself thinking negative things about yourself or your situation, notice it, and distract yourself by thinking of something you enjoy or find beautiful. Depressed thoughts beget depressed thoughts—the opposite is true, too.

➠ Seek help. There is no shame, and much to gain, in seeing a counselor to help you through this difficult time.

DIABETES, TYPE 2

WHAT IS IT?

Formerly known as non-insulin-dependent diabetes, type 2 diabetes is a condition where the blood sugar levels are high. It affects around 250 million people worldwide, mostly in affluent countries where people eat more highly processed and refined food and exercise less. In short, it is a disease of overconsumption. Type 2 diabetes used to be known as adult onset diabetes until recently, when adolescents and even young children have been diagnosed in no small part due to appalling diets. The good news is that if caught early enough, type 2 diabetes can be reversed with diet alone.

SYMPTOMS

☑ The trouble is, there are few, if any, warning signs that you have type 2 diabetes until it is too late. Very often, the first time you are aware

---

BEHIND THE SCENES: HOW DIABETES WORKS

On the face of it, having high blood-sugar levels doesn't sound too serious; however, the body is a finely tuned machine. Or should be. The amount of sugar that circulates in the blood (also known as blood glucose) is kept closely within strict limits. Levels too low can cause hypoglycemia (hypo=low; glyc=sugar; emia=blood) and can result in a coma. Levels too high can cause hyperglycemia (hyper=high; glyc=sugar; emia=blood) and can result in a coma also. A lose-lose situation. If diabetes is not treated, high blood sugar will eventually harm both the large and small blood vessels, resulting in a host of complications including leg ulcers, impotence, gangrene, cataracts, blindness, and/or kidney damage.

Blood sugars rise after meals as glucose is absorbed from the food we eat. All carbohydrates—pasta or pineapple—are made up of glucose molecules held together by chemical bonds. In response to the rise in blood glucose, the hormone insulin is released by the pancreas. Insulin encourages glucose into cells. Cells use glucose to create energy for cell business, whether it be toe-cell business or brain-cell business. At any moment in time,

the amount of glucose circulating in the bloodstream of the average person is a meager 5 grams—or the equivalent of one teaspoon of sugar. The hormones that manage blood sugar levels work constantly to maintain the status quo.

There are two forms of diabetes: type 1 and type 2. Type 1 diabetes is often first diagnosed in those under twenty years old. In this case, the cells that produce insulin in the pancreas are destroyed and these diabetics require life-long insulin injections. Type 2 diabetes is more common, affecting more than 90 percent of cases. It occurs mostly after forty years of age. Unlike type 1, type 2 diabetes manifests as an insulin resistance, where cells resist insulin's invitation to accept glucose. This results in high blood glucose levels. Treatment is via diet or tablets. If left to progress, ultimately, the insulin-secreting cells in the pancreas give up the ghost, as in diabetes type 1, and these people will also need to rely on injected insulin. Type 2 diabetes is predominantly a lifestyle disease brought about by poor eating and exercise habits. If dealt with early enough, it can be reversed.

of a potential problem is via a blood or urine sample. However, the following are some symptoms that your blood sugar levels might be awry.

☑ Feeling unduly tired and fatigued

☑ Feeling excessively hungry or thirsty

☑ Frequent urination

☑ Blurred or failing vision

☑ Erectile dysfunction

☑ Pain or numbness in hands and feet

WHAT CAUSES IT?

❏ Diabetes is indisputably linked to the Western diet and lifestyle. Societies following traditional diets generally do not experience type 2 diabetes. In a nutshell, where there is excess fat, alcohol, and sugar combined with insufficient fiber and exercise, diabetes is more common.

❏ There is a genetic susceptibility. Peruse your family tree.

❏ Obesity is associated with insulin resistance.

❏ Heart disease and diabetes are two sides of the same coin. Those with elevated cholesterol and/or low HDL levels have a higher chance of developing diabetes. And vice versa. Once you have been diagnosed with diabetes, your chance of also suffering heart disease more than doubles.

WHAT TO DO

Diabetes can be a life-threatening condition. If you are taking insulin or tablets for diabetes, it is vital that your doctor is made aware of any changes you are considering to your diet or if you wish to use natural remedies. It is also important to have your blood sugar levels monitored daily.

Diet

❏ Particularly relevant to the diabetic, and those wishing to avoid this fate, is to eat small meals at frequent intervals to sustain blood sugar levels. Eat a small meal containing protein and complex carbohydrates every two to three hours. Examples include hummus on a whole meal cracker, tuna and salad, or a slice of vegetable frittata.

❏ Avoid or severely restrict sugar, coffee, and alcohol. They all have an effect on blood sugar levels.

❏ Fiber is integral to the good diabetic diet, particularly soluble fiber. Many studies have shown that soluble fiber enhances insulin sensitivity, as well as slowing the release of sugar into the bloodstream. Soluble fiber is found in legumes, vegetables, psyllium, chia seeds, nuts, and all other seeds. Avoid refined flour products (e.g., cakes, white bread, biscuits,etc.).

❏ Eat foods with a low- to medium-glycemic index. Avoid high-glycemic index foods. The glycemic index is a ranking of foods based on their immediate effect on blood sugar levels. If you are diabetic, you want foods that will slowly increase blood sugar levels, rather than those which will supply a quick burst of sugar. Foods with a low-glycemic index include bran, oats, buckwheat, pasta, baked beans, lentils, kidney beans, soya beans, apples, pears, peaches, and milk. Foods with a high-glycemic index are best not eaten on their own. High-glycemic foods include most breakfast cereals (except muesli and oatmeal), bread, biscuits, parsnip, potatoes (especially mashed), and candies.

❏ A small glass of dry red or white wine with dinner can help lower blood sugar. Wait until you have your blood sugar levels under control before going overboard with this suggestion.

- Onions and garlic can significantly lower blood sugar levels. Eat daily.

- Other foods that beneficially regulate blood sugar levels include legumes, cinnamon (add a teaspoon to your oatmeal), fenugreek, blueberries, and bitter melon.

- Follow the recommendations for the low-starch diet (see page 245).

- Avoid artificial sweeteners (even the natural ones like stevia). Not because they are bad for you, but because they keep you in the sweet-tooth loop. Most research shows that consuming artificial sweeteners doesn't help you lose weight, in fact the opposite occurs. Philosophically, the aim is to eat nutrient-dense foods. Artificial anything doesn't form part of this equation.

- Reduce red meat and animal fats (including dairy fat). Avoid margarine. A high-fat diet increases your risk of getting diabetes and developing the many complications of that disease. Eat more "good" fats, including fish, avocadoes, olive oil, coconut, nuts, and seeds. Good fat increases satiety—that is, you feel fuller longer. Also, many good-fat foods contain other nutritional prizes such as fiber, vitamins, and minerals.

Remedies

- Herbs for diabetes include goat's rue, gymnema, cinnamon, American ginseng, coleus, codonopsis, licorice, and fenugreek.

- Chromium, magnesium, zinc, vitamin C, vitamin D, EPA, DHA, alpha-lipoic acid, and the B-complex vitamins are all important for insulin response.

- Herbs that can help the circulatory complications of diabetes include ginkgo biloba, bilberry, and ginger.

- Vitamin E prevents and treats many of the complications of diabetes. It is a wise preventative treatment. Take 100 to 500 IU daily.

Other

- If you are carrying excess weight, particularly around the belly, make losing weight and most importantly, inches off waist, your number-one priority.

BODY SHAPE AND DIABETES RISK

People who have the apple-shaped distribution of fat around the tummy, rather than the pear-shaped distribution around the hips, are more at risk of developing diabetes. It is as much about the circumference as the shape of the fruit. For women, you have an increased risk of diabetes (and heart disease) if your waist is larger than 31 inches, and a greatly increased risk if it is over 35 inches. For men, your increased risk is when your waist measures more than 37 inches, and greatly increased risk is over 40 inches. A tape measure may seem a low-tech approach to predicting this serious illness; however, this simple and inexpensive method accurately predicts the amount of visceral fat, or fat in and around the liver. This is evil fat. Formerly, fat was considered to be a benign, and slightly annoying, body tissue that hung around making us look bad. However, some fat, including the visceral variety, is active. In a bad way. It produces inflammatory substances that create insulin resistance, resulting in diabetes. Losing weight is much more important than for just aesthetic reasons.

❏ Exercise is important for diabetes. Firstly, it is vital in any weight-loss program, and secondly, exercise improves insulin sensitivity.

❏ Stress affects blood sugar levels. Learn to chill.

❏ Give up smoking. Nicotine interferes with blood sugar levels and restricts circulation.

AT A GLANCE

DIET

➡ Caffeine, alcohol, and not surprisingly, sugar, all have an effect on blood sugar levels. For the time being, while you are getting your blood sugar levels to a happy place, avoid the two former and forever part company with the latter of these three foods.

➡ Fiber helps to lower blood sugar levels. Make sure every meal you eat is high in natural fibers. It's easy, as most good food is usually high in fiber. Enjoy more legumes, vegetables, nuts, seeds, and whole grains.

➡ Eat a small meal containing protein and complex carbohydrate every two to three hours.

➡ Onions, garlic, legumes, fenugreek, cinnamon, blueberries, and bitter melon can all help regulate blood-sugar levels. Eat them often.

➡ Don't fall into the trap of eating foods that contain artificial sweeteners. There is no proof that they help you lose weight (if that is what you are after) and only serve to keep you on the sweet tooth merry-go-round.

REMEDIES

➡ Herbs for diabetes include goat's rue, gymnema, cinnamon, American ginseng, coleus, codonopsis, licorice, and fenugreek.

➡ Try chromium, magnesium, zinc, vitamin C, vitamin D, EPA, DHA, alpha-lipoic acid, and the B-complex vitamins.

➡ Herbs to help the circulatory complications of diabetes include ginkgo biloba, bilberry, and ginger.

➡ Vitamin E is also important.

OTHER

➡ If you are on the plump side, losing weight is so very important for beating diabetes. It is your top priority.

➡ Exercise improves insulin sensitivity, an important goal. So don't put it off any longer.

➡ The hormones of stress, adrenaline, and cortisol negatively affect blood sugar levels. Although it seems tangential to your condition, managing stress is an important skill to learn.

DIARRHEA

WHAT IS IT?

The Aztec two-step and Montezuma's revenge sound like a heap of fun, unless it's you. Diarrhea is the frequent passing of watery feces, and it's nature's way of ridding the body of toxins. Pronto. If you have been eating or drinking something dodgy, allow nature to take its course. However, if you have a temperature, there is blood or mucus in the stool, or if diarrhea is accompanied by painful cramps and continues for more than twenty-four hours, the cause of your diarrhea needs to be ascertained and treated. Don't delay. In this country, we are lucky that diarrhea is generally considered inconsequential and a minor inconvenience. Elsewhere in the world, diarrhea caused by cholera, typhoid, and dysentery can be a major cause of death.

SYMPTOMS

☑ Frequent loose or watery stools

☑ Abdominal cramps

☑ Light-headedness due to dehydration

WHAT CAUSES IT?

❏ The infamous twenty-four-hour bug that visits and traumatizes schools, nursing homes, and entire suburbs is either viral or bacterial in origin. Often accompanied by vomiting, this diarrhea is usually done and dusted in a day.

❏ Food poisoning is mostly experienced roughly four hours after eating the offending meal.

❏ Unless you are the five-star variety of tourist, travellers often experience diarrhea, usually from E. coli bacteria that appear in different guises around the world. Our intestinal microflora might be used to "homegrown" E. coli but are xenophobic and less able to tolerate foreigners.

❏ Giardia and cryptosporidium are protozoa. They sometimes appear in our water supply and can also be contracted when traveling. Digestive complaints, including burping, bloating, and nausea are symptoms alongside diarrhea that suggest a protozoa infestation.

❏ An antibiotic's job is to kill bacteria. Unfortunately, this will include some "good" bacteria living in our intestines, as well as the intended bad guys. Disruption to intestinal microflora can cause diarrhea.

❏ Excess alcohol places great strain on the body, particularly the liver, which may result in nausea and diarrhea.

❏ Stress increases the output of the fight-or-flight hormone, adrenaline. This hormone, which increases the flow of blood to the muscles for the purposes of fleeing and fighting, is also the hormone that dilates the pupils and increases the heart rate. In this world of fear, digesting food is of little importance. The very frightened animal (or human) will defecate on the spot. Ongoing stress can result in chronic diarrhea.

❏ Certain artificial sweeteners and artificial fats are chemically designed not to be absorbed across the intestine. Due to osmosis, where fluid enters from the bloodstream into the bowel, a common side effect is diarrhea and also what is known as "fecal leakage."

❏ Diarrhea may be the result of a food sensitivity, in particular lactose and gluten intolerance.

❏ Diarrhea is a common symptom of inflammatory bowel disease including Crohn's disease and ulcerative colitis.

- Large doses of vitamin C can cause a bout of diarrhea. As soon as you have a loose bowel movement, you know you've reached your "bowel tolerance" and the tissues are saturated with vitamin C. For most people, this occurs after taking 15 grams (15,000 mg) in a twenty-four-hour period, but some people are more sensitive and react sooner.

- Long-term or chronic diarrhea may be caused by a variety of factors including irritable bowel syndrome (IBS), thyroid problems, cancer, or a reaction to medications. The reason for diarrhea should always be found and treated appropriately.

■ WHAT TO DO

Long-term or chronic diarrhea can be treated in a similar way to an acute episode; however, the cause must be found and treated.

Diet

- Rehydration is key to any treatment for diarrhea. Diarrhea is mostly water, so it is mandatory that you replace lost fluid. Rather than plain water, replace some of the nutrients lost along with the fluid. Adding a little honey or sugar allows for more rapid absorption and will increase your blood sugar levels as they are likely to be low. Some suggestions in addition to plain water include herbal teas with honey, weak black tea with honey, miso soup, an electrolyte replacement drink, chicken or meat broth, or fresh coconut juice.

- Diarrhea is one of the few conditions where roughage is not recommended. The bowel needs less, not more, stimulation. White rice not brown; white cracker biscuits rather than whole meal.

- Rice water is a 3,000-year-old remedy, and even today it is recommended by the World Health Organization. Boil two handfuls of rice with one teaspoon of salt in two liters of water for 20 minutes. Strain and add a tablespoon of honey or sugar to a liter of rice water. Drink a cup every hour or so.

- An "old wives'" tale that is very effective for stopping diarrhea is to grate a raw apple with skin intact, allow some time for it to turn brown, then eat.

- Although fluid replacement is by far the most important remedy, after a day or so, try introducing some solids for nourishment. Cooked white rice is sometimes the only thing you can stomach. It is also bland and not likely to cause further diarrhea. Other possibilities include steamed chicken breast, baked or steamed white fish fillet, bananas, mashed potatoes, and pumpkin or stewed fruit. Plain water crackers with a little Vegemite also fit the bill, replacing lost salt.

- If you have become lactose intolerant as a result of the diarrhea (see Irritable Bowel on page 211), avoid all dairy foods for a week or so. Take some probiotic acidophilus supplements,

LACTOSE AND DIGESTION

Lactose intolerance, the inability to tolerate milk sugar, often occurs after a longish bout of diarrhea. Normally, resident bacteria (of the lactobacillus family) produce lactase, the enzyme that digests lactose. During the digestive mayhem of diarrhea, these lactase-producing bacteria can be wiped or washed out, leaving you unable to digest lactose and causing the symptoms of diarrhea and bloating all over again. With time, the lactase-producing bacteria will recolonize, especially after some judicious probiotic consumption.

and after a week, start with a little good quality plain yogurt, increasing dairy daily until your normal quota is reached.

❏ Avoid foods that aggravate the bowel such as coffee, alcohol, and spicy food.

Remedies

❏ Herbs that can help calm a turbulent belly and reduce diarrhea include ginger, peppermint, chamomile, sage, meadowsweet, raspberry leaf, and cinnamon. Take in tea, tablet, or tincture form.

❏ Acidophilus and bifidus in powder or capsule form is important to re-establish good gastrointestinal microflora.

❏ *Saccharomyces boulardii* is a friendly yeast (as opposed to bacteria) that helps push out the "bad" bugs in the gut. It can be taken in combination with other probiotics, and is particularly helpful if you suspect a villainous bacteria, parasite, or protozoa has taken up residence in your bowel.

❏ To prevent traveler's diarrhea, two weeks before travelling take one teaspoon of probiotics in water, or two capsules with breakfast and one to two garlic tablets after dinner. Continue this when traveling.

❏ Psyllium husks are recommended for both constipation and diarrhea. In the case of constipation, the psyllium swells to bulk up and soften the stool. In the case of diarrhea, the psyllium soaks up excess fluid and helps to slow down the transit through the bowel. Take two to three tablespoons in water twice a day.

❏ Slippery elm powder can soothe an inflamed digestive tract. Particularly good after violent diarrhea. Take one teaspoon twice daily.

❏ Take the homoeopathic remedy podophyllum 30 C if the diarrhea is worse in the morning, looks like pea soup, and involves a lot of flatulence and cramping. Take arsenicum album 30 C if there is a burning sensation around the anus, the diarrhea is watery, and if there is vomiting, anxiety, and/or exhaustion.

Other

❏ Rest as much as possible.

❏ Drink bottled water when travelling or buy an immersion heater to boil water before drinking. If your home water supply is from a tank or might be dodgy, boil before drinking.

❏ If stress and anxiety is the cause of your chronic diarrhea, addressing this is your first course of action.

❏ If there is a diarrhea bug doing the rounds of your neighborhood, take basic hygiene precautions such as washing your hands before preparing food.

❏ Beware salads not made in your own home and peel fruit before eating when traveling.

AT A GLANCE

Diet

→ Replacing lost fluids is the primary treatment for diarrhea. It is easy to become dehydrated with this condition. Rehydrate with a variety of fluids that replace key nutrients as well. Choose from black tea and honey, chicken or meat broth, miso soup, rice water with some added salt, or coconut water.

→ Grated apple allowed to turn brown before eating is excellent for stopping diarrhea.

→ Avoid coffee, alcohol, and spicy food.

→ Stick to bland food for a day or so.

Remedies

→ Herbs for bowels in distress include peppermint, ginger, chamomile, sage, meadowsweet, raspberry leaf, and cinnamon.

→ Acidophilus and bifidus in powder or capsule form are important to re-establish good gastrointestinal microflora.

→ Psyllium husks will help to bulk up and slow down the stool. Take two to three tablespoons twice a day.

Other

→ Rest as much as possible.

→ Drink bottled or boiled water when traveling.

→ If there is a diarrhea bug in your neighborhood, adopting some basic hygiene principles such as regularly washing your hands can be very helpful.

DIVERTICULITIS

WHAT IS IT?

Diverticulosis is a condition whereby small pockets or pouches appear within the colon. If these pockets become inflamed and infected, the condition escalates to becoming a diverticulitis attack. Your -osis has turned into an -itis. In medical terminology, the suffix "osis" refers to a disease or condition, whereas the suffix "itis" is an inflammation of the condition. Diverticulosis is a frequent affliction for those over fifty. The thing is, most people are unaware of it unless a gastroenterologist comments on it after a routine colonoscopy or until a diverticulitis attack occurs.

SYMPTOMS

☑ Tenderness, often on the lower left side of the belly

☑ Severe pain and cramping

☑ Bloating and flatulence

☑ Fever and chills

☑ Nausea and vomiting

☑ Diarrhea

☑ Lack of appetite

WHAT CAUSES IT?

❏ The diverticulitis attack occurs when feces or undigested food become trapped in a bowel pocket causing inflammation and infection.

❏ Diverticulosis is unknown in countries where the diet contains large amounts of fiber (over 50 grams daily) and consists of plenty of vegetables, grains, and legumes, but very little meat, sugar, and white-flour products.

❏ Constipation is a common cause of diverticulosis (see Constipation on page 104).

❏ Poorly fitting dentures or a loss of teeth often results in food that is insufficiently chewed. Seeds and nuts that have a hard coating may travel to the bowel undigested, lodging in a diverticular pouch and causing inflammation and infection.

WHAT TO DO?

Having had a bout of diverticulitis you will most definitely want to prevent another. The following advice is if you are recovering from a recent bout, feel the grumblings of an imminent attack, or wish to avoid any further episodes.

Diet

❏ For the few weeks after an attack, or if you feel any grumblings, avoid chili, pepper, alcohol, and any spicy food as the lining of the bowel will be very tender. Also avoid those foods that may become lodged in the pockets such as nuts and seeds. At this time, raw vegetables and fruit, nuts, seeds, and whole grains are also to be avoided. After the inflammation resolves, these foods are back on the menu again and recommended as they are high in fiber.

❏ In the immediate aftermath, stay on a bland, boring diet for a few days until the inflammation subsides. Yogurt, pureed soups, and even baby food will soothe an angry bowel.

❏ When the bowel is inflamed, turn roughage into softage by pureeing cooked vegetables, legumes, and fruit. In a couple of weeks you'll be back on the hard stuff.

Remedies

❏ Post attack, and to soothe an inflamed bowel at any time, slippery elm is indispensable. It is calming and healing. Take 1 teaspoon in water, yogurt, or mashed banana three times a day.

❏ If you are in pain, it is likely you have an infection. Goldenseal, garlic, andrographis, cat's claw, and echinacea all have antimicrobial powers but if the pain continues for more than a day, antibiotics may be necessary so see your doctor.

❏ The homoeopathic remedy colocynth is for the kind of pain that doubles you over.

❏ Magnesium helps whenever the bowel is cramping. Take 200 mg four times a day during the painful times.

❏ Drink ginger tea made from grated ginger root. If you like, add some other herbs, including lemon balm, peppermint, and/or chamomile. They are all recommended to relax the digestive system.

Prevention

❏ Drink at least 2 liters of water daily. If feces in the bowel become hard and dry there is a greater chance that diverticular pockets will become inflamed.

❏ Fiber is vital to prevent and treat diverticulosis. You need sufficient fiber to bulk the stool, stretch the bowel walls, and sweep out those little pockets so that bits and pieces are not left behind. Eat a diet containing plenty of (well-chewed) fruit, vegetables, whole grains, nuts, seeds, and legumes.

❑ Avoid processed foods and refined carbohydrates such as pastries, cakes, and biscuits.

❑ Chew each and every mouthful of your food at least twelve times. Undigested food can get trapped in the diverticular pockets.

❑ If you have had more than one attack of diverticulitis, it is worthwhile taking some antibiotic herbs on a regular basis. The best of all is goldenseal due to its affinity with mucous membranes, but garlic, andrographis, cat's claw, and echinacea are also superb.

❑ Herbs that are calming and soothing for the colon in general and diverticulosis in particular include ginger, peppermint, lemon balm, licorice, and chamomile. Drink in tea form, alone or combined.

❑ Avoid sugar and refined carbohydrates.

❑ A daily fiber supplement is highly recommended if you have diverticulosis. Psyllium husks, linseeds, and chia seeds are all a good choice. Why not take a combination? You will never regret making slippery elm a daily addition. Add a heaped tablespoon of the mixture to your oatmeal or smoothie, or add to juice.

❑ Nuts and seeds are a great source of soluble fiber. Make sure you chew them well or else enjoy them ground as in the LSA seed mix (linseeds, sunflower seeds, and almonds) or nut butters (almond, cashew, or brazil).

Other

❑ If you are in pain, add some Epsom salts to a warm bath and lie deep enough to cover your stomach, or lay a hot water bottle on your abdomen.

❑ A ginger compress is exceptionally helpful if pain is severe. Into the middle of a kitchen wipe or muslin cloth grate a cupful of ginger. Fold to form a ginger parcel. Place in a shallow bowl and pour over half a cup of boiling water. Leave until bearably hot. Gently squeeze and place on your belly. With cling film, cover the parcel and wrap around your back. Wrap again in a towel, then relax and keep warm for twenty minutes before unpeeling.

❑ Massage a few drops of chamomile or lavender oil on your abdomen to relieve cramping.

❑ As a preventative measure, it is important to strengthen external and internal muscles around the abdominal area. Learn how to switch on your "core" muscles via yoga or Pilates, or learn the technique from a personal trainer.

DIET

➡ After an attack or if your tummy is tender, avoid chili, pepper, alcohol, and any spicy food.

➡ In addition, steer clear of any foods that may lodge in the bowel pockets or further inflame the area such as seeds, nuts, whole grains, raw vegetables, and fruit.

➡ Cook and puree your meals until such time as you have no tenderness.

➡ In general, and to prevent diverticulitis, eat a diet high in fiber-rich foods.

➡ Drink at least 2 liters of water a day to keep the stool soft and prevent constipation.

➡ Avoid sugar.

➡ As a preventative measure, take 1 heaping tablespoon of psyllium husks, linseeds, and/or chia seeds every day.

➡ Chew your food well. Undigested food is a major cause of a diverticulitis attack.

REMEDIES

➡ Slippery elm is your friend. It is healing, calming, and soothing.

➡ Herbs that calm the bowel include peppermint, chamomile, lemon balm, and ginger. Drink as a tea or take in tablet or tincture form.

➡ Herbs to treat and prevent an infection include the poster herb goldenseal, in addition to cat's claw, echinacea, andrographis, and garlic.

OTHER

➡ A ginger compress is exceptionally helpful if pain is severe.

➡ Mix a few drops of chamomile or lavender oil into 20 ml of a base oil such as almond or olive oil. Massage your lower abdomen to relieve cramping.

EAR INFECTION

WHAT IS IT?

The causative germ for an ear infection can be viral, bacterial, or possibly fungal, in which case it becomes the equivalent of "jock itch" of the ear or "ear thrush." Infection of the middle ear (otitis media) and infection of the outer ear (otitis externa), which is also called swimmer's ear, are common conditions that affect adults as well as children, for whom it is the most common reason for a visit to the doctor.

SYMPTOMS

☑ Ear pain or ache

☑ Sense of fullness in the ear

☑ Hearing loss or muffled hearing

☑ Noises such as buzzing and humming

☑ Headache

☑ Nausea

☑ Fever

☑ Itchiness

☑ Discharge, sometimes smelly

✓ For infants, tugging or holding of the ears, irritability, unexplained crying, change in sleeping patterns

WHAT CAUSES IT?

❏ Middle ear infections often occur after or during a cold or flu and are caused by germs travelling up the Eustachian tube connecting the nose and throat to the ear.

❏ Swimming in polluted waters.

❏ Overzealous cleaning of ears.

❏ Underzealous drying of ears.

❏ There is a correlation between people who suffer from hay fever and experience ear infections. Treating the hay fever will go a long way to help prevent future ear infections.

❏ Food sensitivities may contribute to the occurrence of ear infections. Suspect wheat, gluten, dairy, soy, eggs, corn, oranges, tomatoes, or peanuts.

❏ Candida overgrowth may be the underlying cause of frequent ear infections. See page 73 to see if you fit this picture.

❏ External irritants such as hair spray or gel may initiate otitis externa.

❏ Environmental factors such as exposure to cigarette smoke, pollens, and air pollution may also contribute to a susceptibility to ear infections.

WHAT TO DO

Although affecting different parts of the ear, otitis media and externa are often both caused by the same infection and can be treated in the same way. If there is no improvement within a few days, or you suspect the inner ear is involved, see your doctor as you will probably need to take a course of antibiotics.

Diet

❏ Avoid any likely food sensitivities especially dairy, gluten, or soy.

❏ Avoid alcohol as this will swell up the already tender mucous membranes.

❏ Drink lots of clear fluids. Hot broths and soups are ideal.

❏ Avoid sugar. It lowers immunity.

❏ Eat plenty of garlic and onions for their antibiotic properties.

Remedies

❏ Echinacea, eyebright, andrographis, calendula, goldenrod, and goldenseal are antibiotic and anti-inflammatory herbs and are especially good for ear infections. Take them in tablet, tincture, or tea forms; adjust adult dosage when treating children.

MAKING A HERBAL-INFUSED OIL

You can buy infused oil from health food shops or make your own. You will need a handful of one or more of the following fresh or dried herbs: mullein leaves and flowers, St. John's wort flowers, calendula flowers, or chopped fresh (not dried) garlic, and 250 ml of olive or almond oil for base. Adjust herb quantities so that there is a full handful. Place herbs in a glass jar with a lid, and cover the herbs with oil. Make sure they are fully submerged (add more oil if necessary). Seal with lid. Leave in sunlight or in a warm place for three to four days. Alternatively, place flowers and oil in a small saucepan and warm on extremely low heat for two to three hours. Strain through muslin or a kitchen cloth into a sterilized bottle. Keep for up to six months. If you wish, you can add 20 drops of tea tree, lavender, and/or myrrh essential oils.

Ear infections are much more common in babies and young children than in adults. The explanation is anatomical. In early life, the eustachian tube that connects the middle ear to the throat is short and straight. It becomes more angled with age, allowing for better drainage. Until this adjustment, mucus, liquids, and germs have an easier route to travel to the ear.

Glue ear, or secretory otitis media, is a condition where mucus accumulates in the middle ear. It often goes away of its own accord, however deafness can result if left untreated. Chil-dren who experience difficulty with the acquisition of language and/or other learning abilities may in fact be suffering from undiagnosed otitis media. The medical procedure is a myringotomy, where a small hole is made in the eardrum and a grommet is inserted. Grommets are plastic tubes that allow the eustachian tube to open and drain fluid internally. The procedure is uncomfortable and although it solves an immediate crisis, does not prevent glue ear from recurring. The remedies mentioned below will help treat and prevent glue ear.

❑ Cod liver oil capsules are a good preventative. Take one to two daily.

❑ Zinc and vitamin C will boost the immune system and help fight the infection.

❑ Try garlic capsules or tablets in addition to dietary intake.

Other

IMPORTANT: This is not to be done if there is any damage to the eardrum or if you suspect the eardrum is perforated. See your doctor instead.

❑ Applying a few drops of warm oil is a tried-and-true remedy for ear infections. Plain olive or almond oil can be used, or even better, use an oil to which herbs or essential oils have been infused such as St. John's wort flowers, calendula, garlic, or mullein (see below). Warm the oil to blood temperature. This can be done by placing the oil in a small cup or glass then placing it in a sink of hot water. Fill a dropper with the oil and apply 2 to 3 drops into the affected ear(s), stopping the opening with cotton. Do this 3 to 4 times daily for several days.

❑ If a fungal infection is suspected, garlic oil with a couple of drops of tea tree oil is well indicated. Warm a garlic capsule in your hands before piercing and applying.

❑ Don't swim if you suspect an infection. If you are prone to ear infections, wear earplugs whenever you swim and clean them regularly using tea tree oil.

❑ Dry the ear meticulously after showering or swimming. The best way to do this is by using a hairdryer turned to low, held about 18 inches from the ear.

❑ Avoid cleaning your ears with cotton buds. This will tend to push the infection back inside the ear.

❑ To dry out the infection of otitis externa, put 1 or 2 drops of white vinegar and pure alcohol into the ear canal twice a day (this mixture is available at pharmacies). This is a good regular practice if you are a swimmer and prone to ear infections.

❑ Hopi ear candles may help the chronic sufferer by reducing pain and relieving congestion.

They originated from the Hopi Indian tribe of North America and are made from linen, honey extracts, and herbs. Inserted gently into the ear canal, they are then lit. The recipient may hear a mild crackling as the candle burns, drawing excess wax, air, and waste products from the ear. Hopi ear candles are available from some health food shops and from practitioners. Avoid using if the eardrum is perforated and/or if there is any discharge from the ear. Ear candling should feel comfortable. Don't proceed otherwise.

❏ Feed babies in an upright position, so that fluid drains downward and not to the side toward the ear.

At a Glance

Diet

⮕ Middle and outer ear infections can be due to food sensitivities. Possible culprits include wheat, dairy, and soy.

⮕ Drink lots of clear fluids—hot broths and soups are ideal.

⮕ Eat plenty of garlic and onions for their antibiotic properties.

Remedies

⮕ Herbs for infection of the ears include echinacea, eyebright, calendula, goldenrod, and goldenseal.

⮕ If you are prone to ear infections, take one to two cod liver oil capsules daily as a preventative.

⮕ Zinc and vitamin C will boost the immune system and help fight any infection.

Other

⮕ A few drops of warm, herbal-infused oil into each ear works wonders. Use warmed garlic oil or a herbal oil made from mullein, St. John's wort, calendula, or garlic.

⮕ Forget about swimming while you have an infection.

⮕ Dry ears with a hairdryer after showering or swimming. Wet ears are just asking for an infection.

⮕ Ear candles sound odd and look odd, and the crackling sensation as they burn above your head feels even odder. Yet they can be very helpful for a middle ear infection, particularly where there is a lot of congestion.

ECZEMA AND DERMATITIS

WHAT IS IT?

Eczema is an inflammatory skin condition that can present itself in many guises. Eczema can be so mild as to be virtually unnoticeable—such as an inoffensive pink patch—or it can affect you so severely with burning, crusting, and intolerable itching as to make your life a torment.

Part of a family of conditions known as atopic eczema is often an inherited complaint alongside hay fever and asthma. For those affected, many tread the "atopic march," starting with eczema as a baby, moving on to asthma as a child, and hay fever as an adult, with sporadic outbreaks of each condition throughout life. Eczema caused by an allergy to external agents is called dermatitis, although the terms are often used interchangeably.

SYMPTOMS

✓ Itching. Where there is itching, there is scratching. Where there is scratching (particularly with grubby fingernails), there is often also infection. Although not an infectious condition, there is often bacterial or fungal infection alongside eczema, and any treatment ought to attend to this also.

✓ Redness

✓ Dry skin

✓ Swollen patches

✓ Crustiness

✓ Peeling

✓ Oozing

✓ Sores

✓ Bleeding

Although eczema can appear anywhere on the body, the most common places are the:

✓ Hands and feet.

✓ Insides of elbows.

✓ Backs of knees.

✓ Behind the ears.

WHAT CAUSES IT?

❑ Two-thirds of eczema patients have a family history of the condition. It may help to blame your parents.

❑ Stress and worry are major triggers for eczema.

❑ The skin is an organ of elimination. Skin eruptions, including eczema, may occur when the other organs of elimination such as the liver, bowel, lungs, and kidneys are overworked or underfunctioning. This is why many traditional remedies for skin problems also assist these other organs. If you suffer from eczema in addition to constipation, treat the constipation and see if your skin clears. Very often, if the bowel is not processing waste products efficiently, they will be absorbed into the bloodstream and come out on the skin.

❑ Food sensitivities to milk, gluten, wheat, yeast, benzoates, the food additive tartrazine, oranges, eggs, peanuts, and soy foods can commonly cause eczema.

❑ Dysbiosis is the clunky name given to a microbial imbalance within the gut. The number of microbes (mostly bacteria) outnumber cells in the body. When this microbial population, collectively referred to as the microbiome, is out of kilter, many health problems can ensue, including eczema.

❑ Contact dermatitis is a localized eczematous rash that occurs when the skin comes in contact with an irritant. Common substances include detergent, rubber or latex (such as rubber gloves and condoms), nickel in jewelry, perfume, lanolin, dust mites, and some plants.

❏ Certain cosmetics, even "natural" ones, can cause dermatitis.

WHAT TO DO

Although it appears on the skin, in line with naturopathic principles eczema needs to be treated from within as well as attending to the external symptoms. That is, internally by dietary change and/or taking herbs and supplements, and externally by applying soothing lotions and healing potions.

Diet

❏ Avoid sugar like the plague. This measure alone is enough for most eczema sufferers to notice a miraculous improvement.

❏ Avoid possible food sensitivities to such things as milk, gluten, wheat, yeast, benzoates, the food additive tartrazine, oranges, eggs, peanuts, and soy foods. If you are unsure as to what food is your trigger, it is likely to be a food frequently consumed in your diet. Choose one suspect at a time and remove it from your diet for at least two weeks, writing a journal of your symptoms to track improvements. First suspects are gluten and dairy.

❏ Alcohol often exacerbates eczema. Avoid it.

❏ Eczema can be a symptom of an overgrowth of *Candida albicans.* Check out page 73 to see if you fit the profile.

❏ Drink at least 2 liters of pure water daily.

❏ Fish contains the anti-inflammatory omega-3 essential fatty acids. Eat at least three servings of fish weekly. Fish with the highest source of omega-3 fatty acids include tuna, salmon, sardines, mackerel, herring, and pilchards.

❏ Other essential fatty acids are also good for skin health. These are found in avocados, seeds (linseeds, pumpkin, sunflower, sesame), tahini, and tree nuts.

❏ Avoid artificial preservatives, colorings, and flavorings.

Remedies

❏ Evening primrose oil is excellent for eczema. You need to take a fair whack (6 to 10 grams daily) and be prepared to wait three to four weeks for results as it needs to be incorporated into each and every cell wall. Once your eczema has cleared, keep taking 1 to 3 grams daily to keep it in check. Similar results may be achieved with the same dosages of fish oil.

❏ Although eczema is not an infectious skin condition, when scratching breaks the skin's surface it provides an open invitation for germs to enter, further extending the inflammatory cycle. Calendula, echinacea, goldenseal, tea tree, and lavender are antimicrobial and also help the skin to heal. The easiest way to use them is to buy a cream or lotion that already contains one or more of these herbs and apply it several times a day.

❏ Traditional skin-purifying herbs used for eczema include burdock, red clover, calendula, sarsaparilla, and nettles. Drink them in tea form or take as tablets or tincture. Skin complaints often do well with water-based remedies, especially tea. A tea made from these herbs, when cooled, also makes a wonderful hand bath or can be applied as a compress (see Appendix C: Making Remedies).

❏ Probiotics can be very effective in treating eczema. The bugs in your bowel have a lot to do with the health of your skin. A mixture of probiotics that include in their number bifidus and Lactobacillus GG will be most helpful.

- If stress is a factor, as it often is, think about using kava, St. John's wort, zizyphus, withania, or passionflower.

- Vitamins A, D, C, and zinc are excellent for all skin problems. Take daily.

- Herbs to help stop itching include heartsease, aloe vera, nettle, and chickweed. These can be used in a cream or brewed up (alone or together) as a strong tea, added to bath water when cooled or saturate a washcloth and apply to the affected part.

- Eczema is an itchy condition that causes crankiness in the calmest of people. The Bach flower Impatiens will help if your eczema is driving you to distraction.

Other

- If you are prone to eczema, it is essential to keep your skin supple and in good condition at all times. A change in skin quality may be all that is needed to set the eczema ball rolling. Choose any low-allergen body lotion or cream or try jojoba oil as this closely resembles the body's natural sebum. Rub in after bathing. If your hands are affected by eczema, make sure you use a hand cream often throughout the day. The addition of calendula, tea tree, goldenseal, lavender, oats, or gotu kola to any body or hand lotion is a bonus when treating and preventing any outbreak of eczema.

- Avoid soap. Use a stocking filled with a couple of handfuls of rolled oats in the bath or shower instead to calm redness and relieve itching. When saturated with water, the stocking will ooze a silky, milky substance that is magic for inflamed and itchy skin.

- Sweat can aggravate eczema. Shower as soon as possible after exertion.

- Wear cotton gloves to bed in order to stop scratching at night. For babies, put on little mittens or socks.

- As stress is often a major factor, stress management is a key treatment.

- A form of meditation such as creative visualization may assist your recovery. Each day for a few minutes, visualize your skin as rash free. Think swimming in a cool lake under moonlight.

- Avoid synthetic as well as rough-textured or woolen clothing. Cotton and silk are best.

- Wash clothing with low-allergen washing detergents.

- Avoid using strong household chemicals for cleaning, and if you wear gloves, be cautious that rubber or latex is not part of the problem.

- To keep the moisture in, apply a thin layer of barrier cream over the affected area after bathing.

AROMATHERAPY

This blend will be anti-inflammatory, astringent, analgesic, and antiseptic while still being calming, regenerative, and restorative to the affected skin. It may be blended into 20 grams of a light, unscented base cream to which 10 ml of calendula oil has been added. The drops in this blend may also be halved and used as a cold compress.

- 3 drops of myrrh oil—anti-inflammatory, antimicrobial, antiseptic, healing.

- 6 drops of lavender oil—analgesic, antimicrobial, antiseptic, calming, nervine, tonic, vulnerary.

- 2 drops of everlasting oil—anti-allergenic, anti-inflammatory, antimicrobial, antiseptic, astringent, cicatrizant.

- 3 drops of German chamomile oil—analgesic, anti-allergic, anti-inflammatory, antiphlogistic, calming, fungicidal, nerve sedative, vulnerary.

At a Glance

Diet

⇒ Sugar is one of the main offenders for eczema. Stop eating it now and within days your skin will improve.

⇒ Food sensitivities may be the cause of your eczema. Common offenders include milk, gluten, wheat, yeast, oranges, eggs, peanuts, and soy foods.

⇒ A *Candida albicans* overgrowth might be the trigger for your eczema. Check out page 73 to see if you fit the profile.

⇒ Drink at least 2 liters of pure water daily.

⇒ Omega 3-fatty acids and other essential fatty acids are anti-inflammatory, just what you need for this skin condition.

Remedies

⇒ Take 6 to 10 grams of evening primrose oil daily. Evening primrose oil contains anti-inflammatory fatty acids that are particularly good for the skin.

⇒ Although not an infection, skin is often broken with eczema, leaving it open for germs to enter, causing further inflammation. Calendula, echinacea, and tea tree oils are antimicrobial and help skin to heal. Great additions to any skin cream or lotion.

⇒ Probiotics are important for your bowel and your skin. Take a strong probiotic supplement daily that contains bifidus and Lactobacillus GG.

⇒ Stress is often a big factor in eczema. Herbs such as kava, zizyphus, withania, and passionflower can be helpful.

Other

⇒ Keeping your skin well moisturized is important if you are prone to eczema.

⇒ Avoid soap. Use an oat stocking instead (see under Other in main section).

⇒ Visualize your skin feeling smooth and clear.

⇒ Wear cotton, silk, and natural fabrics, avoiding anything synthetic or harsh on the skin.

ENDOMETRIOSIS

WHAT IS IT?

Endometriosis is a condition where endometrial cells (the cells that line the uterus and are shed during menstruation), are found outside the uterus and even outside the abdominal cavity. It is estimated that 10 to 15 percent of women of menstruating age have endometriosis and around 35 percent of infertile women are possibly affected.

SYMPTOMS

☑ Sometimes there are no symptoms.

☑ Painful or heavy periods

☑ Pain during and after intercourse

☑ Pain with bowel movements

☑ Pelvic or lower back pain

☑ Pain and cramping before menstruation

☑ Infertility (the catch-22 is that becoming pregnant is in itself a "cure" for endometriosis)

WHAT CAUSES IT?

❏ There is no official cause for endometriosis.

❏ One theory is that endometriosis is the result of a retrograde or backward flow of menstrual blood.

❏ It is possible that endometrial cells escape during abdominal surgery.

❏ There may be a hereditary link with this condition.

❏ Red-haired women are more likely to develop endometriosis than the rest of the population. Odd.

❏ Women with irritable bowel syndrome (IBS) have a higher chance of also developing endometriosis.

WHAT TO DO

The naturopathic approach is twofold. First, stimulate circulation and drainage from the pelvic region. This will reduce adhesions and scarring as well as stimulate tissue healing and speed up the removal of unwanted endometrial cells. The second is to regulate the hormones and improve liver clearance of excess estrogen. Have patience. Treating any hormonal imbalance takes time. Hopefully within three menstrual cycles you will notice a marked improvement in symptoms.

Diet

❏ Women who eat more fish, fresh fruit, and vegetables have less endometriosis.

❏ Include four servings of fish a week into your diet for the anti-inflammatory omega-3 fatty acids.

❏ Try avoiding gluten for three cycles to see whether your symptoms improve. They often do.

❏ Caffeine, red meat, and deli meats have been found to increase the risk of endometriosis.

BEHIND THE SCENES

Menstrual flow is not a common topic of discussion—even among women—nor is what constitutes a normal amount of blood loss during a menstrual period. For the record, 50 ml is a normal volume, and anything over 80 ml constitutes a heavy period. Just how do you know how much blood you lose? The best way is to assess how often you need to change your pads or tampons. Not desire to change, but need to change. One normal tampon or pad holds around 5 ml of blood, and a large or super size holds 10 ml.

- Decrease deep-fried foods and sugar.

- Include cruciferous vegetables such as broccoli, Brussels sprouts, cabbage, and garlic in your diet. They contain substances that help the liver get rid of excess estrogen.

- Ginger and turmeric are anti-inflammatory; enjoy and use them in your cooking.

Remedies

- Herbs are the most effective treatment for endometriosis. Take a tincture or tablet that contains vitex agnus-castus, paeonia, shatavari, dong quai, wild yam, raspberry leaf, pulsatilla, and/or corydalis.

- Ginger is anti-inflammatory and antispasmodic as well as warming. It is recommended by traditional Chinese medicine, which regards endometriosis as a cold condition. Drink 1 or 2 cups of ginger tea daily or include it in your herbal preparation.

- The essential fatty acids EPO and EPA are very important. Start with 9 grams of a combined supplement daily for two months, then take 6 grams daily for another three months.

- Vitamin E can help reduce scarring and adhesions. Try 500 IU daily.

- Magnesium helps relax the smooth muscle of the uterus, reducing cramps. Take 200 mg three to four times a day as required.

- Take a women's multivitamin with iron, zinc, and B vitamins, especially B_6.

Other

- Exercise can reduce the symptoms of endometriosis.

- Lose weight if needed. Extra body fat can increase estrogen levels, and this will exacerbate endometriosis.

- Stress is a contributing factor to this condition. Learn to relax. Try meditation, tai chi, or yoga.

- While tampons do not directly cause endometriosis, long-term use may make a woman more susceptible to developing the condition.

- Acupuncture has an impressive success rate in the treatment of endometriosis. Use in conjunction with herbs.

- After childbirth, breast-feeding for as long as possible will reduce the chance of endometriosis reoccurring.

WHEN CELLS WANDER

Cells of a kind are designed to band together. Toe cells cuddle up next to one another at the end of each foot, nasal hair cells keep a low profile (hopefully) within their designated nostril, and endometrial cells, side by side, companionably line the wall of the uterus. Except in the case of endometriosis, where endometrial cells fancy themselves as corporeal travellers, leaving the womb to explore new lands elsewhere in the body. Usually they stay locally, within the pelvic cavity, attaching to ovaries, the bowel, and fallopian tubes. However, some cells have grander plans and expat endometrial cells have been found as far afield as the lungs, spleen, and even in the nose. The problem you have with these wanderlust cells is that they, like their stay-at-home cousins, respond to cyclic hormonal signals. Endometrial tissue proliferates when estrogen levels rise and sheds with progesterone withdrawal, leaving blood and endometrial debris at these sites, causing bloating and pain.

Diet

➡ Try a gluten-free diet for three cycles. If your symptoms improve in that time, continue.

➡ Eat fish several times a week.

➡ Enjoy plenty of fresh fruit and vegetables.

➡ Avoid coffee, sugar, red meat, and deli meats.

➡ Include cruciferous vegetables (such as broccoli, Brussels sprouts, cabbage, and garlic) in your diet as they contain substances that can help the liver get rid of excess estrogen.

Remedies

➡ Herbs are excellent for the treatment of endometriosis (see under Remedies in main section).

➡ Take fish oil and evening primrose oil together.

➡ Vitamin E is good for reducing scarring and adhesions.

Other

➡ Keep up or start exercising as it reduces the symptoms of endometriosis.

➡ Lose weight if needed. Extra body fat can increase estrogen levels and this will exacerbate endometriosis.

➡ Acupuncture has an impressive success rate in the treatment of endometriosis. Use in conjunction with herbs.

ERECTILE DYSFUNCTION (IMPOTENCE)

WHAT IS IT?

Few words are guaranteed to strike dread and terror, guilt, and even shame into the hearts of men as easily as "impotence." Maybe that explains the recent name change to erectile dysfunction (ED), which sounds more like a treatable medical condition than a vitriolic insult. Erectile dysfunction affects one in ten men, and 20 to 46 percent of men over forty years of age, so it's a relatively common condition. Maybe it's a man thing, but very few men feel comfortable talking about it.

Erectile dysfunction means the inability to develop or sustain an erection. It is not the same as infertility and is not to be confused with lack of desire or libido. The "gurus" of sexual studies, Masters and Johnson (whose work was first published in the 50s and 60s) believed that both physical and psychological reasons exist for erectile dysfunction—and this is still the current understanding.

Erectile dysfunction is generally viewed as a male complaint, probably because the effect is visual. However, women may also experience impotence, where there is no feeling of stimulation to the clitoris or vagina. Many of the recommendations that follow, particularly the dietary recommendations and herbs, will also help female impotence.

SYMPTOMS

✓ Inability or difficulty in getting an erection

✓ Difficulty sustaining an erection adequate for sexual activity

✓ For women inability to experience a climax

WHAT CAUSES IT?

❑ Smoking. Nicotine decreases blood flow to the peripheral blood vessels, including the penis.

❑ Being overweight. Obesity can lead to diabetes, heart disease, and lowering of testosterone, all causes of ED.

❑ Diabetes is a common cause of erectile dysfunction as it affects both nerves and blood vessels.

❑ Alcohol acts as a depressant on the nervous system: "[Drink] provokes the desire, but it takes away the performance" (Shakespeare).

❑ Atherosclerosis or the thickening of artery walls reduces blood flow to the penis.

❑ Nerve damage or disorders affect nerve pathways.

❑ Hormone imbalance. Testosterone is the hormone of libido in both men and women. If testosterone levels are low, then arousal and performance will be too.

❑ Testicular disease, injury, or infection.

❑ Medical illness including cirrhosis of the liver, kidney failure, and lung disease.

❑ Drugs including some kinds of heart medication, antidepressants, amphetamines, heroin, and tranquilizers.

❑ Masters and Johnson also suggested that erectile dysfunction may also be due to a fear of failure, particularly in terms of sexual performance. Society fosters the stereotype of the "perfect" male: healthy, good-looking, successful, rich, young, and of course, extremely virile. Trying to live up to this unrealistic ideal is impossible, and fear of not succeeding may cause more than heartache.

❑ Mental and physical fatigue and stress.

❑ Depression.

❑ Sexual monotony or boredom. This does not mean that a new partner is needed, but that care, imagination, effort, and communication are required.

WHAT TO DO

There are many modern treatments, ranging from tablets to hormonal injections, implants, microsurgery, and rubber water pumps. Natural remedies can help in certain circumstances. Everyone is different, and each situation requires its own unique solution.

Diet

❑ Go raw. It is easier to feel virile on a diet full of vitality and life force than on reconstituted, processed, and preserved fodder. Eat as much raw food as possible: raw fruit, sprouts, vegetables, seeds, and nuts.

❑ Try a vegetable juice a day filled with raw carrot, beetroot, celery, ginger, parsley, and kale.

❑ Oysters have achieved notoriety as slimy aphrodisiacs, perhaps because they are so high in zinc (an important constituent of semen), which is necessary for the hormonal health of men and women. Half a dozen oysters contain as much as 85 mg of zinc.

❑ Avoid alcohol, coffee, sugar, white flour products, and highly processed food.

Remedies

Before Viagra, the natural world was scoured for aphrodisiacs—from tiger's penis to jackal's bile, from ginseng to horny goat weed. Unfortunately, the area of sexuality is a prime target for scam artists, and there are many "natural" products sold that are as likely to give you "the horn" as a soggy sock in a hailstorm. Nevertheless, there is never smoke without fire, and many herbal aphrodisiacs have retained their reputation for hundreds of years. There must be a good reason.

Natural aphrodisiacs work in three ways. Some restore the balance of the sex hormones, particularly testosterone (which is as important for women's libido as it is for men's). Some assist the adrenal glands, which can be helpful when the problem lies in stress and fatigue, while others improve circulation to the areas concerned. Interestingly, many herbs fulfill all three roles.

❏ Aphrodisiac herbs include panax ginseng, the evocatively named horny goat weed, tribulus, withania, damiana, muira puama, maca, and saw palmetto.

❏ Erectile dysfunction is one of the side effects of certain antidepressants. The herb ginkgo biloba can work very well to combat this problem, for both men and women, and is safe when taken with antidepressant medication. Ginkgo biloba is also good for microcirculation. That is not about the size of the organ, but the size of the blood vessels therein.

❏ Vitamin E can also improve circulation. Take 500 IU daily.

❏ Zinc deficiency is common. Men are more likely to be deficient as approximately 2.5 mg of zinc is lost per ejaculate. Take a supplement daily.

❏ Take a vitamin B complex daily, particularly if you are under stress.

❏ The Bach flower Larch is a good one if you are lacking in confidence in this arena, and crab apple may help if there is an element of shame.

Other

❏ Lose weight if necessary.

❏ Stop smoking.

❏ Exercise is important. It increases energy, improves circulation, and depending on the type of exercise, can increase testosterone levels. Exercise that builds muscle tissue increases testosterone levels. This does not mean for women that they will end up looking like an Arlene Schwarzenegger. Try weights at the gym, boxing classes—anything that improves muscle tone.

❏ Stress and worry are big killers of desire and performance. Learn how to relax.

❏ Acknowledge there is a problem and discuss it openly with your partner. You might be surprised at how liberating just shining some light on this subject can be. If not your partner, talk to a friend, doctor, or counselor.

❏ Sex therapists have a technique to take the fear out of performance anxiety. It encourages a couple to spend more time sensually. They suggest no sex initially. Every few days, spend half an hour every evening massaging each other. Sex is forbidden. The massage is to encourage closeness and intimacy in the relationship and touching without the need for sexual expression. Try this for a month.

❏ Hypnotherapy can also help.

❏ Aromatherapy offers several fragrances to enhance sexuality: the exotic oil of patchouli and jasmine, the intense floral smell of ylang ylang, and the (expensive) pure oil of rose is said to free the true expression of the heart. A few drops of these essential oils may be combined with almond oil for a massage oil, or added to the bath or an oil burner to create a sensual atmosphere.

❏ The sexual organs are located at the sacral chakra (an energy center located along the spinal column). This chakra represents the ability to enjoy pleasure and give to yourself on all levels. The color of the sacral chakra is orange. Perhaps try orange briefs? Or sheets?

❏ Erectile dysfunction may reflect feelings of impotence in other areas of life—work, relationships, money?

Diet

➤ To feel vital and virulent, avoid overcooked, overprocessed food. Eat as much raw food as possible.

Remedies

➤ Aphrodisiac herbs include panax ginseng, horny goat weed, tribulus, withania, damiana, muira puama, maca, and saw palmetto. They are as useful for men as women.

➤ Take circulation-boosting supplements including ginkgo biloba and vitamin E.

➤ Zinc is needed for testosterone. Testosterone is needed for erections. Get some zinc into you.

Other

➤ If you are on the cuddlier side, lose weight. This will increase energy and testosterone levels and reduce your risk of atherosclerosis and diabetes, both causes of ED.

➤ Erectile dysfunction is often as much psychological as it is physical. Seek counseling and start talking about your condition. You will be surprised at how common it is.

FATIGUE

WHAT IS IT?

Many people drag themselves around every day feeling like something the cat brought in. On a scale of 1 to 10 (where 10 is "full of beans"), how would you rate your energy? Anywhere under 7 is just not good enough. Defining fatigue is difficult as it can be hard to put your finger on whether you feel mentally or physically tired, and sometimes, it is a mixture of the two.

SYMPTOMS

☑ Lacking physical energy and psychological motivation

WHAT CAUSES IT?

❏ Fatigue can be due to a flotilla of causes. Depression, postflu or some other infection, overwork, insomnia, anemia, stress, diabetes, chronic fatigue syndrome, low thyroid function, liver disease, hormonal imbalance, can-

cer, a side effect of medication, persistent pain, and many other reasons.

❏ If you have been pushing yourself too hard for too long or burning the candle at both ends, you could be experiencing what naturopaths call "adrenal exhaustion." The adrenal glands, located on top of the kidneys (ad = near; renal = kidney), handle stress by pumping out the stress hormones adrenaline and cortisol. After a period of time, the adrenal glands tire of the incessant strain and exhaustion sets in.

WHAT TO DO

If your fatigue has been with you for more than a couple of weeks and the cause is not obvious (i.e.,, lack of sleep, exams etc.), then it is vital that you have a check-up. A cause must be found. For more detailed information on how to treat the cause, see the relevant chapters in this book.

Diet

❑ When you are fatigued, you can't risk having a poor diet. Eat fresh food, preferably raw, including sprouts, seeds, and "live food" that has not been excessively processed or cooked. Fresh vegetables and fruit are to occupy the main part of your diet.

❑ Avoid sugar, alcohol, and white flour products.

❑ Avoid caffeine. Although it may give you an immediate lift, ultimately, it will leave you more tired. A sure sign of adrenal fatigue is when you "need" a fix of caffeine to keep going. Caffeine causes the adrenal glands to squeeze out a precious few drops of adrenaline, something they can ill afford to do if you have been stressed and fatigued for some time. Avoid coffee, chocolate, cola, guarana, and tea.

❑ Eat every two to three hours to keep your blood sugar levels constant, ensuring that every meal or snack contains some protein.

❑ Juices are an excellent way of obtaining lots of nutrients in a single glass. Drink a daily juice based on raw carrot with beetroot, wheatgrass, parsley, and a touch of ginger added.

Remedies

❑ Take a B complex each morning and another at lunchtime.

❑ Spirulina, wheat grass, and other "green" supplements containing chlorophyll can add a little pep to your day.

❑ Coenzyme Q_{10} (CoQ_{10}) is required to make energy within cells. Although you naturally make CoQ_{10} in your body, sometimes giving nature a helping hand is required.

❑ Herbs for energy include Siberian and Korean ginseng, rhodiola, damiana, and oats.

❑ Royal jelly, with its readily available vitamin B_5 and other goodies, can be a nice pick-me-up. (Note: avoid royal jelly if you are allergic to bee stings.)

❑ The Bach flower Olive is excellent for debilitating fatigue of mind and body, whereas hornbeam will suit if you have that "Monday morning" feeling all week long.

❑ If your blood tests show you are deficient in iron, B_{12}, or another nutrient, then supplement with this until your levels return to a normal range.

Other

❑ Sleep well. You can't possibly feel energetic if you don't get enough sleep.

❑ Exercise increases circulation, allowing more oxygen to get to the brain and the muscles. If exercising gives you more energy the next day, then make exercise part of your routine, especially if it improves your sleep quality. However, if exercising makes you more tired the next day (not just tired muscles), this is a sign you really are exhausted. Rest is your best medicine. (See also Chronic Fatigue Syndrome on page 90.)

❑ Take time out of your normal routine. Put the children into the loving arms of someone else or give yourself some mental health days away from work—whatever is needed. When you have some time to reflect, perhaps the underlying reason for your fatigue will become clear.

❑ Meditation will give you more energy. Make it part of every day.

DIET

→ Even though you are tired, a poor diet is not an option now. Food must be fresh and as unprocessed as possible. Think vegetables, think fruit.

→ Avoid sugar, alcohol, and white flour products.

→ Although you might be hanging out for a double espresso, it is expressly forbidden. Caffeine will only add to your woes, creating a false illusion of energy.

→ Every two to three hours, eat a meal that contains a little protein. This will keep your blood sugar levels steady.

REMEDIES

→ Take a B complex each morning and another at lunchtime.

→ Make it green. Spirulina, wheat grass, and other "green" supplements will increase your energy levels.

→ Herbs for energy include Siberian and Korean ginseng, rhodiola, damiana, and oats.

OTHER

→ Exercise improves energy. Make it part of your routine.

→ Clear your mind; practice meditation. The skill of being still can bring subtle improvements in your day-to-day energy levels.

FLATULENCE

WHAT IS IT?

A fart (flatus) is made up of several gases (hydrogen, carbon dioxide, nitrogen, and the flammable and smelly methane). A certain amount of flatulence is normal (between 200 and 2,400 ml daily). A source of hilarity among small boys, excess flatulence can be a social encumbrance. Two-thirds of the wind you expel is formed by bacteria in the bowel, while the rest is made up of air that you swallow. Excess gas in the abdomen causes bloating. And yes, men do fart more than women.

SYMPTOMS

☑ Abdominal bloating or distension

☑ Cramping or colic

☑ Flatus

☑ Burping

WHAT CAUSES IT?

❑ Poor eating habits can contribute to flatulence and bloating.

❑ Not chewing your food adequately. The first stage of digestion occurs in the mouth, and teeth play an important role in grinding food into smaller bits. When you fail to chew properly, the big bits will pose a challenge further down the digestive tubing. Undigested bits are met by an enthusiastic crowd of microflora in the large bowel, who will consume what you have not digested—and who will thank you with flatulence.

❏ Chewing with your mouth open. Your mother was right, it is rude, but chewing with your mouth agape also allows excess air into the digestive tract.

❏ Eating standing up or eating when you are walking.

❏ Mouth breathers, as opposed to nose breathers, often suffer excessive wind. A key sign is waking up with a bloated abdomen. Mouth breathers are often forced into this situation due to sinus or nasal congestion (see Sinusitis on page 271). Some people become air-gulpers when stressed.

❏ Chewing gum. When you start to chew anything, the digestive system gears up a notch, secreting digestive juices in expectation of food soon coming down the line. Chewing gum sends mixed messages and is a cause of digestive bewilderment, gas, and bloating. Chewing gum immediately after a meal is fine.

❏ Low stomach acid, or hypochlorydria, is a common affliction involving less than optimum hydrochloric acid, which is so important for digestion in the stomach. Signs and symptoms that may indicate low stomach acid include bloating, burping, flatulence, diarrhea, constipation, feeling of overfullness after eating, food allergies, nausea after nutritional supplements, burping after taking oil-filled capsules (such as vitamin E and fish oil), peeling and weak fingernails, dilated blood vessels around the nose, iron deficiency, chronic fungal conditions, and undigested food in the stool.

❏ Antibiotics. Antibiotics kill bacteria, including some of the resident good bugs in the digestive system, leaving some smelly customers behind. The wrong microbiotic crowd in the digestive tract is known as dysbiosis.

❏ Constipation. A slow transit time through the bowel causes a festering of gas-producing bacteria (see Constipation on page 104).

❏ *Candida albicans.* An overgrowth of this fungus is a common cause of bloating and flatulence (see page 73).

❏ Food intolerance can also cause bloating and flatulence. One of the more common examples is lactose intolerance, where there are insufficient quantities of the enzyme lactase. The undigested lactose meanders to the lower bowel where bacteria will digest it and create wind. The other food intolerance that may cause bloating and flatulence is fructose malabsorption (see Candida on page 73).

❏ Stress can muck around with your digestive system.

❏ Sitting still for too long. Get up and move.

❏ Misalignment of your vertebral column can affect the nerves that supply the digestive tract.

WHAT TO DO

My grandfather used to say, "Wherever you may be, let the air go free," and certainly it is healthier to do so rather than try to retain the air. However, the following recommendations will hopefully relieve the problem of excess flatus.

DID YOU KNOW?

Horace Fletcher, an American obsessed with mastication in the 1930s, defined a proper chew as thirty-two times with each mouthful: one chew for every tooth. Obviously, this leaves little time for living between mealtimes! In the twenty-first century, ten thorough chews per mouthful is generally adequate.

Diet

❏ Ban sugar. Bacteria (and yeast) in the gut ferment sugar into gas.

❏ Are you chewing your food sufficiently? Are you paying attention to each mouthful? Fast chewers are bred, not born. Here are a few hints if you find yourself slipping back into your hasty habits.

- Remind yourself to chew *before* sitting down to eat.

- Don't eat while reading or watching TV.

- Write CHEW on a piece of paper and fix it to the fridge or wall.

- Put your knife, fork, or hands down between each mouthful.

❏ Probiotic foods such as yogurt, miso, sauerkraut, kefir, natto, tempeh, and kimchi will introduce beneficial bacteria into the digestive tract.

❏ Avoid high-fructose foods for one week to see if this makes a difference (see page 212).

THE BITTERER THE BETTER

James Green, an American herbalist, said, "the mistake of eliminating the bitter flavor from our daily experience is like eliminating one of the colors of the rainbow." Unfortunately, in the United States, bitter foods are thin on the ground. Grapefruit, chicory, radicchio, endives, cress, olives, hops (say yeah for the cleansing ale), and coffee are the only bitter foods that spring to mind. In England, a salad made from bitter lettuce leaves was traditionally eaten before the meal, rather than with it as we do today. Bitter herbs form the basis of European digestives and aperitifs such as Campari and good old Angostura bitters. In the interest of harmony and health, Chinese cuisine often includes a bitter element, such as bitter melon, said to relieve the body of internal heat.

Taste buds are bundles of nerve endings, located all over the tongue. Their job is to interpret tastes from the chemicals in food, revealing whether food is yuck or yum, and more specifically sweet, salty, bitter, or sour. Bitter buds are found at the back of the tongue, sour to either side, sweet at the tip, and salty in between. Bitter taste buds connect to the vagus nerve, a nerve that stimulates the functioning of the digestive organs, stomach, pancreas, gallbladder, and intestine. One of the main tenets of natural therapies is to improve digestion, and stimulating the vagus nerve will do this—and explains why bitter herbs have been prescribed since Hippocrates.

Symptoms of a digestive system crying out for bitters include bloating, burping, flatulence, and constipation. These symptoms in particular indicate low stomach-acid production. Other signs include peeling fingernails, dry lips, and increased susceptibility to parasitic and fungal infections and a tendency to food poisoning (gastro). As we age, stomach-acid production tends to drop. This inhibits the absorption of nutrients, especially protein, iron, and B_{12}.

Tickling the taste buds with foul-tasting herbal concoctions is a favorite sport among herbalists. The main bitter herbs include gentian, goldenseal, wormwood, St. Mary's thistle, and dandelion root. The idea is to *taste* the bitterness. The bitterer, the better! A teaspoon of herbal bitters in a wineglass of water sipped before dinner will train your digestive system into healthier habits. Bitters enhance your appetite, but will not cause you to overeat.

Note: People with stomach ulcers or women who are pregnant should not take herbal bitters.

- Until your digestion improves, avoid the brassicas (including broccoli, Brussels sprouts, and cabbage) and legumes—both can be difficult to digest. After two or three weeks, introduce these nutritious foods slowly, perhaps two small servings a week.

- Increase bitter foods including radicchio, kale, grapefruit, and cress.

- If you think you may have an overgrowth of *Candida albicans,* in addition to avoiding sugar, restrict yeasts from your diet and follow the recommendations for the candida diet (see page 74).

- Apple cider vinegar and honey in hot water is an old-fashioned remedy for improving digestion. Try two teaspoons of vinegar and one teaspoon of raw honey. Drink a cup of this each morning soon after you wake. (See page 162 for the benefits of apple cider vinegar.)

Remedies

- Take a tablet containing digestive enzymes with each meal. In addition, and sometimes in the same tablet, take some betaine hydrochloride to boost the digestive power of the stomach.

- Herbal bitters can improve stomach-acid production and will alleviate bloating and flatulence. Try one teaspoon in water before main meals (see "The Bitterer the Better").

- Take a strong probiotic supplement each morning.

Other

- Stress management. If you feel your bloating and flatulence increase when you are stressed, learn how to meditate or try some yoga.

- Exercise. At least outside, no one will notice if you fart.

- See an osteopath or chiropractor if you think your back needs adjusting, as your sore back and bloated tummy could be connected.

AROMATHERAPY

Blend the following oils with 20 ml of sweet almond oil, and you will have a fantastic blend possessing antispasmodic, digestive, stomachic, carminative, and therapeutic properties. Excellent for treating heartburn, indigestion, and flatulence, use as an abdominal massage or warm compress.

- 5 drops of mandarin oil—antispasmodic, carminative, digestive, sedative, tonic.

- 2 drops of cardamom oil—antispasmodic, carminative, digestive, stomachic.

- 2 drops of spearmint oil—local anesthetic, antispasmodic, carminative, digestive, stomachic tonic.

Diet

⇒ Restrict sugar from your diet. This alone can reduce your bloating and flatulence by a significant degree.

⇒ Chew your food well. Don't allow partially digested food to travel to the lower bowel where bacteria will feast on it, creating gas.

⇒ Add two teaspoons of apple cider vinegar and one teaspoon of raw honey to a cup of hot water and drink first thing each morning.

Remedies

⇒ With each meal, take a digestive enzyme tablet.

⇒ Each morning, take a strong probiotic supplement to restore your bowel microflora.

Other

⇒ Exercise regularly.

FOOD SENSITIVITY, ALLERGY, AND INTOLERANCE

WHAT IS IT?

Food allergies, unheard of a few decades ago, are now frequently diagnosed or self-diagnosed. Food allergies, food sensitivities, food intolerances—call them what you will. You may as well, because there is still massive confusion about terminology in the medical literature, where the very idea of anyone being allergic to food was pooh-poohed until recently. While the debate and semantics continue, there does, however, seem to be an increase in people's reactions to foods, broadly broken down as follows:

1. Food allergy—immune mediated
2. Food sensitivity—immune mediated
3. Lactose intolerance—nonimmune mediated
4. Fructose malabsorption—nonimmune mediated
5. Chemical sensitivity—nonimmune mediated

TYPE 1: FOOD ALLERGY

This is a true allergy, recruiting antibodies produced in the body known as immunoglobulin E (IgE). As quickly as seconds to minutes after the ingestion of the culprit food, a violent reaction occurs—the results of which can be fatal. Common allergens in this group are crustaceans, eggs, fish, milk, peanuts, soybeans, and tree nuts—although any food can be a potential trigger. You don't even have to eat the offending allergen: a chaste kiss on the lips has been known to cause an anaphylactic reaction.

SYMPTOMS

☑ Hives

☑ Asthma attack

☑ Swelling of the airways including throat, lips, and tongue

☑ Drop in blood pressure

- ✓ Feeling lightheaded
- ✓ Anaphylaxis—a shutdown of the heart and lungs

WHAT CAUSES IT?

- ❏ Leaky gut hypothesis. In theory, the barrier between the intestine and the bloodstream should be virtually impenetrable. Only the smallest of molecules should be able to cross over. So, when there are larger particles in the bloodstream, the immune system responds as if there is a pathogen (e.g., virus, bacteria) and responds as such. However, the particle in question is a fragment of partially digested food, not a pathogen.

- ❏ Starting young. For a few months after birth the baby's digestive tract is relatively "leaky," allowing bigger than normal molecules to cross from the intestine to the bloodstream. One reason for this leakiness is to allow antibodies from mother's breast milk to pass freely and kick start the infant immune system. Therefore, from an evolutionary point of view, human babies are meant to drink only mother's milk for some time. In industrialized countries such as our own, babies are often weaned at six months (if not earlier), when the digestive tract is still allowing the passage of large molecules. Often the first foods we start babies on include cow's milk, soy foods, orange juice, and wheat —all major players in the food allergy stakes.

- ❏ A susceptibility to allergy can be inherited.

- ❏ The straw that breaks the camel's back. In the normal course of events, our immune system is able to deal with a certain level of sensitivity to food allergens. However, when the immune system is under challenge—during stress, infections, or not eating or sleeping well—the food sensitivity becomes the "straw that breaks the camel's back" and a "new" food allergy appears. This explains why people in their thirties, forties, and fifties can suddenly become "allergic" to a food to which they have never previously reacted.

- ❏ Familiarity breeds contempt. Today's supermarkets offer a vast range of options, yet every week our shopping trollies are predictably full of the regulars—even the cat gets the same tuna tidbits in jelly. What did you have for breakfast? Chances are it was the same as yesterday, and the day before that. Human beings are creatures of habit. The foods that are most often implicated in food allergies include wheat, milk, oranges, eggs, peanuts, and tomatoes. It is no coincidence that some of these foods form the basis of many people's diets.

  Our digestive tract was not designed for such dietary monotony and has not changed substantially for hundreds of thousands of years—unlike our diet. Before the advent of agriculture about 10,000 years ago, we roamed the countryside nibbling on anything and everything we could get our hands on: flowers, seeds, roots, fruits, insects, and mastodons. Our ability to eat from a wide variety of foods substantially improved our survival prospects. If, for example, our diet had consisted solely of mastodon chops, when the mastodons snuffed it, so would we. Humans have always been masters of adaptation.

- ❏ Addictive allergy. Sometimes a food allergy does not cause a reaction, but suppresses one. This phenomenon, called an "addictive allergy," is when the allergic molecule attaches to receptor sites in the brain, much like our very own brain chemicals called endorphins, which act as natural opiates. If deprived of these chemicals, the receptor sites will remain empty and addictive symptoms may result such as craving the food, irritability, and mood changes. Milk is a common addictive allergy. If you are particularly devoted to a food and cannot bear the thought of life without it, quite possibly, that food is the problem.

WHAT TO DO

Due to the potential severity of reactions to these foods, strict avoidance of these foods is the only way. Don't touch them with a ten-foot pole. (Although it has been known for children to grow out of them, they should always be regarded with extreme caution if and when these foods are reintroduced into the diet.) If prescribed by your doctor, it is recommended that you carry your EpiPen with you at all times. Should you encounter the food by chance, a quick jab of adrenaline with the EpiPen will open up airways and potentially save your life. ("Epi" is short for epinephrine, the other name for adrenaline.)

TYPE 2: FOOD SENSITIVITY

The type 2 reaction is also immune mediated, but not as dramatic as type 1. Symptoms can take hours or days to appear after the food has been ingested, which can make these food reactions more difficult to identify. Common foods in this group include eggs, soybeans, fish, crustaceans, peanuts, milk, wheat, tree nuts, and sesame seeds.

WHAT CAUSES IT?

See type 1.

SYMPTOMS

☑ Digestive system: mouth ulcers, chronic diarrhea, constipation, duodenal ulcer, flatulence, gastritis, irritable bowel syndrome, cramping, mucus on stools.

☑ Urinary system: chronic cystitis, bed-wetting.

☑ Immune system: chronic infections such as colds and frequent ear infections.

☑ Mental/emotional: anxiety, depression, hyperactivity, inability to concentrate, insomnia, irritability, mental confusion, personality change.

☑ Muscular/skeletal: joint pain, tender muscles.

☑ Respiratory tract: asthma, chronic bronchitis, wheezing, itchy nose or throat, sinusitis.

☑ Endocrine: diabetes, thyroid problems.

☑ Skin: acne, eczema, hives, itching, skin rashes.

☑ Weight: weight gain, weight loss.

☑ Other: rapid heartbeat, water retention, bloating, fatigue, headaches, migraines, hypoglycemia.

WHAT TO DO

Diet

❑ Avoid the suspect food(s) for a month (also known as the four-week allergy program). Be strict. Using wheat as an example, obvious foods to exclude are bread, pasta, and pastries, but many processed foods also contain wheat, such as soups and crumbed foods. Look for allergy-based recipe books and websites to help with planning meals.

❑ Keep a diary of your symptoms starting a week before you begin the program so that you can accurately compare before and after. Mention all physical and psychological symptoms, even if they don't appear to relate to the allergy. It is advisable to record other influences such as weather changes, emotional upsets, and menstrual period. This diary will be invaluable in assessing the degree of allergy.

❑ When the month is up, it is time to take the "challenge." Eat a portion of the suspected allergy food three times on the same day. For example, if wheat is the suspected allergen, have toast and Wheaties for breakfast, a sandwich for lunch, and pasta for dinner. Refrain from the food for two days after the challenge as symptoms such as eczema may take that long to reappear.

❏ Recovery. Once you have ascertained that a particular food is a problem, continue fairly rigorous avoidance for a further three months. It is necessary to "heal" the gut to prevent further allergic substances from passing over the intestinal barrier. Additionally, it is wise to stabilize the immune system.

❏ After three months on the program, start to reintroduce the allergen very slowly. No more than one serving every four days. Again, record any reactions in your food diary.

Remedies

These remedies are designed to help in several ways: to improve the digestive process, support the immune system, and repair and fortify the intestinal wall.

For Your Digestion

❏ Take one teaspoon of herbal bitters in a small glass of water and sip before dinner. Herbal bitters stimulate the bitter taste buds. This in turn stimulates the vagus nerve, which helps improve the functioning of the entire digestive system. It also increases stomach acid, which can help properly break down protein structures.

❏ If your digestive system is on the weak side (that is, you experience burping, flatulence, bloating, constipation, or diarrhea), take one digestive enzyme tablet and one betaine hydrochloride tablet with each meal.

❏ Take probiotics. In addition to the repair of your digestive tract, the good microflora will also help digestion.

For Your Immune System

❏ Echinacea is known as an immune-system modulator. Perfect for when the immune system is underactive or overactive as it is in the case of allergies. Take 500 to 1,000 mg of echinacea twice a day in tablet or tincture form. Other herbs that can help include those for allergies, such as albizia and baical skullcap.

- Lactoferrin is an iron-containing protein that is found in colostrum, the first breast milk, and has excellent gastrointestinal and immune system benefits.

- Avoid coffee, sugar, and alcohol. These put extra stress on an already fragile immune system.

For Repair and Fortification of Your Intestinal Wall

- Glutamine is an amino acid that helps repair intestinal cells.

- Probiotics are necessary to create a healthy intestinal environment, decreasing intestinal permeability. The probiotics you choose need to contain at least *lactobacillus* and *bifidobacterium spp.*

- Zinc is needed for cellular repair.

- Herbs that help inflammation include ginger, turmeric, and aloe vera, and those that repair include goldenseal, calendula, and aloe vera.

TYPE 3: LACTOSE INTOLERANCE

WHAT IS IT?

Not an immune-mediated reaction at all, lactose intolerance is the result of a missing enzyme, lactase. Lactose intolerance is one of the most common food intolerances in the world. In fact, 20 percent of Caucasians are affected and more than 60 percent of some other ethnic groups including Asians and Africans. This reflects the fact that dairy foods in general, and milk in particular (which has the highest amount of lactose), are not universally consumed.

Lactose intolerance can be diagnosed via a hydrogen breath test, but just removing dairy from your diet for a few days will give you an idea as to whether this is a problem for you.

BEHIND THE SCENES

Lactose is milk sugar, a double sugar comprised of galactose and glucose joined together by a chemical bond. In the healthy intestine, certain bacteria create an enzyme called lactase. Lactase has the ability to break the bond between galactose and glucose, and send the two merrily on their way across the intestinal wall into the bloodstream. (Galactose gets converted to glucose somewhere on this journey.) Without lactase, lactose is unable to be absorbed and will, via osmosis, draw fluids from the body causing diarrhea and bloating—classic lactose intolerance symptoms.

WHAT CAUSES IT?

- Common in those of Asian, African, and Mediterranean descent.

- A bowel infection of viral, bacterial, or parasitic origin often creates lactose intolerance as the lactase-producing bacteria are wiped out by the infection.

- Bowel surgery.

- Gluten intolerance.

- Preterm infants are often lactose intolerant.

There are two kinds of milk-sensitivity problems. The first is to lactose, or milk sugar. This is a deficiency of the lactase needed to break down and digest lactose. The second is a casein sensitivity. Casein is a major protein in milk products. This is more of an immune response type 2 reaction.

SYMPTOMS

- ☑ Abdominal pain
- ☑ Abdominal bloating
- ☑ Flatulence
- ☑ Diarrhea

WHAT TO DO

Diet

❏ For a month, avoid all food containing lactose—milk (cow, goat, and sheep), yogurt, ice cream, ricotta and cottage cheese, and cream. Hard cheese and butter have negligible amounts of lactose.

❏ After a month of avoiding lactose and taking the probiotic supplement, begin by eating a small amount of milk product. The first one to try would be a spoonful of good quality natural yogurt. Each day, increase your intake in small amounts of different dairy foods, for as long as you are symptom free.

Remedies

❏ Take probiotics, especially *Lactobacillus spp.*

TYPE 4: FRUCTOSE MALABSORPTION

WHAT IS IT?

Fructose malabsorption is the most recent food sensitivity on the scene. Researched by Australian dietician Sue Shepherd, fructose malabsorption is the difficulty in digesting fructose, a sugar found in fruits and vegetables. If not adequately digested, fructose (and fructose-like molecules) travel down the intestine where they ferment. Many people with irritable bowel syndrome (IBS) respond well by decreasing fructose foods from their diet. Fructose malabsorption can be detected by a hydrogen breath test.

A diagnosis of fructose malabsorption is a controversial one, as fructose-containing fruits and vegetables have been part of mankind's diet since God was a boy, and fruit and vegetables happen to be extremely good for you in all other ways, being chockful of vitamins, minerals, phytonutrients, antioxidants, and fiber while still being low in calories. It is more than likely the problem has arisen in recent times as food manufacturing has increased the amount of fructose added to processed foods. This, combined with dysbiosis (the wrong bugs in the wrong place in your gut), has predisposed some individuals to this condition.

SYMPTOMS

☑ Reflux

☑ Constipation and/or diarrhea

☑ Bloating

☑ Flatulence

☑ Abdominal pain

☑ Vomiting

☑ Depression

BEHIND THE SCENES

Our immune system is programmed to respond to substances foreign to, or not recognized by, the body. These substances are often bacteria or viruses, which are made up of molecules of protein. When a protein molecule that our body does not recognize manages to escape our defense systems, the immune system is placed on alert. This happens in the case of hay fever. When a person inhales pollen (a protein), it causes an allergic reaction—often sneezing and mucus production. Food allergy is similar, except the allergic substance, known as an allergen, is absorbed across the intestinal wall during the course of digestion. For the person with an allergy to milk, when a fraction of the milk protein (casein) is absorbed, their immune system will react.

WHAT TO DO?

Diet

❑ Avoid or reduce the following foods: fruit juice, tinned and dried fruit, grapes, guava, apple, coconut milk and cream, honeydew melon, mango, nashi pear, papaya, pear, quince, star fruit, tomato, watermelon, Lebanese cucumber, sweet potato, tomato paste, relish, sweet and sour sauce, BBQ sauce, fructose corn syrup, fructose, honey, fortified wines, globe artichokes, asparagus, garlic, green beans, onions, leek, shallots, and wheat.

The preceding list includes some very beneficial foods, and it would be a nutritional crime to be bereft of them for life. The best way to tackle the problem, if your symptoms are indeed made worse by these foods, is to remove them from your diet for a month while improving your intestinal microbiome with a course of probiotics and perhaps some digestive enzymes with each meal. Once all symptoms have abated, gingerly begin to reintroduce fructose-rich fruit and vegetables (leaving aside the processed fructose products) and hopefully, you will once again be able to enjoy these nutritious foods.

Remedies

❑ Take a probiotic supplement daily.

❑ Take a digestive enzyme tablet with each meal.

TYPE 5: CHEMICAL SENSITIVITY

WHAT IS IT?

Common chemicals that people may be sensitive to include:

❑ Histamine (red wine, soy sauce).

❑ Salicylates (spices, herbs, berries).

❑ MSG (packet soup).

❑ Sodium benzoate (prunes, tea, soft drinks).

❑ Sulphites (dried fruit, processed meats).

FOR KIDS

Treating food allergies in children is much the same as for adults: take out the offending food and improve immunity. Some children "grow out" of their food allergies and are able to tolerate the food after a year or so. When patients come to see me with possible food allergy symptoms, I always quiz them to see if they had allergies as a child. If they were allergic to a specific food, then chances are they might be again.

Taking good food out of a child's diet is problematic. Firstly, you need to ensure that any of the positive nutrients that the particular food supplied is replaced in some way (e.g., in the case of dairy, the calcium and protein). Secondly, a restricted diet places a strain on the family, most often mom who needs to find new recipes and school lunches. And finally, having a food allergy is difficult socially. Some children can be cruel, and not being able to eat the same foods as your peers and/or being seen as different may negatively affect your youngster's psyche. Nevertheless, sometimes it is necessary to take the hard road. Supplements for children are similar (except ditch the bitters); just adjust the dosage to suit.

SYMPTOMS

- ☑ Difficulty in breathing
- ☑ Wheezing
- ☑ Headache
- ☑ Nasal congestion
- ☑ Runny nose
- ☑ Skin rash
- ☑ Hives
- ☑ Itching
- ☑ Swelling of the hands, face, and feet
- ☑ Inflammation of the eyes
- ☑ Stomach pain
- ☑ Nausea
- ☑ Burning or itching sensation in the mouth
- ☑ Flushing of the skin
- ☑ Diarrhea
- ☑ Blood pressure changes (both high or low possible)
- ☑ Dizziness and fainting
- ☑ Fluid retention (edema)

WHAT TO DO

These reactions are not immune mediated.

Diet

- ❑ As these reactions are not immune mediated, try to avoid these chemicals as much as you can.

Testing

No testing method, laboratory or other, is 100 percent accurate in diagnosing a food allergy. However, a cytotoxic blood test, whereby a sample of blood is analyzed for IgG antibodies to specific foods may be undertaken.

The "gold standard" for diagnosing a food allergy is the method of food avoidance and challenge. This requires strictly eliminating the suspect food from your diet for two weeks. After this time, there should be a noticeable reduction in symptoms and the suspect food should stand out like a sore thumb. Mostly, it will be a food that you eat every day, like wheat, oranges (orange juice), or milk (cheese, etc.).

Note: People with a type 1 reaction should never undertake this challenge as it can be life-threatening.

AT A GLANCE

Good Foods

➠ Foods you are not allergic to. Try to rotate them anyway.

Foods to Avoid

➠ Foods containing the allergen plus coffee, sugar, and alcohol.

Remedies

➠ Echinacea, probiotics, digestive enzymes.

➠ Lifestyle changes.

➠ Stress management.

➠ Mind-body alignment. A food allergy could represent a conflict within. Who or what in your life are you allergic to?

FUNGAL INFECTIONS

WHAT IS IT?

Various forms of fungi take up residence within and on our bodies, particularly in warm moist areas such as between the toes and in the vagina, as well as on skin and nails. Fungi are a primitive vegetable, although officially, fungi have been bequeathed their own kingdom. If you don't have a green thumb and can't grow a vegetable to save yourself, it must be good to know you can grow some kind of vegetation closer to home. Or maybe not. The most common fungal infections include ringworm, athlete's foot, jock itch, thrush, and onychomycosis, the medical term for manky toe- and fingernails. Two common fungi are *Candida albicans* and *Trichophyton rubrum*. Fungi are spread by spores, so it is easy for the whole family and the dog to catch. Most fungal conditions are superficial and not a serious threat to your health. They should clear up within days, except manky toenails, which tend to take far longer.

SYMPTOMS

Symptoms differ according to the specific fungus and where it is located on the body.

Skin (includes jock itch, ringworm, tinea of the feet)

- ☑ Itching
- ☑ Blisters
- ☑ Redness
- ☑ Round, red ring with clear patch in center (ringworm)
- ☑ Burning
- ☑ Flaking
- ☑ Peeling and cracking

- ☑ Pale white patches, often on the upper arm that don't tan in the sun

Nails

- ☑ Discoloration: white, cream, yellow, and even green
- ☑ Thickening
- ☑ Cracking and peeling

Other

- ☑ Thrush
- ☑ Sinusitis
- ☑ Itchy ears
- ☑ Sometimes a fungal infection can coincide with other conditions including eczema and psoriasis.

WHAT CAUSES IT?

- ❏ Working in occupations where you are constantly exposed to water such as dishwasher in a restaurant or bartender (where there is a double whammy of yeasty beer and water).

- ❏ Communal showers such as in swimming pools, gyms, and boarding schools.

- ❏ Damp houses are a major health threat. Rising damp and rooms that never see the light of day will promote fungal growth and spores that infiltrate your home and body.

- ❏ If your immune system is under par, you are more likely to suffer from all sorts of infections, including fungal.

- ❏ If you have recurrent fungal infections, your problem may be more systemic (see Candida, page 73).

- ❏ A history of taking antibiotics can set you up for fungal infections.

WHAT TO DO

Diet

❏ Eat lots of garlic for its antifungal properties. Raw is better than cooked.

❏ Caprylic acid (found in coconut oil) has anti-fungal properties. This does not mean that coconut cream pie is back on the table—cook with coconut oil and enjoy shredded coconut in muesli.

❏ Avoid the following (and see page 74 for more details on the candida diet)

- Sugar (including sugar added to foods—for example, cakes, soft drink, biscuits, most breakfast cereals, malt, molasses, honey, and golden syrup).

- Fruit juice, grapes, dried fruit, melons (papaya, watermelon, rock melon).

- Yeasted bread, sour dough, pizzas.

- Yeast spreads.

- Beer, wine, fortified wine, liqueurs, sparkling wine, champagne.

- Yellow cheese (camembert, brie, etc.), blue cheese.

Remedies

❏ Garlic is a brilliant antifungal agent. Double up with it in food as well as a supplement. Take one or two garlic capsules made from freeze-dried whole garlic after dinner each night.

❏ Other herbs with antifungal properties include goldenseal, tea tree, eucalyptus, cinnamon, clove, thyme, oregano, barberry, olive leaf, and calendula. Take in tablet or tincture form.

❏ A fungal infection is a sign the immune system is not doing its job adequately. Take a combined tablet of echinacea, vitamin C, zinc, and the bioflavonoids.

❏ Restore microbial harmony. Take one or two capsules of probiotics each morning.

Other

❏ If skin or nails are involved, apply an essential oil alone or in a cream. Test on a small area of skin first, just in case you have a reaction. The first oil to try is tea tree, and nine times out of ten it will work wonders. Depending on the variety, some fungi don't respond as effectively to tea tree as other oils. The next one to try is the essential oil of thyme. Still no joy? Others to try are clove, eucalyptus, cinnamon, and lavender in that order. Keep applying for a week after all symptoms appear to be gone, just to make sure. Nail infections are the most stubborn. Use a pipette or some implement that will get the oil under the nail bed as much as possible.

❏ After swimming or bathing, dry meticulously between the toes, under the breasts, and any hard-to-reach area. Use a small towel or hairdryer.

❏ Don't leave soggy speedos or sportswear on for longer than necessary.

❏ Wear shoes or thongs to local pools and public washing areas.

❏ Wash clothes, towels, and bed linen in hot water to kill the fungus. Add a few drops of tea tree or thyme oil to the final rinse.

❏ Fresh air and sunshine work wonders for blankets, duvets, and pillows.

❏ If your house is damp, you can be certain there are fungi. If you are renting, move. If you own your damp house, then your health will benefit from attending to the problem. Maybe a new damp course needs to be put in. At the very least, invest in a heavy-duty dehumidifier for affected rooms.

- Could your pet have a fungal infection? If you have noticed your dog or cat (mouse or ferret) scratching, they may have a fungal infection. Wash them with a tea tree–based pet shampoo. Pet bedding should also be aired in the sunshine as much as possible.

- Paint an iodine solution (available from the chemist) between the toes. Being next to purple toes probably causes the fungus to drop dead from embarrassment as much as from the antifungal effect of iodine.

- Colloidal silver applied directly onto fungal bits also works well.

- Apple cider vinegar contains malic acid, a competent antifungal agent. Make sure it is traditionally made and still contains the "mother" apple! Add 20 ml of apple cider vinegar to a cup of warm water and rinse the affected area (scalp, groin, skin) with it.

- Don't share bed linen or towels.

AROMATHERAPY

Athlete's Foot

Mix the following blend into a cup of corn flour and put into a container with a shaker lid. It can be used after a shower directly onto the affected area or alternatively, the powder can be shaken into the sock or sprinkled directly into the shoe. Sprinkle a few drops into a bowl of warm water and soak the feet until the water becomes too cool. (Always make sure to dry feet thoroughly after soaking or bathing.)

- 4 drops of myrrh oil—fungicidal, antimicrobial, antiseptic

- 5 drops of lemongrass oil—deodorant, fungicidal, analgesic

- 6 drops of Cypress oil—deodorant, antisudorific

General Fungal Infections

- Use 6 drops of the following blend in a cool compress or blend with 15 grams vitamin E cream, adding 5 ml calendula-infused oil and apply as needed.

- 3 drops of lemon eucalyptus oil—fungicidal, deodorant.

- 4 drops of tea-tree oil—fungicidal, refreshing, immune-stimulant.

- 3 drops of geranium oil—fungicidal, anti-inflammatory, deodorant, tissue repairing.

DIET

➡ Garlic is antifungal. Raw is best. Add to salad dressings or bruschetta.

➡ Avoid sugars, fruits, alcohol, and yeasts that will exacerbate symptoms (see above).

REMEDIES

➡ Take garlic capsules and/or antifungal herbs. Take in tablet or tincture form.

➡ Take probiotics each morning.

OTHER

➡ Tea tree oil is remarkably antifungal. Add directly to affected areas. Other oils that have an antifungal effect include thyme, clove, eucalyptus, cinnamon, and lavender.

➡ Wash clothes, towels, and bed linen in hot water, rinse with a few drops of tea tree oil added to the water, and line dry in the sunshine.

➡ If your house is damp, move.

➡ After showering, apply some diluted apple cider vinegar to the affected parts. (Apple cider vinegar contains malic acid, which has antifungal properties.)

GALLSTONES

WHAT IS IT?

"Fair, fat, fertile, and forty" is the ditty medical students still learn to describe women most at risk of gallstones. Unflattering, perhaps, but accurate. Up to 30 percent of people have gallstones, many of whom are unaware of the fact until it is revealed by a routine scan of the upper abdomen. That is, until a gallstone becomes stuck in the duct leading from the gallbladder. Owee.

SYMPTOMS

☑ The majority of people experience no symptoms until a stone gets caught in the bile duct.

☑ A stone stuck in the bile duct causes agonizing pain and complications including pancreatitis. Infection of the liver can be life-threatening.

☑ Nausea and vomiting

☑ Fever

☑ Clay-colored stool

☑ Sharp cramping or dull pain

☑ Pain in the right or the middle of the abdomen

☑ Pain can be referred to the right shoulder blade.

☑ Jaundice; skin and whites of eyes turn yellow

WHAT CAUSES IT?

❏ Being overweight increases your risk of gallstones by 600 percent.

❏ A low-fiber and high-fat diet places you at risk. Gallstones are unheard of in countries with high-fiber and low-fat diets.

❏ Certain foods can trigger an attack, especially eggs and fatty food.

- There is an increased risk for pregnant women and those taking the oral contraceptive pill.

- Gallbladder attacks can occur after sudden weight loss.

- Gallstones are in your genes.

WHAT TO DO

The surgical removal of the gallbladder (cholecystectomy) is a routine procedure via keyhole surgery. The gallbladder is not an essential organ; however, it's nice to retain all your original bits and pieces if possible. If they do not pose an immediate threat, you can live quietly at peace with your gallstones, especially by following the recommendations below.

Although many cholecystectomies are very successful and patients are trouble-free thereafter, there are a certain percentage of people who have difficulty digesting fats after the operation. Many of the suggestions below can help.

Diet

- Drink plenty of water. At least 2 liters a day. This is most important to keep the bile from becoming too concentrated.

BEHIND THE SCENES

The gallbladder, a pear-shaped sac, stores and concentrates bile produced by the liver. Bile is part waste product (residue of red blood cells) and part digestive juice. After a meal, the gallbladder contracts, forcing bile to be excreted into the small intestine via a narrow tube called the bile duct. Gallstones as small as grains of sand can pass through the bile duct into the intestines without touching the sides, and larger stones won't fit into the bile duct—it's the in-between-sized stones that are the troublemakers.

- First thing each morning, drink a cup of hot water with the juice of half a lemon squeezed into it. Good for liver, good for gallbladder, good for you.

- Eat plenty of high-fiber foods including vegetables, legumes, and whole grains.

- Restrict high-fat foods including yellow cheese, butter, and margarine, fatty cuts of meat, chicken skin, deli meats (such as salami and other lunch meats), highly spiced foods and pastries, biscuits, and cakes. The gallbladder constricts more with high-fat food. Interestingly, the good fats found in nuts, seeds, fish, and avocadoes don't pose a threat.

- Eat steamed or raw vegetables, fruit, brown rice, oats, whole meal breads, fruit, chicken without skin, and fish.

- Increase bitter vegetables in the diet such as rocket, kale, and artichokes. Bitters stimulate the liver to create more bile and improve bile flow.

- Foods that are particularly good for the gallbladder include turmeric, artichoke, dandelion root, grapefruit, pears, and lemons.

- Your daily vegetable juice should combine carrot, beetroot (including the leaves), and cucumber.

- Develop a hankering for dandelion tea; it is good for both liver and gallbladder health.

Remedies

- The old liver and digestive remedy works well for gall bladders too—take a teaspoon of herbal bitters in water before dinner.

- Choleretics are herbs that help the liver produce bile and optimize the proper functioning of the gallbladder. Choleretic herbs include St. Mary's thistle, globe artichoke, turmeric, chelidonium, calendula, ginger, and peppermint.

Take a tincture or tablet of one or more of these herbs once or twice a day.

❏ Peppermint is not only choleretic, but also prevents cramping. Take one or two capsules of peppermint oil daily and drink peppermint tea.

❏ Lecithin can aid fat digestion. Add two tablespoons to your cereal or take four capsules daily.

❏ If your diet is not fiber rich, take a soluble fiber supplement daily. Choose psyllium, pectin, oat bran, chia seeds, or ground linseeds, or a combination.

❏ If you experience cramping, crush a magnesium phosphate tablet in water and sip every ten minutes.

Other

❏ Lose weight if necessary. Being overweight increases your risk of gallstones.

❏ To treat the painful abdominal symptoms, apply a heat pack to the area. A ginger or castor oil compress will add to the soothing effect.

❏ Acupuncture is an effective treatment for gallbladder disease.

❏ The liver is the organ of anger, the gallbladder is the organ of resentment, and bile represents bitterness. Is it possible you may have a buildup of these emotions?

❏ The Bach flowers Willow and Chicory are good for resentment issues

---

DID YOU KNOW?

The old chestnut that keeps being rolled out for gallstones is the "olive oil and lemon juice flush" that claims to dissolve gallstones. Literally. Not only will this not dissolve gallstones, it may likely cause a gallbladder attack. Not to be done at home. Or anywhere.

AT A GLANCE

DIET

➡ To prevent bile from becoming too concentrated, thereby increasing the risk for stones to form, make sure you drink at least 2 liters of water a day.

➡ A fiber-rich diet is key to preventing gallstones. Whole grains, vegetables, and legumes all fit the high-fiber bill.

➡ A high-fat diet increases your risk, so decrease dairy foods, deli meats, pastries, and fatty cuts of meat.

➡ Rocket, kale, artichokes, turmeric, grapefruit, pears, and lemons are all good for the liver and gallbladder.

REMEDIES

➡ Take a tincture or tablet of one or more of the herbs that support the functioning of the liver and hence the gallbladder once or twice a day.

➡ Add a fiber supplement.

OTHER

➡ Being overweight increases your risk of gallstones. Lose weight now.

➡ Acupuncture is an effective treatment for gallbladder disease.

➡ Deal with negative emotions such as anger, resentment, and bitterness.

GLANDULAR FEVER (MONONUCLEOSIS)

WHAT IS IT?

Catching a kissing disease sounds like fun. Well, it's not. Not remotely fun. Caused by the Epstein-Barr virus, glandular fever is a common infection in children and teenagers. It often cruelly strikes students at the end of their schooling, around the time of important exams and assessments. Also called acute mononucleosis, an episode of glandular fever can last a couple of weeks, or symptoms can linger for months and sometimes years. Glandular fever is thought to be a possible precursor to chronic fatigue syndrome. That threat alone is enough to treat this kissing disease very seriously.

SYMPTOMS

☑ Swollen lymph glands in the neck, underarms, and groin

☑ Swollen tonsils

☑ Sore throat

☑ Fever

☑ Fatigue

☑ Loss of appetite

☑ Headache

☑ Night sweats

☑ The spleen and liver can also be affected by glandular fever.

WHAT CAUSES IT?

❏ The Epstein-Barr virus is spread by saliva, so in addition to kissing, you can catch it by sharing cutlery and crockery, or being downwind from someone sneezing or coughing.

WHAT TO DO

If you treat your glandular fever with the recommendations below, and make sure you rest well, then there is every reason to expect you will be fighting fit within a couple of weeks.

Diet

❏ If your appetite has reduced, don't force yourself to eat big meals. Your appetite will return as soon as your body is ready to digest more solid sustenance. But the meals you do eat need to be nutritious. Lean meat, chicken, and fish. Plenty of fresh vegetables and fruit.

❏ It is important to consume plenty of fluids.

❏ Soup is good but avoid those based on cream, cheese, or milk. Make a broth from vegetable, fish, chicken, or beef stock and add vegetables, onions, beans, and garlic.

❏ Drink fresh vegetable and fruit juices. Vegetables to include are carrots, celery, parsley, beetroot, kale, and ginger and for fruit, try berries, pineapple, oranges, grapefruit, and mandarin.

❏ Avoid sugar. Studies have shown that within a few minutes of sugar consumption, lymphocyte activity is reduced markedly. Lymphocytes (white blood cells) are major players in the immune system. Sugar also tends to increase mucus. A little raw honey is better and soothes a sore throat.

❏ Calendula is a plant that is good for the immune and lymphatic system. If you grow this colorful flower, use some petals in your salads and sandwiches.

Remedies

❏ Herbs to support and strengthen the immune and lymphatic systems are mandatory. Choose from andrographis, echinacea, cat's claw, baptisia, calendula, poke root, goldenseal, and/or olive leaf, and take twice a day in tablet or tincture form. If you are using the gargle mentioned below, you don't need this mixture as well. Use one or the other.

❏ If your throat is inflamed and sore, add 5 ml of poke root, calendula, echinacea, goldenseal, and/or myrrh to 30 ml of water. Gargle three times a day and swallow. This will probably be one of the worst experiences of your life. As mentioned above, if you are using this gargle, you don't need to take tablets or tinctures as well.

❏ Vitamin C and zinc are important to keep your immune system in good shape. Take two to three times a day.

❏ The herb poke root (*Phytolacca decandra*) is specific for swollen glands and is marvelous when treating glandular fever. Poke root is quite strong so only take 10 to 15 drops three times a day. Best mixed with the other immune and lymphatic herbs mentioned previously. Poke root is not easy to come by, so you might need to consult a herbalist.

❏ Calendula is another herb for the lymphatic system and is particularly suited to glandular fever. Drink calendula tea or mix it with other herbs including echinacea, ginger, and peppermint.

❏ If the infection has passed and you still feel fatigued, take a (long) course of the adaptogen herbs. The stalwarts of the herbal materia medica, adaptogens help the body recover after illness, restoring energy and physical resilience. Many of these herbs also support immunity. Choose from Siberian ginseng, withania, rehmannia, licorice, and/or panax ginseng. (For more on adaptogens, see Chronic Fatigue on page 90.)

❏ If the liver has been affected (ascertained by a blood test), keep away from fatty foods and drink juices made from a combination of carrots, celery, and beetroot. The juice of half a lemon in the morning in hot water is good for the liver. So are the herbs St. Mary's thistle, dandelion root, and globe artichoke.

Other

❏ Go to bed. To make sure your bout of glandular fever does not end up as chronic fatigue syndrome, take the advice from one of Australia's leading herbalists, Kerry Bone. He recommends that as soon as you have got some extra energy, GO TO BED. Keep your energy as a reservoir for recovery. This is particularly difficult information for normally active teenagers to hear, but it is so important for recovery.

❏ Don't exercise. As mentioned above, any extra energy should be kept in reserve for recovery. Try a gentle stroll or stretch, no more.

❏ The Bach flower Olive is appropriate if you are horribly tired, and hornbeam if feeling just weary.

❏ Before this illness, were you inclined to take on too much? Did you have a tendency to burn the candle at both ends? If so, take this as a warning, and don't push yourself so hard in the future.

DIET

➟ Don't force yourself to eat if you are not hungry. But make sure what you do eat is nutritious. Lean meat, chicken, fish, fresh vegetables, and fruit.

➟ Avoid sugar.

➟ Keep up your fluids; soups and juices are a good idea.

REMEDIES

➟ Take herbs for glandular fever as a gargle (and swallow) three times a day if you have a sore throat, otherwise take in tablet or tincture form.

➟ Vitamin C, zinc, and the bioflavonoids will boost your immune system. At a time like this, boost away.

➟ If you are still fatigued after a couple of weeks, take adaptogen herbs. These herbs help the body recover after illness.

OTHER

➟ Take rest. There is a tendency to underestimate the ferocity and tenacity of glandular fever. It is wise to take weeks away from work or school, rather than days. Be warned. Unless treated well, glandular fever has been known to come back to haunt you.

GLUTEN INTOLERANCE
(CELIAC DISEASE AND GLUTEN SENSITIVITY)

Celiac (pronounced "see-lee-ak") disease was not identified until 1950 (even though symptoms have been observed since ancient Roman times), whereas gluten sensitivity has only been described in medical literature in the last decade or so.

Celiac disease and gluten sensitivity are two conditions that lie along a spectrum. Both conditions involve a protein called gluten, which is found in a variety of grains including wheat, rye, spelt, barley, triticale, kamut, and oats. Celiac disease often presents with tummy symptoms, the classic being diarrhea, and is considered more serious than gluten sensitivity. For ease of reading, both will be referred to in this chapter as gluten intolerance.

For those with a gluten intolerance, gluten causes the intestinal wall to become inflamed. This happens when nutrients from food cross from the bowel to the bloodstream via little projections (villi) that line the intestines. The inflammatory effect of gluten flattens the villi, compromising the absorption of precious nutrients including zinc, iron, and others. If you are unknowingly gluten intolerant and eat gluten on a regular basis (and who doesn't?), long-term nutritional deficiencies may result in a range of health problems.

In addition to reduced nutrient absorption, permeability across the intestinal wall is increased (meaning larger food fragments are able to pass through to the bloodstream, thus creating food allergies). This means that the symptoms of gluten intolerance can be confused with other food sensitivities. Difficult. To add insult to injury, due to the inflammation of the intestinal wall, inevitably there will be disruption to the microbiome, the bacterial population that live in the bowel. Some of these bacteria create useful substances—for example, the enzyme lactase, which is needed to break down lactose (milk sugar). A dearth of lactase-producing bacteria explains why many people with gluten intolerance are also lactose intolerant and unable to tolerate dairy foods. Once gluten is removed from the diet, allowing the intestinal wall to repair, and the microbiome time to recover, you will be able to enjoy dairy foods once again.

SYMPTOMS

- ✓ Diarrhea
- ✓ Constipation
- ✓ Abdominal bloating
- ✓ Tummy pain
- ✓ Fatigue
- ✓ Sinusitis
- ✓ Asthma
- ✓ Brain fog
- ✓ Eczema
- ✓ *Dermatitis herpetiformis* (an eczema-type skin condition)
- ✓ Itchy ears
- ✓ Joint and muscle pains
- ✓ Mouth ulcers
- ✓ Weight loss
- ✓ Hair loss
- ✓ Iron-deficiency anemia

To find out whether or not you are a fully certified celiac, a biopsy or small sample of the inside of your intestine needs to be taken to see if the villi are damaged. A blood test for celiac disease

OATS AND CELIAC DISEASE

For years, oats were tarred with the gluten brush. It appears that in the early days of gluten identification, samples of oat flour were taken from the same mills that processed wheat grain (the wheat gluten had contaminated the oat sample). However, there is still a hitch, as one in seven celiac sufferers may in fact be intolerant of the protein in oats as well. The Celiac Society of America lists oats as suitable on their list of foods whereas the Celiac Society of Australia recommends that celiac sufferers don't eat oats, just in case. When you are first exploring whether gluten intolerance may be a problem for you, eliminate oats alongside the gluten-containing grains. If your symptoms resolve, oats should be the first grain to resume eating.

is also available, but a 100-percent diagnosis relies on the intestinal biopsy. Gluten sensitivity may not show up on a biopsy or blood test. The best way to ascertain if gluten is the cause of your health problems is to eliminate it from your diet for a month. This is enough time for the villi to regrow. If your symptoms abate significantly in this time, it's likely that you have an intolerance to gluten.

WHAT CAUSES IT?

- ❏ Gluten intolerance is believed to be an autoimmune disease, one of a mysterious assortment of conditions that include rheumatoid arthritis, ulcerative colitis, and multiple sclerosis (MS).
- ❏ There is a large genetic link with celiac disease.
- ❏ Gluten is ubiquitous in our diet—an overconsumption of gluten-containing grains has possibly created this sensitivity.

- Celiac disease is diagnosed most commonly at infancy, as one would expect, after the introduction of grains to the diet. The other most commonly diagnosed time is for women in their thirties. The reason for this late-in-the-day occurrence in women could be due to stress acting as the last straw on a fragile immune system.

- There may be a link with thyroid disease and gluten intolerance.

WHAT TO DO

The remedy for gluten intolerance is dietary abstention. For the newly diagnosed, the following recommendations will help restore health and microbial equilibrium to your intestines.

Gluten-Free Diet

The person with severe celiac disease needs to avoid all gluten—even the mere speck of gluten in dressings and sauces can initiate symptoms. This is a lifelong dietary sentence. After a couple of months of a gluten-free diet, however, those with gluten sensitivity can cautiously reintroduce gluten-containing foods. Oats, with their dubious gluten credentials, are to be introduced first, followed slowly, slowly by the other gluten-containing grains.

Avoid

- Our society is enamored with gluten. Everywhere you look there's bread, pasta, bagels, croissants, biscuits, and cakes. Look closely at labels, and you will also find wheat flour (containing gluten) hidden in sauces, soups, and a multitude of processed foods.

- Avoid grains containing gluten such as wheat (this includes bulgur, semolina, and couscous), spelt, rye, barley, triticale, kamut, and oats.

- Avoid foods containing by-products of these grains such as beer, ale, lager, malted drinks, malted or flavored milk drinks, instant tea, coffee substitutes, malt vinegar, malt, wheat starch, mustard, pickles, soy sauce, gravy mixes, seasoning "rubs," hydrolyzed vegetable protein (HVP), texturized vegetable protein (TVP), licorice sweets (real licorice root is okay), pastries, scones, cakes, biscuits, crackers, pasta, hokkien noodles, bread, oatmeal, baked beans, frozen french fries (which may be coated in wheat flour), and battered food.

- For the first month of your gluten-free diet, also avoid dairy foods as they contain lactose (milk sugar). Due to a possible lack of lactase (see above), it is likely that you will have symptoms in response to lactose, and this will only confuse things. After a month off all gluten, slowly start to reintroduce dairy foods, including milk, yogurt, and cheese.

Include

- Any packaged food with "gluten free" written on the label can go in your shopping cart.

- Allowed grains include rice (brown, basmati, jasmine, rice cakes, rice noodles, risotto), buckwheat (don't be fooled by the name), corn (polenta, corn cakes, popcorn), millet, amaranth, wild rice, quinoa, and chia seeds.

- All legumes (lentils, chickpeas, etc.), fruits, vegetables, meats, fish, eggs, nuts, and seeds.

- Wine, gin, tea, and coffee.

Recommended Diet for Repairing the Intestinal Wall

- Prebiotic foods can provide the right food for probiotic microflora vegetables—asparagus, Jerusalem artichokes, leeks and onions, legumes such as baked beans, chickpeas, and lentils, and supplementary fibers including psyllium, pectin, guar gum, and slippery elm.

- Probiotic foods can restore beneficial microflora. Nondairy probiotic foods include miso, sauerkraut, kefir, natto, tempeh, and the Korean delicacy kimchi. After a month, you can start including dairy-based probiotic foods such as kefir and yogurt.

- Avoid sugar. You don't want to encourage the wrong bacteria.

- Include one or two raw vegetable juices a day. Add carrot and cabbage, as they are both healing for damaged tissue.

- Add turmeric (fresh or dried) as an anti-inflammatory.

- Fresh garlic will help increase immunity.

Remedies

The following recommendations will help to heal the intestinal wall. They only need to be used in the month following the cessation of gluten-containing foods. Cells lining the intestinal wall are some of the fastest growing cells in the body, and therefore don't take too long to be restored to robust good health.

- As above, a good quality probiotic supplement is required for the first month. Many of the best probiotic supplements are produced on a culture of milk. For most people, there is not enough lactose to cause a reaction; however, there are nondairy probiotics available.

- Slippery elm powder can soothe and repair the intestinal wall (as well as being a prebiotic). Try one teaspoon in water or mashed banana twice a day.

- Aloe vera helps to heal. Drink 10 ml of aloe juice daily (less for children).

- Glutamine is an amino acid that helps heal intestinal cells. It is often combined in supplements containing aloe vera and slippery elm.

- Lactoferrin is a protein that improves immunity, particularly of the intestine. Perfect for gluten intolerance. It can be found in colostrum supplements or in combination with other nutrients. Even though colostrum is a dairy food, this amount is unlikely to trigger any symptoms.

- Herbs that can heal and calm the intestinal lining include meadowsweet, chamomile, peppermint, and lemon balm. Take as tablet, tincture, or better still, as a herbal tea.

- Vitamin A is necessary for healing the damaged intestinal wall. Take as a supplement or preferably in the form of cod liver oil.

- Zinc can help the repair of cells. Take a liquid zinc supplement daily.

- If you are low in iron, take a liquid iron supplement daily. (Note: If you are taking both zinc and iron supplements, take them eight hours apart. Taken together they reduce each other's absorption.)

Other

- There are celiac-support and information groups in the real world and online.

- There are many gluten-free recipes available in print and online.

Diet

➡ For the first month, avoid all gluten-containing grains and food made from them such as wheat, rye, barley, spelt, triticale, and oats. Your life as you have known it is now over. Eat anything (within reason) that says "gluten free" on the package, and eat corn, rice, quinoa, and chia freely.

➡ If you have been diagnosed with celiac disease, you will need to remain gluten free. If you suspect you are gluten sensitive, then cautiously reintroduce gluten-containing foods. When you experience a recurrence of symptoms, you know you have gone a sandwich too far.

➡ Eat prebiotic foods to encourage beneficial microflora.

➡ Eat probiotic foods to restore beneficial microflora.

➡ Avoid sugar.

➡ Raw vegetable juice containing carrot and cabbage are healing to the intestinal wall.

Remedies

➡ Take a probiotic supplement daily to begin the intestinal restoration of the microbiome.

➡ Take liquid iron and zinc—at least eight hours apart for better absorption.

➡ Glutamine, aloe vera, and slippery elm can help repair the intestinal wall.

Other

➡ Join a celiac group online to gather more information.

➡ Buy a gluten-free recipe book.

GOUT

WHAT IS IT?

Gout conjures up images of a hefty King Henry VIII with copious jowls, lolling around in an ermine coat, tucking into a pie of roast swan washed down with a few pints of ale. However, gout can strike even the most humble of folk. An arthritic condition affecting mainly men, gout is caused by a higher than normal concentration of uric acid in the blood. Often the first attack hits the big toe, although uric acid crystals may deposit in other joints and tendons. The pain can be so intense that even the weight of a bed sheet can bring on a cold sweat.

SYMPTOMS

✓ Pain in one or more joints, often the big toe, but may also affect the ankle and knee.

✓ Pain appears very suddenly.

✓ The affected joint can be warm and red.

✓ The pain can be throbbing or crushing, and is often excruciating.

✓ Tophi is not the collective noun for coagulated bean curd, but are the harmless lumps below the skin around joints that can occur in long-term sufferers of gout.

WHAT CAUSES IT?

❏ If you suffer from gout, there is a 25 percent chance someone else in your family has it, too.

❏ Triggers include excess alcohol (particularly beer and spirits), purine-rich foods (see below), and cold weather.

❏ Some medications can be triggers for an attack of gout.

❏ Conditions that increase the risk of gout include obesity, diabetes, and heart and kidney disease.

WHAT TO DO

Diet

❏ Reduce foods high in purines, including offal or organ meats (liver, heart, spleen, intestines), and sweetbreads (thymus, pancreas), red meat, poultry, deli meats, shellfish, crustaceans, yeast, herring, sardines, mackerel, anchovies, asparagus, mushrooms, and spinach.

❏ A juice made of $2/3$ carrot, $1/3$ celery, a knob of ginger, and several sprigs of parsley can help the kidneys to excrete uric acid and reduce inflammation.

❏ Naturopathically, gout is thought of as an acidic condition. Reduce acid-forming foods (i.e., sugar, grains, and meat), and increase fruits and vegetables (see Appendix E: Acid-Forming Food).

❏ Reduce alcohol. It increases uric acid levels and inhibits excretion. Moderate amounts of wine are acceptable; however, beer and spirits are to be avoided.

❏ Drink 2 liters of water daily to dilute uric acid as much as possible.

❏ A popular remedy is the cherry cure. Cherries contain anthocyanidins that help lower uric acid. Eat 250 to 500 grams of cherries (fresh, frozen, or canned) each day or drink a cup of pure cherry juice. Strawberries and blueberries also contain anthocyanidins, so if cherries are not available, eat these berries instead.

❏ Turmeric and ginger are anti-inflammatory. Add them to your food.

❏ Drinking soft drinks is associated with gout. Switch to water.

Remedies

❏ Taking 10 ml of fish oil daily is excellent for any inflammatory arthritic condition, including gout. Once inflammation has eased, reduce to 5 ml daily. (Fish oil is okay, but oily fish are not, and are mentioned in the purine list above. The purines are a protein derivative, so don't appear in the oil.)

❏ Folic acid works on gout in the same way as the commonly prescribed medicine allopurinol (a xanthine oxidase inhibitor). Take 400 mcg of folic acid along with a B complex each day. The evidence for folic acid is controversial; however, the recommended dose is not exceptionally high and is worth a trial.

❏ The bioflavonoids, especially quercetin, are effective anti-inflammatories. Take in large doses until pain subsides. (Note that in supplements, often the bioflavonoids are combined with vitamin C. In this instance, vitamin C is to be avoided, so find a supplement with the bioflavonoids alone.)

BEHIND THE SCENES

Uric acid is a derivative of purines in food. Purines, namely adenine and guanine, are found in certain protein foods, and are the nitrogen-containing structures called bases found in our DNA.

❑ Herbs that are helpful for gout include nettle leaf, dandelion leaf, boswellia, couch grass, juniper, willow bark, gravel root, parsley, celery seed, birch, turmeric, and ginger. Take in tincture, tablet, or tea form.

❑ Vitamin C in large doses should be avoided. The vitamin C competes with uric acid excretion, causing a sudden spike in uric acid and symptoms. Doses under 250 mg should pose no threat, but over 3 grams a day is likely to trigger an attack. Food that is rich in vitamin C, such as berries and citrus, do not pose any threat as they do not contain the megadoses of vitamin C that you can only obtain by supplementation.

❑ Gout is an arthritic condition. The traditional apple cider vinegar and honey in hot water each morning is a nice way to start the day.

❑ The tissue salts silica and natrum phosphoricum (nat. phos.) help remove and neutralize uric acid in the tissues.

Other

❑ Lose weight if necessary. Overweight is associated with diabetes and heart disease, both risk factors for gout.

❑ Regular exercise has been associated with the reduced risk of gout.

❑ Rub affected joints with juniper oil.

❑ Acupuncture is a good adjunctive treatment.

AROMATHERAPY

Add 6 to 8 drops of this detoxifying blend to a warm bath with Epsom salts or blend with Arnica, St. John's wort, and sweet almond oil and massage into the affected area.

❑ 4 drops of coriander seed—analgesic, antioxidant, soothing

❑ 3 drops of carrot seed—diuretic, depurative

❑ 4 drops of grapefruit—diuretic, cleansing, stimulating

❑ 3 drops of juniper—diuretic, purifying

AT A GLANCE

Diet

➠ Avoid or reduce foods containing purines, which may trigger an attack.

➠ Drink plenty of water to dilute the uric acid.

➠ Drink vegetable juice daily (especially the carrot, celery, parsley, and ginger juice recommended above).

➠ Increase fruits and vegetables; decrease meat, sugar, and grains.

➠ Cherries, blueberries, and strawberries contain anthocyanins, which can be very good for gout. Eat them daily.

Remedies

➠ Folic acid is a very effective remedy for relieving and preventing gout.

➠ Take fish oil daily. It contains the anti-inflammatory omega-3 fatty acids.

➠ Take quercetin, an anti-inflammatory bioflavonoid, as directed above.

Other

➠ Being overweight may contribute to gout.

➠ If not too painful, rub the affected joint with juniper oil.

GUM DISEASE

WHAT IS IT?

If you've noticed you're a little longer in the tooth lately, the cause may well be gingivitis—the first sign of periodontal disease. Periodontal means "around the tooth" and refers to any disorder of the gums and jawbone. Although located in the mouth, periodontal disease has more global health implications. The inflammatory toxins created by the bacteria responsible are involved in heart disease, diabetes, and even miscarriages. If you don't attend promptly to gum disease, your path may be strewn with discarded teeth. Yours. There are many natural methods for the treatment and prevention of gum disease.

SYMPTOMS

☑ Bright red or purple gums

☑ Swollen gums

☑ Bleeding gums, particularly when brushing teeth

☑ Gums tender to the touch

☑ Bad breath

☑ Bad taste in the mouth

WHAT CAUSES IT?

❏ Gingivitis is initiated by dental plaque, a biofilm produced by bacteria that coats the teeth and gums. A slothful approach to dental hygiene will increase the growth of plaque, and hence gum disease.

❏ The first sign of scurvy is bleeding gums. Although this blight of eighteenth-century sailors is less common nowadays, many people do not eat sufficient vitamin C on a daily basis, creating a subclinical scurvy effect.

❏ Faulty dental work.

❏ Mouth breathing. Breathing through the mouth dries up saliva—our first line of defense against bacteria. Saliva contains antibacterial enzymes and acids.

❏ Tobacco smoking is associated with susceptibility to periodontal disease because smoke decreases oxygenation of the gum cells.

❏ Hormonal changes during pregnancy.

❏ Eating too many soft foods. Vigorous chewing increases circulation to the gums.

WHAT TO DO

Diet

❏ Avoid sugar. Bacteria thrive on sugar. Bacteria produce plaque. Plaque causes gum disease.

❏ The polyphenols in green tea are effective against the bacteria behind gum disease. Drink two to three cups a day.

❏ Eat foods rich in vitamin C daily such as citrus, berries, broccoli, capsicum, and kiwifruit.

❏ Chewing crunchy food like raw apples, carrots, seeds, and nuts can help in the prevention and treatment of gingivitis. It's a case of use it or lose it—or should that be chew it or lose it? Chewing on fresh, crunchy food massages the gums, increasing the blood flow to the area and boosting local immune response. Chew each mouthful well. One study showed that eating a raw apple has been found to be 30 percent more effective than an immediate brushing. Chewing also increases the flow of saliva.

❏ Spending five minutes chewing gum containing xylitol after each meal will also do the trick. Xylitol is a naturally occurring compound that has an antibacterial action. Particularly effective against the bacteria responsible for tooth decay (*strep mutans*), it can also reduce the likelihood of gingivitis.

Remedies

❏ Herbs that can help promote blood flow and healing to the gums include bilberry, ginkgo, and prickly ash in tablet, tincture, or tea form.

❏ Various herbal toothpastes contain gum-healing and -strengthening herbs such as sage, thyme, echinacea, ratanhia, and myrrh.

❏ Grapeseed extract and resveratrol are two antioxidant-rich supplements that can help keep gingivitis at bay.

❏ Vitamin C plays a vital role in maintaining collagen, the grist of gum tissue. If your diet is lacking in fresh fruit and vegetables, gingivitis could be a very early indicator of scurvy, the classic vitamin-C deficiency disease. Take 1 grams of vitamin C daily, but not the chewable tablets as the ascorbic acid can affect dental enamel. Take in powder or standard tablet form with added bioflavonoids.

❏ CoQ_{10}, a coenzyme vital for improving oxygenation to all cells, is an outstanding treatment for gingivitis. Take two capsules (50 mg) daily, until symptoms clear, then one capsule daily as a preventative. A clever way to get the CoQ_{10} straight to the site of the action is to squeeze the contents of a capsule onto your gums and massage in using your finger or a soft brush. Even once a week will help.

❏ Gingivitis indicates a bacterial problem, so take all the usual natural antibiotics to boost immunity such as vitamin C, zinc, andrographis, cat's claw, olive leaf, echinacea, and garlic.

❏ Rinse and spit with dilute colloidal silver.

❏ Propolis mouthwash is antiseptic and slightly anesthetic. Use it once or twice a day until the problem is resolved.

Other

❏ Take your teeth to a dentist for a checkup and thorough cleaning every six months to keep teeth free of plaque.

❏ Floss after every meal.

❏ Electric oscillating toothbrushes are twice as effective at loosening plaque than conventional hand-held brushes. Check with your dentist or dental hygienist as to the best brush for you, and don't be too humble to ask for instructions on proper brushing technique—being an enthusiastic scrubber may not help your cause.

❏ Gum massage improves circulation and can help the healing process. Try a vigorous gum massage twice a day for three to four minutes with your finger, a soft brush, or a well-chewed twig. With a little pressure, slowly press down in regular small circles, covering an area over both gum and teeth. You can massage with various unguents such as distilled extract of witch hazel, cooled sage tea, diluted apple cider vinegar, sea salt, the white portion of a lemon peel, or a drop of tea tree or eucalyptus oil.

❏ Dip your toothbrush in a solution of $1/2$ hydrogen peroxide, $1/2$ water, then dip it in baking soda and smear the mixture along the gum line and into all the crevices between the teeth and gums.

❏ Buteyko breathing emphasizes nose breathing, rather than mouth breathing. Breathing through your mouth decreases saliva, which contains enzymes and substances that are antibiotic, deactivating the bacteria causing dental plaque and gum disease. (See Appendix F: Buteyko Breathing.)

Diet

⇨ Avoid sugar. Sugar feeds the very bacteria that cause gum disease.

⇨ Eat foods rich in vitamin C daily.

⇨ Chew your food well. It will massage the gums and stimulate the flow of saliva that contains bactericidal enzymes.

⇨ Green tea contains polyphenols that protect against gum disease. Drink two to three cups a day.

Remedies

⇨ Herbs for gum disease include bilberry, ginkgo, prickly ash, andrographis, cat's claw, olive leaf, echinacea, and garlic.

⇨ Take a tablet of vitamin C along with bioflavonoids.

⇨ CoQ_{10} is brilliant for treating gingivitis. Take daily. You can also massage the contents onto your gums.

⇨ Propolis mouthwash is antibacterial. Use it once or twice a day.

Other

⇨ Buteyko breathing reduces mouth breathing. Mouth breathing creates the environment for more plaque-forming bacteria that cause gum disease. Nose breathing is best.

⇨ Good dental hygiene is key to preventing and treating gum disease. This includes regular visits to the dentist, together with brushing and flossing at least twice a day. Promise?

HAY FEVER

WHAT IS IT?

If three sneezes in a row is a sign of good luck, ten sneezes is more likely to mean your luck has run out—and you probably have hay fever. Also known as allergic rhinitis, hay fever occurs when an allergen gets up your nose, in your eyes, or even in your food, and your immune system overreacts in a fit of sneezing and itchiness.

SYMPTOMS

☑ Itchy eyes, nose, upper palate, throat, face
☑ Runny nose
☑ Teary eyes
☑ Puffiness under the eyes
☑ Dark circles under the eyes, especially toward the nose
☑ Sneezing
☑ Irritability
☑ Fatigue
☑ Loss of smell
☑ Headaches

WHAT CAUSES IT

❏ Hay fever is part of the allergic group of atopic conditions that include asthma, sinusitis, and eczema. The atopic group are largely inherited.

Sift through your family tree, and you'll find a relative with one or more of these conditions. If not, take a close look at the milkman.

❏ Common allergens include dust, pollen, mold, animal dander (fur, etc.), food additives and preservatives, detergents, the ubiquitous dust mite, and cockroach droppings.

❏ Seasonal hay fever, as the name suggests, is an allergy to seasonal allergens. It flares up when those plants are in flower and pollen becomes airborne.

❏ Several foods can provoke a hay fever response, including dairy, wheat, eggs, citrus, corn, peanuts, wine, nuts, and shellfish.

WHAT TO DO

Diet

❏ If you sneeze and splutter at grasses, pollens, and dust (airborne allergens), the chances are high (about 80 percent) that you may have a food sensitivity as well. If you avoid eating the foods that you are sensitive to, you will decrease the load on your immune system and the hay fever symptoms should abate. The first foods to investigate are wheat and dairy. If you know you are sensitive to grasses, think about choosing wheat as your first food sensitivity simply because it too is a grass.

❏ Drink at least 2 liters of clear fluid a day to allow the mucus to drain. Hay fever increases your risk of infected sinuses, so keep those fluids up.

❏ Avoid alcohol as it swells the mucous linings, which are already inflamed. You may also be sensitive to the histamines in red wine.

❏ Increase foods containing vitamin C, a natural antihistamine, such as citrus, papaya, kiwifruit, strawberries, pineapple, guava, rock melon, broccoli, cauliflower, Brussels sprouts, and capsicum.

❏ Garlic and onions have mucus-clearing and antibiotic properties.

❏ Raw honeycomb is a curious and delicious remedy. The theory behind it is that if you are allergic to pollens, then the tiny amount of bee-preserved pollen in the honeycomb will act as a kind of vaccine. Take a teaspoon of honeycomb each day. Try honeycomb from local bees as it will more likely contain the pollen you are sensitive to. Raw local honey will also contain some natural anti-allergy substances.

❏ Avoid dairy products if they tend to increase mucus production.

❏ There may be a link between a high-salt diet and hay fever as there is with asthma and sinusitis. Reduce added salt in your diet and packaged food that often contains high levels of salt.

Remedies

❏ If your hay fever is a seasonal thing, start using a few of these remedies six weeks prior to as well as during the sneezing season, which is often the change of season from winter to spring. If you suffer all year around, take the remedies for as long as you need.

❏ Herbs that help reduce hay fever symptoms include eyebright, albizia, horseradish, goldenrod, and goldenseal.

❏ Quercetin, the bioflavonoid, acts like an antihistamine, and can work well when taken in conjunction with vitamin C.

❏ Vitamin C on its own is an excellent natural antihistamine. Take 2 grams during the hay fever season three times a day. (Adjust for children's dose.)

❏ Evening primrose oil taken throughout the year can decrease your allergic response. The itching and redness of the mucous membranes that line the throat and nose caused by hay fever is due to the release of inflammatory substances such as histamine that are released in response to an allergen. If the mucous membrane cells themselves are less likely to react, then hay fever symptoms can also get less and less. The essential fatty acid DHGLA, found in evening primrose oil, is particularly anti-inflammatory. Initially you will need to take eight to nine evening primrose capsules (or the equivalent of 8 to 10 ml of evening primrose oil) to ensure that all cell membranes incorporate DHGLA. Once benefits are noticed, possibly after a couple of months, dosage can be lowered to two to three capsules a day. Halve the dose for children.

❏ Propolis and bee pollen products work similarly to the honeycomb described above, acting as a kind of vaccine.

Other

❏ God's gift to sinus and hay fever sufferers is the Neti pot.

❏ Buteyko breathing also works brilliantly for hay fever. Sneezing and spluttering are considered forms of "overbreathing'—a big no-no as far as the Buteyko technique is concerned. To stop a hay fever attack, this technique can work a treat. Firstly, close your mouth. Then take a small breath in, followed by a small breath out. Block

---

NETI POT

Nasal irrigation, intranasal douche, or nose bidet—using a Neti pot is never going to sound elegant. Looking like the lovechild between a teapot and Aladdin's magical lamp without the genie, the Neti pot is the gadget used to practice *jala neti*, an ancient yogic purification and cleansing technique. A godsend for sinus sufferers, the Neti pot flushes warm salty water through the nasal passages, allowing mucus to drain out of the body and with it, unwanted bacteria, viruses, dust, and pollen. Salt has the additional effect of reducing any swelling of the lining of the sinuses, preventing further mucous production, killing some bacteria, and preventing sinus pain.

Traditionally made from silver or copper, Neti pots are now available in a variety of materials. Ceramic (looks pretty but can break), glass (if breaks could be dangerous), and plastic pots (light and won't break, but are high on the yuk factor). Stainless steel pots are popular as they are easily cleaned, nontoxic, and unbreakable.

USING A NETI POT

Into the Neti pot, mix 500 ml of warm water with 1 teaspoon of non-iodized sea salt. Tradition says that the mixture should be as warm as your blood and as salty as your tears. Stand over the sink or in the shower, holding your head to the left side, tilted slightly down. Slowly pour half the water up your right nostril. Within a couple of moments, your left nostril should drip, then flow. Give a gentle snort to clear out the remaining water and repeat on the other side. With practice, the process will actually feel pleasant. Counterintuitively, if the water stings, the reason may be insufficient salt.

Using a Neti pot has scientific street cred, proving in studies to be as effective for sinusitis as corticosteroids, a commonly used medication for sinusitis. Using a Neti pot regularly may be effective for long-term (chronic) sinusitis and hay fever as well as for those exposed to nasal irritants in their work. Avoid using a Neti pot if there is serious congestion and infection, allowing the condition to ease before recommencing.

your nose with your thumb and forefinger. Hold for as long as possible, shaking your head slowly from side to side. When you feel like you are about to burst, release the nose, but keep the mouth closed. Yes, of course you look like a loony. But as long as it works, right? Repeat a couple of times. If you are a mouth breather, try to breathe through your nose at all times.

❏ Where possible, avoid or reduce known allergens such as chemicals, mold, and dust in your home and work environment.

❏ Allergy desensitization is a long-term commitment but is very effective. First, an allergy specialist will determine the exact nature of your allergens by pricking the skin of the forearms with tiny amounts of the offending substances. Depending on the extent of your allergy, a welt of varying size will appear. Depending on the ilk of your practitioner, either vaccine or homoeopathic dosages of the allergen may be dispensed, either as drops or via regular injection.

At a Glance

Diet

➠ If you are allergic to grasses, you may also be reacting to wheat in your diet, as wheat is another grass. Try eliminating it from your diet for a month and see if your hay fever symptoms improve.

➠ Increase foods high in vitamin C, which has natural antihistamine properties.

➠ Drink at least 2 liters of clear fluid a day to allow the mucus to drain.

➠ Alcohol causes the mucous membranes lining the airways to swell. With hay fever, they are already swollen, so drink less alcohol.

➠ Local raw honey and honeycomb contains small amounts of the pollen that you may be allergic to. Homeopathically, eating some of the honey product will build up your resistance and reduce your symptoms in a similar way to how a vaccine does. Do be careful about administering any bee product due to some people's extreme allergic reactions.

Remedies

➠ Vitamin C and the bioflavonoid quercetin have natural anti-inflammatory and antihistamine properties. Perfect for hay fever.

➠ Herbs that can help reduce hay fever symptoms include eyebright, albizzia, horseradish, goldenrod, and goldenseal.

➠ A course of evening primrose oil will reduce the sensitivity of cells lining the airways and their reaction to allergens. This effect can take months, but is well worth the effort.

Other

➠ Use a Neti pot every morning as a preventative. The saline from the Neti pot drains the sinuses and astringes the mucous membranes.

➠ Buteyko breathing is an effective treatment for hay fever.

➠ Allergy desensitization, whereby minute amounts of the allergen are injected or taken under your tongue is another effective long-term strategy for treating hay fever.

HEADACHES AND MIGRAINES

WHAT IS IT?

The "ache" part of a headache is not derived from the brain, which feels no pain itself, but from highly sensitive nerve endings within the walls of the arteries (blood vessels) that supply blood to the brain. Pain registers when these arteries constrict or dilate.

Whatever causes this change to the arteries, causes the headache. Headaches are rarely life threatening, but can make your life miserable. The odd painkiller is fine for the odd headache, but if you suffer headaches every week or more often, the cause should be sought and remedied.

WHAT CAUSES IT?

Headaches are very much a symptom rather than a disease. Figuring out the cause is fundamental to determining a cure. Headaches can be due to a number of factors or triggers listed below, and very often are multifactorial. One or maybe two triggers may not be enough to cause a headache; however, the third trigger may be the proverbial straw that breaks the camel's back. If your headache doesn't neatly fit into any of the following categories, and if pain persists, as they say on TV, see your doctor.

STRESS AND TENSION HEADACHE

This very common type of headache occurs from emotional or physical stress. Either way, if the muscles of your shoulders and neck tense up, the thin layer of muscle over the scalp can be tense too. Tension headaches are often felt from the neck up and over the back of the head.

WHAT TO DO

❑ Have a back and shoulder massage every week. In addition, learn some stretches to relax your neck and shoulders when stress occurs—don't wait for the tension to build up. One simple method is to sit or stand with your back straight. Tuck your chin in and look down to your left foot, while dropping your right shoulder. Increase the stretch by gentle pressure of your left hand pulling down. Reverse sides.

❑ A glass of alcohol may relieve a tension headache temporarily as it dilates blood vessels, but don't depend on this as your regular treatment.

❑ Magnesium, 200 mg taken three times daily (less for children) can relieve muscle spasm, or try a tablet of magnesia phosphate (mag. phos.) and potassium phosphate (kali. phos.) tissue salts each hour for the duration of the headache.

❑ Add two handfuls of Epsom salts and seven drops of lavender oil to a bathtub full of warm water, and soak your tension away.

❑ Rub a couple of drops of lavender or rosemary oil into your temples.

❑ Put your feet in a tub of hot-as-you-can-stand water with a few drops of lavender oil. On your forehead and back of your neck place a cool, damp facecloth. Keep still for fifteen minutes.

❑ Press the acupuncture point *He-Gu,* or "Joining of the Valleys," which is situated at the vortex between thumb and first finger. Dig deep into this spot with the opposite thumb, and massage in a tight circle for about a minute. Then, for another minute, massage the scalp deeply as a good hairdresser does when shampooing you. Do another minute of *He-Gu* on the other hand and finish off with a final minute on the scalp. Your headache should disappear within four minutes.

❏ Herbs to help with stress and tension headaches include valerian, vervain, St. John's wort, passionflower, skullcap, and lavender. Take in tea, tablet, or tincture form. A tea will work the quickest.

❏ Buteyko breathing will help a stress headache as it helps to relax smooth muscle. Smooth muscle lines blood vessels, including in the head. (See Appendix F: Buteyko Breathing.)

❏ See Stress on page 276.

LOW BLOOD SUGAR HEADACHE

This type of headache disappears a few minutes after eating. Often felt as a dull throb at the temples, if you have a headache, feel dizzy, or become irritable when you miss meals, it is likely that your blood sugar levels are low.

WHAT TO DO

❏ Eat small meals every two to three hours. Make sure there is some protein with each meal.

❏ Avoid caffeine and sugar; they cause havoc to blood sugar levels.

❏ With each meal, take a supplement containing a combination of chromium, zinc, magnesium, manganese, and B vitamins to restore blood sugar balance.

DEHYDRATION HEADACHE

Yes, it can be this simple. Is your mouth dry? Have you been drinking coffee all day and not enough water? Try the skin pinch test. Pull the skin on top of your hand so it is all bunched up.

If it takes longer than a couple of seconds to go back into place, you probably are a little dehydrated.

WHAT TO DO

❏ To quickly rehydrate, drink some water with a little apple or pear juice added.

❏ Drink at least 2 liters of fluid a day, more on hot days and when you exercise.

FOOD CHEMICAL SENSITIVITIES HEADACHE

Certain food chemicals, natural and artificial, can cause headaches. These headaches can be a little tricky to diagnose, as they can occur up to seventy-two hours after consuming the suspect substance.

WHAT TO DO

❏ Try avoiding the suspected allergen for a couple of weeks. The following is a list of likely suspects.

• Aspartame, an artificial sweetener, is a combination of the amino acids phenylalanine and aspartic acid. There have been reported instances of migraine after consuming products containing aspartame. Check the nutritional information on anything containing artificial sweeteners.

• Nitrates in food can cause the "hot-dog headache." Nitrates are used to preserve meat and maintain its rosy hue, even though the animal last drew breath years ago. Nitrates are common in salami, sausages, deli meats, hot dogs, pastrami, and smoked salmon.

• Vasoactive amines are derived from amino acids, and though most people have the enzyme that breaks them down, those who have less of the enzyme seem more likely to react to foods containing them. Vasoactive amines include histamine and tyramine, and are found in aged cheese, chicken liver, pickled herring, deli meats such as salami, sour cream, and red wine.

- MSG, occurring naturally in some foods but added to others such as takeout, can also be a common headache trigger.

HANGOVER HEADACHE

Hangover headaches are a common side effect of drinking too much alcohol. We get hangovers for various reasons. The first is dehydration. Alcohol is a diuretic, which means it causes us to wee prolifically. As urine is mostly water, the water has to come from somewhere in the body, including the bloodstream and the brain. The second cause of hangovers is a buildup of acetaldehyde, a substance released as alcohol is broken down. *Ipso facto,* the more alcohol you have swimming around, the more hangover-causing acetaldehyde there will be. The third cause of hangovers is due to a group of chemicals called congeners. Congeners are added to certain kinds of alcohol to enhance flavor and color. In general, the darker the color, and the less expensive the alcohol is, the more congeners there will be. Vodka and gin have less congeners than dark rum, brandy, bourbon, and scotch. Top-shelf liquors have less congeners than house brands. Sometimes it pays to be a snob.

WHAT TO DO

❏ Try to match each alcoholic drink with a glass of water to avoid dehydration and the worst of the hangover symptoms.

❏ Avoid fizzy and sweet alcoholic drinks. The fizz increases the rate of alcohol absorption, and the sweetness masks the taste of the alcohol so you are likely to drink more than normal. Fruit daiquiris are prime offenders.

❏ When you get home, drink a diluted sports drink to top up your electrolyte levels.

❏ The hair of the dog is not recommended unless you are a masochist or obsessive pet fancier.

❏ If you know you will drink more than perhaps you should, take the following supplements the day before and the day after: St. Mary's thistle, B vitamins, zinc, and magnesium.

"YOUR NECK IS OUT" HEADACHE

Very commonly, headaches occur when there is a misalignment of the neck or back.

WHAT TO DO

❏ Seek advice from your osteopath, massage therapist, chiropractor, or physiotherapist.

❏ Be aware of your posture throughout the day, in the car, at work, watching television.

❏ Natural anti-inflammatories including turmeric, quercetin, and ginger can work well. Take every second hour when pain is severe and make that appointment with your body worker.

CAFFEINE WITHDRAWAL HEADACHE

Caffeine withdrawal headaches (CWHs) are throbbers. While drinking more than four cups of coffee each day increases your risk of headaches by 20 to 30 percent, it's when you decide to quit that the real humdinger of a headache hits. But it's only temporary. In general the CWH only lasts twenty-four hours, but some can extend for days.

WHAT TO DO

❏ If you want to quit caffeine (coffee, cola, and tea), don't go cold turkey. Reduce gradually.

❏ Drink plenty of water and if necessary, take a

pharmaceutical painkiller, as this headache is a one-time-only occurrence.

❏ The tissue salt iron phosphate (ferrum. phos.) is good for a throbbing headache.

❏ The homeopathic remedy coffea is also good for this type of headache.

HORMONAL HEADACHES

Occurring most often in the days leading up to menstruation, these headaches can be brutal. Some women notice headaches when taking the oral contraceptive pill or hormone replacement therapy. If you are not sure whether your headache is due to hormones or not, put a note in your diary every time you get a headache. After three months a cyclic pattern will emerge if your headache "qualifies" as hormonal.

WHAT TO DO

The following can be helpful:

❏ Vitex agnus-castus tincture or tablet each morning.

❏ Black cohosh is good for headaches during menopause.

❏ Take 3 grams evening primrose oil a day throughout the month.

❏ In addition to a women's multivitamin, take B_6 and magnesium.

❏ Try the homeopathic remedy pulsatilla.

HYPERTENSION HEADACHE

The problem with high-blood pressure (hypertension) is that very often you don't know you have it. However, one of the few symptoms that people notice is a headache, sometimes described as "fullness in the head."

WHAT TO DO

❏ Decrease salt in your diet.

❏ Lose weight if necessary.

❏ Increase exercise.

❏ See High Blood Pressure on page 192.

❏ Buteyko breathing may help reduce blood pressure and hypertension headaches.

SINUS HEADACHE

Sinus headaches are felt above and behind the eyes, and become worse if you bend forward. Press firmly on the eyebrows and cheekbones. If this feels painful, inflamed, or infected, sinuses may be the problem.

WHAT TO DO

❏ Use a Neti pot each morning.

❏ Take a tablet containing garlic, horseradish, eyebright, goldenseal, goldenrod, and/or vitamin C.

❏ Drink lots of clear, hot fluids, including 2 cups of fenugreek tea a day.

❏ Avoid milk products if they add to your sinus congestion.

❏ If you are a chronic sinus sufferer, Buteyko breathing will help.

❏ See Sinusitis on page 271.

CONSTIPATION HEADACHE

The bowel is a major organ of elimination. If elimination is slow, as happens with constipation, toxic substances can be released into the bloodstream, resulting in, on this occasion, a headache. These are dull headaches, and are often associated with a bad taste in the mouth, bad breath, and coated tongue.

WHAT TO DO

❏ Drink at least 2 liters of fluid a day.

❏ Eat fiber-rich food (fruit, vegetables, legumes, whole grains), and take a soluble fiber supplement such as psyllium husks.

❏ Exercise daily.

❏ Take magnesium if your constipation is due to stress.

❏ See Constipation on page 104.

LACK-OF-SLEEP HEADACHE

Most of us need a good eight hours of uninterrupted sleep each night.

WHAT TO DO

❏ Californian poppy, valerian, passionflower, and kava are all good for insomnia.

❏ Pray that your infant starts sleeping through the night.

❏ See Insomnia on page 206.

EYESTRAIN HEADACHE

Eyestrain is an often-overlooked cause of headache. If you have blurred vision and light sensitivity, it is more than likely that your headache is eyestrain related.

WHAT TO DO

❏ Supplements helpful for eyesight include beta-carotene, lycopene, vitamin C, lutein, and zeaxanthin.

❏ Foods good for eyesight include dark green leafy vegetables, Asian greens, kale, spinach, sweet corn, egg yolk, mandarins, tangerines, oranges, persimmons, orange capsicum, carrots, rock melon, broccoli, processed tomato products (e.g.,tomato sauce, sun-dried toma-

toes), watermelon, pink grapefruit, papaya, and guava.

❏ Have your eyes checked by an optometrist.

❏ Make sure you take regular "screen breaks" away from your computer, and increase your font size and screen resolution to reduce the strain.

❏ Try the *He-Gu,* or "Joining of the Valleys," pressure-point method (see Stress and Tension Headache above).

❏ Practice eye exercises daily. Focus on your finger when it is a couple of inches away from your face; keep your sights on the finger as you take it to arm's distance. Bring the finger in again, then follow with your eyes as you take the finger left and right as far as your field of vision. Then up and down. Try to do this exercise twice a day.

MIGRAINE

Migraine is a different animal altogether than a headache. In the grip of a migraine, all you want to do is lie in a dark and quiet room. Migraines can throb (sometimes on only one side of head), and may occur with nausea or vomiting. Visual disturbances and ultrasensitivity to light are other common symptoms.

Although more dramatic than the humble headache, once you have identified the various triggers, migraines can be well managed, or at least minimized.

WHAT TO DO

❏ Hormones often play a role in migraine headaches. Vitex agnus-castus and black cohosh are a good place to start.

❏ A migraine may be triggered by certain foods such as aspartame, cheese, oranges, chocolate, and red wine.

For a small percentage of sufferers, feverfew may help to prevent migraines. Take a tablet, or small leaf, every day for a month. Feverfew, taken at this preventative dose, is safe to use for the rest of your life.

Acupuncture can help some migraine sufferers.

Buteyko breathing will help if the blood vessels are constricted. (See Appendix F.)

AT A GLANCE

The remedies you choose should relate to the triggers you consider likely causes of your headache. Following are some general recommendations.

DIET

Eat small meals every two to three hours to keep blood sugar levels steady.

Avoid possible trigger foods, including nitrates found in deli meats, aspartame found in some artificial sweeteners, aged cheese, oranges, chocolate, and red wine.

Drink at least 2 liters of fluid daily to avoid getting dehydrated.

Eat fiber-rich food including legumes, seeds, nuts, and vegetables to avoid constipation.

Reduce salt to decrease risk of high blood pressure.

REMEDIES

Magnesium is excellent for any muscle tension—the cause of many headaches.

Vitex agnus-castus and black cohosh will help any hormonal headache.

Kava, valerian, passionflower, skullcap, vervain, lavender, and St. Johns wort will help if your headache is due to stress.

OTHER

Make a beeline for your body worker. Very often headaches are due to muscular-skeletal imbalance. Chiro, physio, massage—whichever modality and practitioner you prefer.

Rub lavender oil into each temple.

The acupuncture point *He-Gu,* or "Joining of the Valleys," can help reduce the pain of most headaches.

HEMOCHROMATOSIS

WHAT IS IT?

Hemochromatosis is a case of too much of a good thing. While iron-deficiency anemia is the most common nutritional deficiency, people with hemochromatosis have the opposite problem—they absorb too much iron. The excess iron can be deposited in the body, especially the liver, but also joints, testicles, and heart. Eventually, hemochromatosis can lead to liver disease and even liver failure. It may increase your risk of developing heart problems, diabetes, and testicular atrophy. Excess iron can oxidize in the body causing free radical damage. Diagnosis is made via blood tests and also genetic testing to see if you are at risk; this is worthwhile if you know you have a relative with this condition, as symptoms often are not revealed until later in life.

WHAT CAUSES IT?

❏ A relatively common genetic disorder, hemochromatosis affects around 1 in 300 Caucasians of European descent.

❏ Hemochromatosis can also occur from long-term alcoholism and other health conditions.

SYMPTOMS

Symptoms often appear later in life: for men in their forties and fifties and for women ten to fifteen years later after years of menstruation has reduced the total iron load in the body.

☑ Fatigue is a common symptoms of hemochromatosis, the same symptom as anemia.

☑ Bronzing or darkening of the skin (rusting from within!)

☑ Loss of body hair

☑ Low libido

☑ Abdominal pain

☑ Weight loss

WHAT TO DO

Diet

❏ If you love to tuck into a juicy T-bone steak, you might need to redirect your affections to snapper or better still, lentil burgers. Reduce or avoid iron-rich food such as liver, liverwurst and pate, beef, lamb, duck, venison, goat, the darker cuts of turkey and chicken, mollusks—oysters, clams, mussels—and yes, blood sausage (black pudding) is out. While non-heme iron is less well absorbed (see Anemia on page 10) continue to eat, but don't go crazy on the following iron-rich foods:

- Dried fruit—prunes, raisins, dates.
- Dark leafy green vegetables—kale, bok choy, gai lan, spinach.
- Legumes—lentils, kidney beans, soy beans.
- Seaweed.
- Parsley.
- Blackstrap molasses.

❏ Drink tea (black or green) with meals as this will further reduce iron absorption.

❏ Citrus fruit and berries are excellent sources of vitamin C, which helps iron absorption. Enjoy these delicious fruits, but eat them one hour before or two hours after meals to reduce absorption of iron. Same goes for orange juice.

Note: If you are undergoing regular venesection (blood taking—see below in "Other") to reduce your iron levels, you may not need to adhere to the above suggestions. Your doctor will be keeping an eye on your iron levels via blood tests.

❏ Reduce or avoid alcohol to lessen the load on the liver.

❏ Avoid raw seafood as it may contain bacteria, including *Vibrio vulnificus* and *Salmonella enteriditis* that thrive in an iron-rich environment.

❏ Turmeric is an excellent liver tonic and is anti-inflammatory, the perfect combination for this condition.

Remedies

❏ Take a zinc supplement as zinc competes with iron for absorption. Make sure you take the supplement at meal times.

❏ Take an antioxidant supplement that does not contain vitamin C. The excess iron in the body has a tendency to oxidize and cause free radi-

cal damage. As curcumin (the therapeutic substance in turmeric) is antioxidant, perhaps choose an antioxidant that also contains this.

❏ Avoid any supplement with vitamin C as this increases iron absorption

❏ Avoid any supplement containing iron.

Other

❏ Often venesection, also known as phlebotomy, taking blood in 500 ml units, is the best way to treat hemochromatosis. If you are also able to donate your blood, this doubles the good. Generally venesection occurs relatively frequently until your blood levels are acceptable, then less frequently. Make sure you hydrate with water before and after treatment. Also take some arnica if you are prone to bruising.

❏ Don't use cast-iron cookware.

AT A GLANCE

Diet

➥ Reduce iron-rich foods including liver, liverwurst and patê, beef, lamb, duck, venison, goat, the darker cuts of turkey and chicken, mollusks—oysters, clams, mussels. From the plant kingdom, reduce your intake of prunes, raisins, dates, and dark leafy green vegetables such as kale, bok choy, gai lan, spinach. Also leave out legumes/pulses such as lentils, kidney beans, soya beans. Other things to eat less of include seaweed, parsley, and blackstrap molasses.

➥ Drink tea (black or green) with meals as this will further reduce iron absorption.

➥ **NOTE:** If you are undergoing regular venesection (blood taking) to reduce your iron levels,

you may not need to adhere to the above suggestions. Your doctor will be keeping an eye on your iron levels via blood tests.

Remedies

➥ As zinc competes with iron for absorption, take a zinc supplement with meals containing iron-rich foods.

➥ Avoid supplements containing iron and vitamin C.

Other

➥ Avoid using cast-iron cookware.

➥ If you are having venesection, make sure you drink at least 500 ml extra fluid that day.

HEMORRHOIDS

WHAT IS IT?

If you have a distended and painful varicose vein on your leg, you can expect sympathy and offers of support from your friends. If the exact same problem is in your bottom, everyone thinks it's funny. Except you. Hemorrhoids, also known as piles, are veins and other tissue inside the anus that have become distended and weakened.

SYMPTOMS

☑ Bright red blood on the toilet tissue, stool, or within the toilet bowl

☑ Itching of the anus

☑ Pain in and around the anus

☑ Aching and throbbing in and around the anus

☑ Pain during bowel movements

☑ Tender lumps around the anus

☑ Soiling or "skid marks" on underpants

WHAT CAUSES IT?

❏ Long-term constipation is the cause of many a hemorrhoid. Years of straining to pass hard stools will distend the tissue in question. Hemorrhoids are virtually unknown and constipation is nonexistent in countries where people eat a low-meat, high-fiber diet.

❏ Being overweight or pregnant can cause piles as the flow of blood from veins from the lower body is restricted.

❏ Babies can cause rectal strife if their birth takes hours of straining.

❏ Lifting loads that are too heavy or using an incorrect lifting technique can cause hemorrhoids. "Roids" of both kinds are not unknown to body builders.

❏ Whether they are present in the anus as hemorrhoids, or on the legs as varicose veins, a tendency toward weak veins is hereditary.

❏ Long periods of time standing or sitting (especially on hard chairs) will increase the risk of hemorrhoids. If you must sit for work, ensure your chair is well padded. For both sitting and standing, take short breaks regularly.

❏ When you were young, did your grandmother warn you not to sit on cold concrete? And did you anyway? Oh, the reckless things we do as children.

❏ Sitting on the toilet reading the newspaper is also not recommended.

WHAT TO DO

Diet

❏ Keeping the stool soft and easy to pass is the best way to prevent hemorrhoids. Increase whole grains, nuts, seeds, vegetables, fruits, dried fruits, and legumes.

❏ Also increase the foods containing the group of bioflavonoids that help strengthen the blood vessels, such as red grapes (especially the skin and pips), green tea, and all berries.

❏ Reduce red meat, sugar, and refined-flour products.

❏ Buckwheat contains the bioflavonoid rutin, which strengthens veins.

❏ Drink plenty of fluids, at least 2 liters a day.

❏ Eat a few prunes or prune juice daily.

Remedies

❏ Herbs that can strengthen the connective tissue of veins include horse chestnut, gotu kola (a great repairer of tissue), grapeseed, ginkgo biloba, and butcher's broom. Take these in tincture or tablet form. Particularly if you also have varicose veins, these herbs will serve you well in the future.

❏ The following nutrients can all improve the health and strength of the walls of veins: quercetin, vitamin C, rutin, resveratrol, pine bark, and grapeseed extract. Find a supplement that contains a group of these.

❏ Try the topical application of herbs such as witch hazel, calendula, gotu kola, and horse chestnut. Either make a strong tea, dilute into a tincture, or find them in a cream. Apply after each shower and bowel movement.

❏ The gentle fiber slippery elm comes into its own in the treatment of piles. It helps to heal the inflamed tissue around the anus. Take three tablets or one teaspoonful of the powder twice a day. If you are pile prone, slippery elm should also become part of your life.

❏ Fiber supplements including psyllium husks, chia seeds, and linseeds will help to bulk and soften the stool. Take a heaped tablespoon each day in water, in your breakfast cereal or in a smoothie. Take with a large glass of water.

❏ Cooling aloe vera gel can give soothing and healing relief. If you grow an aloe plant, peel off the outer skin and cut the pulp into small oblong suppositories. Wrap them in plastic wrap and pop them in the freezer. Unwrap and insert before bed each night for a week. Tea tree suppositories are available at healthfood stores and work in a similar way.

❏ An old-fashioned but still very effective treatment is an application of castor oil and honey around and just inside the anus. Heat a teaspoon of each, mix well, and apply while still warm. Apply at night, wearing a protective pad to bed to prevent marking the bed sheets.

❏ One of the tissue salts, calcium fluoride (calc. fluor.), can also strengthen vein walls and is a good long-term remedy.

❏ A vitamin C supplement with bioflavonoids will also help build up the strength of the veins.

Other

❏ Replace that cheap, rough toilet paper for soft toilet tissue, and even better, moisten slightly with water. Pre-moistened toilet paper is also available.

❏ If your job requires long periods of sitting or standing, at the end of each day lie with your legs up the wall, bottom raised on a cushion. This will make the blood return to the upper body.

❏ Exercise is important to keep the blood moving; however, avoid pushing heavy weights at the gym.

❏ Straining on the toilet doesn't help the situation. The Western style of toilet is not designed the way nature intended us to defecate—squatting has been the favored position for millennia. It activates the abdominal muscles and causes the rectum and anus to widen out, making a more efficient funnel shape. Try putting a few old phonebooks or blocks on either side of the toilet so that your knees are slightly raised. Or look for the commercially marketed plastic shapes, which fit around the toilet.

❏ Kegel exercises can help bring awareness to and strengthen the muscles in the pelvic area. Practice these very simple movements daily to treat existing hemorrhoids and prevent the formation of future ones.

If you see blood on your toilet paper, stool, or in the toilet bowl, chances are high that it is from a hemorrhoid. However, there is a possibility that the blood can be due to another cause. Take your nether regions to the doctor, who has seen it all before, to confirm whether it is a simple hemorrhoid or if further investigation is required.

AT A GLANCE

DIET

→ Keeping the stool soft and easy to pass is the very best way to prevent hemorrhoids.

→ Increase whole grains, nuts, seeds, vegetables, fruits, dried fruits, and legumes, and reduce red meat, sugar, and refined flour products.

→ Red grapes (especially the skin and pips), green tea, and all berries contain nutrients that strengthen vein walls.

→ Drink plenty of fluids, at least 2 liters a day.

REMEDIES

→ Herbs that help strengthen the walls of the veins also help treat and prevent hemorrhoids. These include horse chestnut, gotu kola, grape seed, ginkgo biloba, and butcher's broom.

→ Applying healing and calming herbs as a cream or suppository to the site such as aloe vera, gotu kola, calendula, and/or tea tree will all help to soothe and heal.

→ Slippery elm is excellent for relieving the pain of hemorrhoids.

→ If you are prone to constipation, take a single daily supplement or a combination of psyllium husks, chia seeds, and linseeds.

OTHER

→ Use soft toilet tissue to avoid irritating the area.

→ Exercise regularly to improve circulation.

→ If you need to lift heavy objects, learn how to lift properly, as straining is not only an excellent way to hurt your back, but can also create a fine set of hemorrhoids.

→ If you see blood on toilet paper, in a stool, or in the toilet bowl, take your nether regions to the doctor.

HIGH BLOOD PRESSURE

WHAT IS IT?

High blood pressure or hypertension is a symptom rather than a disease, but it is a symptom that must be treated, as having high blood pressure increases your risk of heart disease fourfold. High blood pressure increases your chance of dying from a stroke, heart attack, kidney disease, or heart failure, which is enough reason to think about and actively pursue treatment. Blood pressure is the measurement of force of the blood against the artery walls as the heart pumps the blood around the body. It is gauged by two numbers, systolic and diastolic, measured in millimeters of mercury, mmHg (e.g., 120/80). The systolic (siss-toll-ic) or the "top" reading measures the force of blood on arteries when the heart beats, while the diastolic (dye-as-toll-ic) or "bottom" reading records force of blood on arteries between beats, the resting pressure. Both top and bottom readings are important, but when the diastolic reading is very high, it is particularly worrisome as it shows the pressure of blood in the arteries is high even when the heart is at rest.

Blood pressure varies from moment to moment. In general, it is higher during the day than at night, winter than summer, and as you get older.

Normal blood pressure is less than 120 systolic and less than 80 diastolic.

Prehypertension is 120–129 systolic and 80–89 diastolic (time to start looking at lifestyle and diet).

Hypertension is more than 130 systolic and more than 90 diastolic (treatment is necessary).

The opposite to high blood pressure is low blood pressure (hypotension). Symptoms can include fainting, light-headedness, and confusion. Hypotension may be caused by dehydration, certain medications, or be a symptom of severe allergy. If there are no symptoms, hypotension is often not treated, and seen as much preferable to having hypertension, which poses a greater risk to your health.

SYMPTOMS

High blood pressure is often asymptomatic—in other words, has no obvious symptoms you are aware of, and as high blood pressure has such serious potential repercussions—that is, dying—it is best to at least know you have it. Have it checked when you are visiting your health professional or buy a relatively inexpensive digital sphygmometer (blood pressure machine) for home use. This is a good investment if you already know you have high blood pressure, so you can keep a close eye on your treatment progress. Some symptoms of high blood pressure include:

- ☑ Headache
- ☑ Feeling of fullness in the head
- ☑ Face going red
- ☑ Buzzing or noise in the ears
- ☑ Nosebleeds
- ☑ Fatigue
- ☑ Confusion

WHAT CAUSES IT?

- ❑ Atherosclerosis increases blood pressure. As the artery wall thickens and hardens, this has a mechanical effect on increasing the pressure of blood flowing through.
- ❑ Kidney disease.
- ❑ Thyroid disease, particularly high thyroid.

- Certain medications have high blood pressure as a side effect.

- Most often there is no obvious cause for blood pressure to be high; this is called essential hypertension.

Although not causative, the following factors increase your risk of having high blood pressure:

- Being overweight or obese.

- A family history of hypertension.

- Smoking tobacco.

- Having diabetes.

- Stress or anxiety. Adrenaline, the stress hormone, increases blood pressure.

- Getting older—men over fifty-five years of age, and women over sixty-five years of age have a higher risk.

- Being physically inactive.

- High blood fats (cholesterol, triglycerides), which will show up on blood tests.

- High salt diet. Some people are salt sensitive, meaning it can increase their blood pressure.

- Dehydration. The heart will work harder if there is not enough blood in the body.

WHAT TO DO

Diet

- Salt. Compared to the hunter-gatherer diet, on which our physiology evolved, the modern diet has ten times the amount of sodium. Sodium is part of the molecule sodium chloride, better known as salt. Salt is added to processed and packaged food to enhance taste and as a preservative: deli meats, packaged soups, premade sauces, takeout, snacks, and breakfast cereal. Once in the body, sodium has an osmotic effect, drawing water into the body, increasing

blood pressure. Many studies have shown that decreasing salt in the diet decreases blood pressure, in particular the well-known DASH (Dietary Approaches to Stop Hypertension) research of the late 1990s. The older you get, the more salt sensitive you become. The best way to lower salt in your diet is not by choosing "low salt" processed foods, but by ditching processed foods altogether. If you make your own food (and it's not as time consuming as you think; a salad or stir-fry takes minutes to prepare) you are in charge of exactly how much salt is added or not. If you have high blood pressure, your goal is to consume less than 6 grams of salt daily (the average is 9.5 grams). Food labels declare sodium levels rather than total salt. Read as mg of sodium per 100 grams of food. A low-salt food is one that has less than 120 mg sodium per 100 grams food; 5 grams of salt contains 2000 mg of sodium. Your daily sodium levels should be less than 2,400 mg.

- Potassium. A lot of attention has been placed on decreasing sodium levels. But increasing potassium in your diet will also likely decrease your blood pressure. It's a ratio thing. Ideally we should be eating twice the amount of potassium as we do sodium. We eat four times less potassium than our hunter-gatherer forebears. Potassium-rich foods include all fruits and vegetables, but in particular bananas, citrus fruit, apricots, avocado, parsley, and potatoes, as well as almonds, cashews, pecans, sunflower seeds, sesame seeds, sardines, parsley, kelp, and kidney beans.

- Garlic helps to lower blood pressure. Eat it raw or cooked.

- Calcium also has a blood pressure–lowering effect. Eat calcium-rich foods. (See Appendix D, Food Sources.)

- Caffeine. If you don't usually drink caffeinated beverages, a double-shot macchiato is likely to shoot your blood pressure through the roof. However, if you regularly enjoy coffee, your body generally will have developed a tolerance for caffeine. This tolerance reaches its limit at around five cups of coffee per day. Also, some people can be very sensitive to caffeine; if you have high blood pressure, stay away from caffeine and see if this makes a difference to your blood pressure.

- The omega-3 fatty acid EPA, found in fish, has shown in a small way to decrease blood pressure. Eat three servings of fish weekly, particularly the oilier fish, including mackerel, salmon, and sardines.

- The DASH research mentioned previously found that people who increased their whole grains, fruit, vegetables, and fish intake while decreasing sugar, red meat, and fatty foods had a decrease in blood pressure. Then again these dietary recommendations will go a long way to helping most health problems.

- Drink at least 2 liters of fluid daily to avoid dehydration.

Remedies

- Magnesium, potassium, and calcium will all do their part to help decrease blood pressure. It might serve you well to take an extra supplement of magnesium as it helps to relax muscle and is a stress reliever. Artery walls are made of muscle, and the magnesium will help to widen the diameter of the blood vessel, thereby reducing blood pressure. If you find your blood pressure is not better after two to three months, then don't continue and try something else.

- Garlic is so good for all cardiovascular problems including high cholesterol and atherosclerosis. It also helps to reduce blood pressure. Eat as much as you can, as well as taking it in supplement form. Make sure it has high allicin levels, as this is the effective constituent. Enteric-coated garlic tablets are available if you don't want to have garlic breath.

- Herbs can be very useful in lowering blood pressure. These include *Coleus forskohlii,* valerian (as it helps to reduce stress hormones and relaxes muscle), olive leaf (long before olive leaf became popular for coughs and colds, it was used for hypertension), and hawthorn. Hawthorn is a traditional heart tonic as well. Dandelion leaves are useful as a diuretic, which has a blood-pressure-lowering effect.

- If stress is part of your high blood pressure, then herbs to help stress and anxiety will help enormously. These include valerian, St. John's wort, kava, valerian, oats, passionflower, vervain, kava, lemon balm, zizyphus, magnolia, and chamomile.

- Fish oil, 3 to 6 grams daily, has some effect on lowering blood pressure. Absolutely recommended if you also have high cholesterol levels. And make that a trifecta if you suffer from arthritis too.

Other

- Buteyko breathing slightly increases carbon dioxide levels in the body (see Appendix F, Buteyko Breathing). This, in turn, helps to dampen the sympathetic nervous response (the one fuelled by adrenaline), which will in turn relax the muscle surrounding blood vessels and reduce blood pressure. Professor Buteyko was actually studying blood pressure when he developed his breathing technique.

- Manage your stress.

- Regular exercise, particularly aerobic exercise, such as jogging and cycling, has been shown to lower blood pressure. Exercise for twenty to sixty minutes three times a week.

❏ Meditation. Many studies have shown that meditation decreases blood pressure. Find a class or an app and practice.

❏ Lose weight. Losing ten pounds can decrease systolic measurement by 4.5mmHG and diastolic by 3.2mmHG.

AROMATHERAPY

For high blood pressure combine:

❏ 4 drops of bergamot—excellent for stress-related conditions.

❏ 4 drops of neroli—calming and tonifying.

❏ 2 drops of ylang ylang—hypotensive; soothes palpitations.

This will be soothing and calming on both the nervous and circulatory systems.

❏ For low blood pressure combine:

4 drops of pine—hypertensive, circulatory stimulant.

4 drops of rosemary—reduces palpitations, circulatory stimulant, hypertensive.

2 drops of ginger—circulatory stimulant.

This is a blend that will be both warming and stimulating to the circulatory system.

Either of these blends can be used in a full body massage if added to 20 ml sweet almond oil, in bathwater if combined with Epsom salts; in a vaporizer (you will need to halve the number of drops used), or a personal perfume mix into 20 ml of jojoba oil.

AT A GLANCE

DIET

⇒ Lose the salt. Don't shake it on your meals, and reduce consumption of processed and packaged foods that often contain obscene amounts of salt. Aim to eat less than 6 grams of salt a day or 2,400 mg of sodium.

⇒ Increase potassium-rich foods. Increasing the ratio of potassium to sodium in the body will help lower blood pressure. Potassium-rich foods include all fruits and vegetables, especially bananas, citrus fruit, apricots, avocado, parsley, and potatoes, as well as almonds, cashews, pecans, sunflower seeds, sesame seeds, sardines, parsley, kelp, and kidney beans.

⇒ Caffeine may increase blood pressure in those people sensitive to it. Avoid caffeine for a cou-

ple of weeks and see if you feel better or your blood pressure decreases. If so, on either count, desist. Decaffeinated is fine.

⇒ General recommendations that help to decrease blood pressure include reducing sugar and red meat and increasing whole grains, fresh fruit and vegetables, and fish in your diet.

⇒ Avoid dehydration. Drink at least 2 liters of fluid daily.

REMEDIES

⇒ Take a magnesium supplement morning and night. Magnesium, the great muscle relaxer, will help to relax the muscle that lines blood vessels. Magnesium also helps with stress.

⇒ Potassium and calcium supplementation may also be helpful.

- If you have other risk factors for heart disease including high cholesterol and/or atherosclerosis, then taking fish oil and garlic supplements makes good sense, as these work to help lower blood pressure as well.

- Herbal remedies can be taken to help reduce blood pressure, including coleus, hawthorn, olive leaf, and valerian.

- Adrenaline increases blood pressure. If you are stressed, very likely this has a negative impact on your blood pressure. Choose from one or more of the following antistress herbs: St. John's wort, kava, valerian, oats, passionflower, vervain, kava, lemon balm, zizyphus, magnolia, and chamomile.

OTHER

- Buteyko breathing reduces the stress response, thereby helping to reduce blood pressure. Practice some of the techniques or take a course.

- Take up yoga, tai chi, or macramé. Whatever does it for you to reduce your stress levels.

- Every few pounds you lose will help reduce your blood pressure. Why not start or increase your aerobic exercise?

- It doesn't matter what style of meditation you prefer. It helps to lower blood pressure. Dust off that meditation cushion and find a class in the real world or online.

INFERTILITY

WHAT IS IT?

Some people live out their lives without feeling the urge to procreate. Others are consumed by an incredible longing, and cannot imagine life without the experience of rearing children. Infertility is defined as the inability to conceive a baby after a year of unprotected sex or the inability to maintain a pregnancy to term. A few decades ago, becoming pregnant used to be as easy as falling off a log, and often as unplanned. In industrialized countries today, however, infertility is on the increase, affecting around 15 to 20 percent of all couples.

SYMPTOMS

☑ Inability to become pregnant or carry a baby to term.

☑ A range of emotions. For couples wanting to conceive, the diagnosis of infertility can be an emotional bombshell. Feelings range from denial, anger, depression, and guilt to feelings of inadequacy.

WHAT CAUSES IT?

❏ Certain health conditions can affect fertility, including cystic fibrosis, celiac disease, mumps, diabetes, and chronic bronchitis.

❏ Chemotherapy, cortisone, and some heart medications may also have a detrimental effect.

❏ Smoking, excessive alcohol, and the use of marijuana and cocaine have all been shown to damage sperm.

❏ Stress and infertility are linked, particularly for women.

Men

❑ Up to 40 percent of infertility is due to the male partner.

❑ Low sperm count and motility (the ability of sperm to move under their own steam) is a major cause of infertility. The *British Medical Journal* reports that the average sperm count has dropped over the last 50 years from 113 million per ml in 1940 to 66 million per ml in 1990.

❑ The cause for this type of interference with sperm health is unclear. Some studies blame mobile phone use, others suggest an increase in hormonal disruptors found in the environment, particularly the amount of degrading plastic in oceans and landfills.

❑ Low sperm count, motility, and agglutination (where sperm stick together) have been linked to exposure to chemicals, including pesticides, lead, cadmium, arsenic, and solvents.

❑ A varicocele is a relatively common cause of male infertility. A varicocele is basically a varicose vein in the scrotum that causes poor blood flow, and apparently feels like a small sac of worms. Varicoceles are treatable by surgery.

❑ Infection of the prostate gland or the testicles is another cause of male infertility.

❑ Obesity is associated with male infertility as testosterone production is decreased and scrotum temperature is increased.

❑ Occupations with the largest infertility rates include welders, painters, taxi drivers, truck drivers, and bakers.

Women

❑ Women who are extremely overweight often have problems conceiving due to hormonal imbalances.

❑ Additionally, underweight women, particularly those suffering anorexia nervosa, are often low in estrogen and may not be ovulating at all.

❑ Gynecological problems may be to blame, including endometriosis, fibroids, and polycystic ovarian syndrome.

❑ For sperm to survive and conception to occur, the vaginal mucus needs to be a certain pH (a little bit acidic).

❑ Sometimes an "antisperm" antibody is produced, rendering the sperm useless.

❑ Women over the age of forty find it more difficult to conceive as fewer eggs remain. Human physiology favors younger mothers.

WHAT TO DO

It takes around 75 days for sperm to mature and roughly 100 days for ovum to be ready to be fertilized. To give it your best shot (pardon the pun), both partners should be on their very best healthy behavior for at least three months prior to conception. The remedies (herbal as well as vitamin and mineral supplements) recommended below are fine to take even if you are pregnant and don't know it yet. However, there are several herbs and supplements that are not recommended during pregnancy. If in doubt, the wisest course of action is to check with your practitioner before taking any remedies.

Diet

Women

❑ Caffeine is out. This includes your cup of coffee, as well as cola and that irresistible chocolate bar. There have been several studies, including one reported in the medical journal *The Lancet,* which found that as little as a cup of coffee a day reduces a woman's chance of conceiving; two to three cups a day reduces your chances by 25 percent. So it is worthwhile cutting it out completely.

Men and Women

❑ Reduce alcohol. For men, alcohol is often implicated in erectile dysfunction. If this is a problem for you, desist (from drinking). Note, however, that many babies are conceived after a celebratory glass of bubbles, or a relaxing holiday meal that involves some pinot noir. Moderation is key.

❑ Protein is important. Make sure both partners eat adequate amounts of protein foods, including eggs, fish, chicken, red meat, nuts, seeds, and legumes.

❑ Eat a diet rich in antioxidants (see below).

❑ Omega-3 fatty acids are important for fertility for both men and women. Oily fish is of course recommended, but as there is a risk of ingesting methyl mercury with some of the larger fish, such as marlin, swordfish, and bluefin tuna, stick to sardines and salmon. Other sources of omega-3 fatty acids are walnuts, linseeds, and chia seeds.

Oxygen—Friend and Foe

We have come to know oxygen as a handy little molecule that helps us stay alive, but when oxygen is altered chemically, it may oxidize certain substances to form free radicals. Free radicals are thought to be at least partially responsible for heart disease and cancer. Factors that add to this unfortunate state of affairs include radiation (from the sun, mobile phones, x-rays, etc.), carcinogens (like cigarette smoke, benzene, diesel exhaust), pesticides, and the general process of aging. Oxidative damage is a fact of life.

Free radicals wreak havoc in the body, including—and this is the scary part—the DNA found in the central nucleus of cells. DNA is the blueprint or recipe for the creation of new cells. If the recipe is changed, new cells are created with a difference or mutation. Most often, the immune system gobbles up these mutated cells but sometimes they survive and divide in a manner not originally intended (e.g., forming a tumor). The number of potentially damaging hits to DNA per cell per day is about 100,000, and there are over 100 trillion cells per human. Considering this kind of bombardment, it's a wonder we have time to make a cup of tea (although tea does contain lots of antioxidants), let alone repair and protect all these cells from free-radical damage.

In response to free-radical damage, our body manufactures antioxidants, including superoxide dismutase and catalase. In addition, your diet provides you with antioxidants. That is if your diet is a good one. In the last few years, there has been a flurry of scientific research into antioxidants. Not a week goes by without another antioxidant being identified, often from the plant world. Which only goes to prove; never underestimate a vegetable.

You may already be familiar with antioxidants such as vitamins A, C, and E as well as zinc and selenium. In fact, a run-of-the-mill multivitamin and mineral supplement is a good source of antioxidants. However, don't rely solely on supplements for your antioxidant intake. For a start,

ANTIOXIDANTS

Since the mid-1990s, antioxidants have been a buzzword in the fields of both nutrition and medicine. Antioxidants are of interest to nutritionists and naturopaths (because most antioxidants are found in food), and for medicine (because antioxidants help prevent certain diseases such as heart disease, cancer, and possibly osteoarthritis and autoimmune conditions). The discovery of antioxidants and what they do in the body has transformed the old-fashioned message of eating fresh fruits, vegetables, and whole grains into scientific good sense.

new antioxidants are being found all the time in simple everyday foods. For example, catechins (good for preventing heart disease and cancer) are found in tea (green and black) and red wine. Lycopene (which helps prevent prostate cancer) is found in cooked tomatoes. Coincidentally, many of the substances that make plants brightly colored are antioxidants. Other plant antioxidants that are good for the liver include silymarin (in milk thistle) and curcumin, which is found in the yellow Indian spice turmeric. Finally, the detoxifying and antioxidant substance indole-3-carbinol is found in abundance in broccoli, Brussels sprouts, and cabbage.

We can't stop all free-radical damage, but we can help the body help itself. As a safeguard against the damage of free radicals, it is really important to eat plenty of fresh fruit and vegetables, particularly the strongly colored varieties. If you wish to go further, take antioxidant supplements, perhaps one that contains a combination of vitamin, mineral, and plant antioxidants.

The following foods rate very highly on the oxygen radical absorbance capacity (ORAC) scale, a technique developed by the National Institutes of Health in Bethesda, Maryland. There are some limitations to the ORAC rating; for example, it doesn't say exactly *which* antioxidants are in the food, only that there *are* antioxidants. Additionally, it is not a reflection of how well these antioxidants are absorbed by the body. Nutrition is a new science, and no doubt in the future a more exhaustive format will be developed. In the meantime, know that the following foods are high in antioxidants and extremely good for you.

- Berries (strawberries, blueberries, raspberries, cranberries)
- Plums, prunes
- Cherries
- Red grapes
- Apples
- Artichokes
- Nuts (walnuts, pecans, almonds, hazelnuts)
- Legumes (pinto beans, lentils, kidney beans, soy)
- Spices (turmeric, pepper, sumac, cumin, cinnamon, cloves)
- Cocoa
- Garlic
- Herbs (parsley, oregano, basil, thyme)

Remedies

- Good fertility herbs for men include damiana, Korean ginseng, saw palmetto, tribulus, withania, and ginkgo biloba. These herbs will assist in sperm production and motility.

- Good fertility herbs for women include dong quai, shatavari, peony, rehmannia, withania, chaste tree, and false unicorn root.

- Raspberry leaf, often recommended in the later stages of pregnancy, has also traditionally been prescribed for women early in pregnancy to help prevent miscarriage.

- Vitamin C and the bioflavonoids are important for both sexes. They are necessary for the maintenance and strength of healthy blood vessels, including the tiny capillaries within the endometrium that line the uterus, which is important in the prevention of miscarriage. In addition, vitamin C can reduce sperm agglutination. Take 1 gram of vitamin C daily, with added bioflavonoids.

- Stress can be a cause of infertility. One of the physical manifestations of stress can include muscle tightness and spasm. Consider that the tiny fallopian tubes (which carry the fertilized egg to the uterus) are lined with muscle tissue.

Now picture two stressed fallopian tubes: they will be tightened and narrowed. Magnesium is an excellent muscle relaxer.

❏ Zinc is a most necessary mineral in the field of fertility. It is of primary importance to the hormonal well-being of both men and women. Low sperm count has been linked to a zinc deficiency. Men need to take a zinc supplement in addition to their multivitamin.

❏ Vitamin E has a reputation as a fertility vitamin. It helps with hormonal imbalances and with circulation.

❏ The amino acids taurine and arginine are both important in the formation and viability of sperm. If you suffer from herpes, take a lysine supplement as well, just in case the extra arginine triggers an attack.

Other

❏ Tight-fitting trousers and underpants are out for men. They will cut the circulation to and increase the temperature of the scrotum, reducing the sperm's chance of being viable. In addition, forgo long hot showers and electric blankets.

❏ Massage or bathe with a few drops of rose oil. Although true essential oil of rose costs a bomb, it has a fine reputation both as an aphrodisiac and for improving fertility.

❏ There is a relatively small window of opportunity for the sperm to fertilize an egg, and intercourse is recommended at this time. Generally this is around days thirteen to fifteen of a woman's menstrual cycle—the time of ovulation—although it has been known for fertilization to occur any time up to a day or so before the period is due. Many women can tell that they are ovulating because their vaginal discharge becomes a little thicker, clear, and slightly sticky—in fact, like egg white. There are also body temperature changes at this time. If you have trouble determining when you ovulate, seek the advice of a naturopath who specializes in the area of natural fertility.

❏ Stop smoking. Smoking increases free-radical damage within the body. Most women stop smoking anyway when they are trying to conceive, as the risks to the unborn child are many including low birth weight, a risk factor for poor health. However, men should also consider taking this step, as smoking reduces circulation, and improved circulation in the reproductive area is what we are aiming for.

❏ There is some evidence to even suggest certain positions during intercourse can increase the likelihood of conception. One suggestion is to place a pillow under the woman's hips. Another factor that can increase the chances of conception is female orgasm, as contractions that develop as a result of orgasm can help transport sperm further into the cervix.

❏ We do live in polluted times, but try, where you can, to reduce plastics and chemicals in your environment (e.g., pesticides, solvents, and chemical-based cleaning products).

❏ If your relationship is bearing the brunt of your desire to have a baby, see a counselor, or at least talk it out with friends and family. The less stressed you are as a couple, the more likely conception is.

❏ Bach flowers are helpful for the full gamut of emotions you may be feeling. Gorse is good for despondency,

❏ Trust that your baby knows the right time to make his or her entrance on this planet.

DIET

→ Women should consider giving up coffee and other caffeinated drinks. Studies show that caffeine can reduce the chance of conceiving.

→ It is recommended that men and women drink no more than one or two standard alcoholic drinks a day.

→ For both partners, eat sufficient protein (eggs, fish, chicken, red meat, nuts, seeds, and legumes), a diet rich in antioxidants (berries, legumes, vegetables, herbs, and spices) and omega-3 fatty acids (fish—except for marlin, swordfish, and bluefin tuna—walnuts, linseeds, and chia seeds).

REMEDIES

→ Good fertility herbs for men include damiana, Korean ginseng, saw palmetto, tribulus, withania, and ginkgo biloba.

→ Good fertility herbs for women include dong quai, shatavari, peony, rehmannia, withania, chaste tree, and false unicorn root.

→ Vitamin E and zinc are both important for the reproductive health of both men and women.

OTHER

→ Trying to conceive can be stressful on relationships. Seeing a counselor may help.

→ If possible, reduce the amount of chemicals you use at work or home.

INFLAMMATORY BOWEL DISEASE (IBD)

WHAT IS IT?

Inflammatory bowel disease (IBD) doesn't just mess with your bowel; it plays with your head. Symptoms appear randomly and viciously, not only causing pain and discomfort, but also affecting your mood and wiping out your energy for days at a time.

The two main forms of IBD are ulcerative colitis and Crohn's disease. They are discussed here together as many of their symptoms are similar, as is the naturopathic treatment.

Ulcerative colitis is a disease primarily of the colon (large intestine), and rarely affects the small intestine. Crohn's disease, however, is not fussy, affecting all the way along the bowel from the small intestine on into the colon, albeit in an erratic manner, skipping bits here and there.

Inflammatory bowel disease is marked by periods of remission and exacerbation. It is important you become well acquainted with your inner beast. Does he (she?) react badly to stress, alcohol, or pasta? Watch and learn how to tame your beast, and even when times are good, play nice, and don't tempt fate.

SYMPTOMS

☑ Urgent need to have a bowel movement

☑ Diarrhea

☑ Bleeding on the stool, toilet paper, or in the bowl

☑ Fever

☑ Abdominal pain

- ✓ Malaise
- ✓ Fatigue
- ✓ Depressed mood
- ✓ Mucus (more common with ulcerative colitis) on the stool or toilet paper
- ✓ Mouth ulcers (only with Crohn's disease)
- ✓ Anal fistulas (only with Crohn's disease; an anal fistula is a small tunnel that forms between the anal canal and the skin, usually close to the anus, which is caused by an abscess that forms within the bowel wall).

WHAT CAUSES IT?

- ❑ Genetics plays a role, so search your family tree. The incidence of IBD is slightly higher within the Jewish population.

- ❑ Dysbiosis, otherwise known as bad bugs in your gut.

- ❑ Viral trigger. Although not necessarily a cause, there is some evidence that a virus may trigger the onset of IBD. There may be a long hiatus between having the virus (e.g., measles) and suffering the disease, so there may not seem to be an obvious connection.

- ❑ Again, while not a cause, stress can initiate the onset and is almost always behind exacerbations of this disease.

- ❑ There is debate whether or not IBD is an autoimmune condition. If so, this explains why they are triggered by events such as viruses and stress. This is something that is often noted by people with other autoimmune conditions such as multiple sclerosis and rheumatoid arthritis.

- ❑ Curiously, smokers and those who have had their appendix removed are less likely to suffer from ulcerative colitis.

WHAT TO DO

Diet

For When There Are Symptoms of Intense Pain, Bleeding, and Mucus

- ❑ When symptoms are in full flight, the best thing to do is fast for a day or so, drinking only water or juice. This allows the bowel to rest and recover.

- ❑ Although high-fiber foods are recommended to keep the bowel healthy, in times of pain and bleeding, you need food that is not going to rub or chafe the inflamed bowel wall: white rice, peeled and mashed potatoes, sweet potatoes, and pumpkin; stewed and peeled pear and apple (stew with a little honey, not sugar), and banana; good quality unsweetened yogurt (unless you are lactose intolerant); soups made from beef stock, chicken stock, or miso are excellent, pureed if necessary; steamed chicken breast, white fish, eggs, and tofu are good sources of protein.

- ❑ Avoid red meat (the stock is fine), dairy foods (except unsweetened yogurt), salads, raw vegetables, corn, uncooked fruit, nuts, seeds, whole-grain products, chili, spicy food, coffee, and alcohol.

- ❑ Avoid sugar. Not just sugar added to tea and coffee, but sugar in packaged foods, like breakfast cereal, fruit yogurt, and of course, biscuits, pastries, and cakes (see below).

- ❑ Avoid gluten. Even if you are not gluten intolerant it can increase inflammation. Avoid wheat, rye, oats, and barley.

- ❑ Drink herbal tea using a combination of ginger, peppermint, chamomile, meadowsweet, and/or lemon balm.

For When There Are No, Few, or Mild Symptoms

❏ Avoid sugar like the plague. Sugar feeds the bad bugs of the bowel. As your bowel microflora (microbiome) is already in disarray due to this disease, the last thing you should do is encourage more malevolent microflora. This includes sugar in packaged foods as well as adding sugar to coffee, tea, and so forth.

❏ Fiber is very important for the health of the bowel. Fiber allows for regular bowel movements and also provides fuel for the good bugs, which in turn improves the health and integrity of the bowel wall itself. Vegetables, fruits, nuts, seeds, and legumes are all to be eaten and enjoyed on a regular basis.

❏ Avoid or reduce gluten in your diet. Many people with IBD have gluten intolerance.

❏ Eat prebiotic and probiotic foods. Prebiotics include asparagus, Jerusalem artichokes, leeks and onions, legumes, such as baked beans, chickpeas, and lentils. Probiotics include yogurt, miso, sauerkraut, kefir, natto, tempeh, and the Korean delicacy kimchi (see below).

❏ Increase foods rich in omega-3 for their anti-inflammatory properties: fish, linseeds, chia seeds, and walnuts.

PREBIOTICS AND PROBIOTICS

Naturopaths have long proselytized that illness begins in the gut and good health starts with a healthy digestive tract. Hippocrates didn't hold back when he claimed that "death sits in the bowel." There are ten times more bacteria within the digestive system than there are cells in the body. Known as microflora, this internal ecosystem weighs four pounds and makes up most of the dry weight of feces. Before reaching for a bottle of antiseptic, it is good to know that many of these bacteria are beneficial to our health. The good guys are referred to as probiotics and breed in the bowel. They can be found in food or taken as a supplement. Every person's assembly of microflora is unique to him or her, akin to their fingerprint or DNA. How long before we see this featured on *CSI*?

Only a few of the more than 500 different species of bacteria found in the bowel have been studied in depth. Some are known to create vitamins such as K, B_5, B_9, and B_{12}. Others help improve the absorption of magnesium, calcium, and iron. The good bugs defend their turf from pathogenic intruders, which is why a timely course of probiotics before travelling can prevent a bout of Delhi belly or Montezuma's revenge. A large percentage of the immune system is located bowel-side, and probiotics are important for the maintenance and regulation of immunity, helping prevent coughs, colds, and more serious infections. In addition to IBD, other conditions that respond well to probiotics include diarrhea, irritable bowel sydrome (IBS), colon cancer (preventative), and even eczema and asthma.

Prebiotics is food for probiotics. Prebiotics are found in certain vegetables (especially asparagus, Jerusalem artichokes, leeks, and onions), legumes such as baked beans, chickpeas, and lentils, and supplementary fibers including psyllium, pectin, guar gum, and slippery elm.

Foods from many cultures include foods that contain probiotics including yogurt, miso, sauerkraut, kefir, natto, tempeh, and the Korean delicacy kimchi. To seed and maintain a healthy microbiome, probiotic foods need to be consumed several times a week.

- Avoid trans-fatty acids and deep-fried foods; they may cause further inflammation.

- Have a carrot and cabbage juice in the ratio of 2:1. Carrots contain beta-carotene that converts to vitamin A, a healer of epithelial cells, and cabbage contains a substance known as S-methylmethionine, which is effective in the treatment of ulcers.

- Mucopolysaccharides are substances that improve wound healing and tissue regeneration for the inflamed digestive tract lining. Foods containing mucopolysaccharides include oysters, tripe, shellfish, aloe vera, slippery elm, pig's feet, wheat germ, okra, and cactus (spikes removed).

Remedies

The following remedies can be taken in conjunction with prescription medication. The best scenario is when you can work with your doctor or specialist to reduce prescription medication as symptoms improve.

- Fish oil is brilliant for reducing the inflammation of IBD. A large dose is needed (10 to 15 ml daily, less for children), and you will need to wait a few weeks for it to take full effect. Keep taking it even after the symptoms have abated.

- Probiotics are needed to restore harmony to the bedlam within. Don't stint when buying probiotics that include any and all of the following: *Lactobacillus casei, Lactobacillus plantarum, Lactobacillus acidophilus, Lactobacillus GG, Escherichia coli nissle 1917, Bifidobacterium longum, Bifidobacterium breve, and Bifidobacterium infantis.*

- When you experience diarrhea and bleeding, and particularly if ulceration is affecting the small intestine as is the case with Crohn's disease, your absorption and retention of nutrients will be compromised. A daily multivitamin tablet is recommended—even better if you can find a multivitamin in a liquid form as this will be more readily absorbed.

- Herbs to help IBD include aloe vera, marshmallow, licorice, chamomile, calendula, peppermint, cat's claw, andrographis, and echinacea.

- If you have experienced a lot of bleeding, you may be low in iron. If this is the case, take a gentle liquid herbal iron tonic.

- Vitamin A and zinc are needed for the health and repair of the mucous membrane lining the bowel.

- Glutamine is an amino acid that is excellent in repairing and feeding cells that line the bowel.

- Psyllium husks are very effective for this condition. Not only do they absorb excess fluid and slow down transit time, helping to reduce diarrhea, psyllium husks are also an excellent prebiotic.

- Aloe vera is healing and calming to inflamed mucous membranes. Take a dose morning and night.

- Slippery elm powder is both healing and a prebiotic.

- Magnesium is excellent for muscle spasm. Take to ease and avoid abdominal cramps.

- If you experience bloating and/or flatulence or notice undigested food in your stool, take one digestive enzyme with each meal.

Other

- Stress is the wild card with IBD. It is *the* major trigger. Whatever causes you stress—whether it be work, study, relationships, travel—if you can change the stressor, do it. Otherwise you must learn how to change your way of handling stress. Try counseling, meditation, prayer. Find the method that works for you.

- Corticosteroids are a common medical treatment for IBD. Long-term use of steroids can affect your bone density, however. Get this checked.

- IBD can be very severe—bad enough to warrant surgery to resect parts of, or the entire bowel itself. If your IBD is in this category you might want to consider radical treatment: a water fast. Fasting allows the bowel to heal undisturbed by the passage of food and the taxing effort of digestion. This approach does not suit everyone, of course. A proper fast needs to be longer than five days and up to several weeks, and must be supervised, with blood pressure and urine samples taken daily. There are only a few centers that cater to fasting.

- Regular gentle exercise such as walking or swimming.

- Given that stress is a major trigger with IBD, it is not too long a bow to draw to say you hold your stress in your guts. Belly breathing not only reduces stress, but also relaxes the bowel itself. Belly, abdominal, or diaphragmatic breathing is the way we were meant to breathe. Over time, and especially for anxious people, breathing travels further up the body. Look at a dog or young child at rest—they are belly breathing. Initially, lie on your bed with a pillow beneath your head and knees. Place your hands palm down on your lower belly. Breathe in through your nose, counting slowly to three or four. Feel your tummy rise with the breath. Breathe out just as slowly, allowing the belly to drop. Once you feel comfortable with this, progress to doing this seated, and then try to belly breathe all the time.

At a Glance

Diet

- Follow the suggestions above for your diet when there are symptoms of intense pain, bleeding, and mucus, or for when there are no, few, or mild symptoms.

Remedies

- The omega-3 fatty acids in fish oil make it fabulous for reducing the inflammation of IBD but need to be taken in large amounts (10 to 15 ml) for the long term.

- A good quality probiotic supplement will go a long way to repopulate the bowel with health-giving microflora.

- Glutamine helps to repair and nourish the cells lining the bowel.

- Psyllium husks are prebiotic and help to stop diarrhea.

Other

- Stress is a major trigger in IBD. Find out what your stressors are, and avoid them if possible. Additionally, find out how to manage your stress. Try meditation, yoga, tai chi. Whatever, just do it.

- Fasting, under supervision, is a radical approach to healing IBD that might appeal to some.

INSOMNIA

WHAT IS IT?

Insomnia is characterized by a difficulty in falling and remaining asleep. Although Leonardo da Vinci and Margaret Thatcher apparently thrived on less than a handful of hours, the average adult requires seven to nine hours solid sleep a night. Why do we need so much? Sleep deprivation places significant stress on the body, releasing the silent stress hormone cortisol, which over the long term has serious health implications. Studies show that insufficient sleep is responsible for an increased risk of motor vehicle accidents, depression, substance abuse, diabetes, heart disease, lowered immunity, poor concentration, and even obesity. A good night's sleep is powerful medicine.

SYMPTOMS

- ☑ Trouble falling asleep
- ☑ Waking during the night and having trouble getting back to sleep
- ☑ Nonrestorative sleep (i.e., not feeling refreshed when you wake up)
- ☑ Feeling tired or falling asleep during the day

WHAT CAUSES IT?

- ❑ Worrywart-ism and stress are the most common causes of insomnia. Worrying thoughts can assert themselves the moment your head hits the pillow or can wake you during the night.

- ❑ Some mothers never recover from nighttime waking to feed and care for their babies, becoming hypervigilant at the slightest disturbance. This poor sleeping pattern continues even after the reasons for your insomnia have left home and have families of their own.

- ❑ Poor sleep patterns may appear after a traumatic event such as an accident, robbery, assault, divorce, childhood sexual abuse, or the death of someone close.

- ❑ Depression and/or anxiety can impact sleep, often causing early morning waking (around 3 A.M. to 4 A.M.), when it is difficult to go back to sleep.

- ❑ Factors in your environment may also cause insomnia such as a lumpy mattress, a fidgety bed companion, a bed companion who snores, a flickering streetlight, or a neighbor with a drum kit.

- ❑ If you suffer from sleep apnea or snoring, these will interfere with the quality of sleep.

- ❑ Shift work can destroy many people's chances of sleeping well. Even after returning to normal working hours, sleep patterns can be disturbed.

- ❑ Our bodies follow the circadian rhythms that operate on a twenty-four-hour clock. For instance, between 5 P.M. and 9 P.M., your body temperature and pulse rates are higher than at any other time, and urine production is lowest from 1 A.M. to 5 A.M. These patterns occur at the same time during the twenty-four-hour clock irrespective of whether you are working, partying, or traveling.

- ❑ Although alcohol can send you to sleep, it can also interfere with your sleep cycles.

- ❑ While the human growth hormone is secreted during sleep throughout life, growing children have the greatest requirements—a one-year-old requires approximately fourteen hours of sleep a day while a five-year-old needs around twelve hours. Children as young as six months can take sleeping remedies.

WHAT TO DO

Diet

❏ Low blood-sugar levels might be the cause of your sleep problems if you tend to wake after a few hours sleep. Then again, if you wake up at 1 A.M. to raid the fridge and scoff down leftover chocolate cake, low blood sugar is definitely your problem. The solution is to eat a small meal before going to bed. In the old days this meal used to be called supper, and it is well overdue for a comeback. Supper should contain a little protein and carbohydrate to sustain blood sugar levels. For example, hot milk and honey and an oatmeal biscuit, or cheese and crackers, or a small bowl of chicken and vegetable soup.

❏ Although a snack is recommended, avoid eating a heavy meal within three hours of going to bed. A roast dinner with the works will take several hours to digest, causing your digestive system to work hard when it should be snoozing.

❏ Avoid caffeine in coffee, tea, chocolate, guarana, and cola. Energy drinks often contain staggering amounts of caffeine. Some people are so sensitive to caffeine that even a morning cappuccino affects their sleep that night. Caffeine only affects some people's ability to sleep, so if you find avoiding it doesn't makes any difference, and you love your coffee, then don't deprive yourself unnecessarily.

❏ Limit after-dinner drinks to a small cup of herbal tea or warm milk. Getting up to go to the toilet during the night is bound to disturb sleep unless you have terrific sleepwalking skills.

❏ Warm milk, honey, and nutmeg is a traditional remedy that works well because milk contains tryptophan and calcium. Tryptophan converts to the soothing neurotransmitter serotonin, and calcium relaxes muscles. Honey is soothing, and also helps the tryptophan cross the blood–brain barrier to be converted to serotonin. Nutmeg has a slight sedative effect. Or maybe it works well because grandma said it did. Turkey, figs, dates, and bananas also contain tryptophan.

BEHIND THE SCENES

A good night's sleep is comprised of five or more sleep cycles, each lasting approximately ninety minutes. Each cycle has various stages. Stage 1 is a light sleep where you drift in and out of consciousness and can be wakened easily. During this stage, people may experience sudden muscle contractions preceded by a sensation of falling. Stage 2 is when the brain waves slow down, and Stage 3 is when your deepest sleep is experienced—no eye or muscle movement is detected. This is when some children (and adults) experience bed-wetting, sleepwalking, or night terrors. Stage 3 is also when the human growth hormone (HGH) is secreted. HGH is responsible for growth in children, explaining why children need more sleep. In adults, HGH stimulates the immune system, increases muscle and bone mass, enhances cell repair, and promotes fat loss. Some scientists claim that HGH is the ultimate "antiaging" hormone. No wonder we need our beauty sleep. Following Stage 3 is REM (rapid eye movement) sleep, where dreaming occurs. REM sleep lasts only about five to ten minutes. As people age, in addition to less sleep, they tend to wake at the transition between non-REM and REM sleep. A person deprived of REM sleep becomes moody and depressed.

- Though a nightcap may have an initial sedative effect, alcohol interferes with those important sleep cycles. You are less likely to have a refreshing sleep and may wake up in the morning more tired than when you went to bed. Alcohol is also a diuretic, so it is likely to wake you to go to the toilet during the night.

Remedies

- Valerian, chamomile, kava, passionflower, Californian poppy, hops, skullcap, lemon balm, and vervain are all somniferous (sleep-inducing) herbs. Take one or a combination in tablet form or in a tincture or tea before bed. Valerian is a wonderful sleeping herb for most people. However, for a small percentage, it can have a "paradoxical" effect, that is, the reverse of what is intended. If this happens to you, then always avoid valerian and choose from some of the other herbs.

- If your sleeping problems are due to anxiety or stress, taking some of these herbs during the day can also help. They won't make you sleepy during the day, as no herb is able to override the body, but they can calm down the nervous system, affording a better night's sleep at the end of a less-stressed day.

- The nature of your errant sleeping patterns determines when you take your herbal medicine. If you have problems getting to sleep, then take a dose after dinner and another just before you hop into bed. However, if you wake during the night, forget the dinner dose, and take it straight before bedtime, and have another tablet or dose handy if you wake during the night. Many times the first waking is one and one-half hours or three hours after falling asleep. This equates to sleep cycles 1 and 2. The trick is to send you into a deeper sleep for the first cycle, so you are less likely to wake in between. Check with your practitioner, but you might need to take a larger dose to encourage this deeper sleep state for the first cycle.

- A vitamin B complex taken each morning is good for the nervous system. Don't take it at night as it may be overly stimulating.

- Calcium and magnesium are soothing minerals. Taken at night, they can help you sleep.

- A homoeopathic remedy for sleep is coffea 30. Take 7 drops before bed each night.

- Melatonin is the natural sleep chemical produced by the body to induce sleep. It is at its peak at nighttime. Melatonin can also be used to promote sleep, and is often used by frequent fliers to reset their body clock. Your doctor can prescribe melatonin. Homoeopathic melatonin is available over the counter and works well for some.

- Bach flowers useful for insomnia include Mimulus (for fears that can be described, which is good for worrywarts), Aspen (for fears of unknown origin and for fear of letting go), White Chestnut (for thoughts that go around and around in the mind), and Rock Rose (for nightmares and night terrors).

Other

- Routine is vital. Rise at the same time every morning (regardless of the number of hours slept) and go to bed at the same time each night.

- Exercise. A physically tired and exercised body is more likely to sleep. Even though you might feel tired, it's your mind that is tired, not your body. Choose a regular time to exercise, which is not too close to bedtime, preferably in the morning.

- Your deepest sleep, in the early hours of the morning, is also when the body reaches its lowest temperature. Having a warm bath or shower before bed not only relaxes tense muscles, but by heating the body, your internal thermostat kicks in trying to lower basal temperature, lulling the body into believing it should be deeply asleep.

❏ A couple of handfuls of Epsom salts in a warm bath will help muscles to relax and assist in a restful night's sleep. Epsom salts are made from magnesium sulphate. Taken internally, Epsom salts can cause diarrhea (hence the phrase "goes through you like a dose of salts"), but absorbed through the skin, Epsom salts can have a relaxing effect.

❏ When you first go to bed, start belly breathing, and do it again if you happen to wake through the night. Belly breathing, or diaphragmatic breathing, switches on the parasympathetic, or calming, nervous system as opposed to the sympathetic, or fight-or-flight, nervous system. Place hands palm down on your lower belly. Breathe in and out through your nose, counting slowly to three or four (whichever is more comfortable). Feel your tummy rise with the in breath. Breathe out just as slowly, allowing the belly to drop.

❏ Create a sleep-inducing environment. This might mean moving your bed to a room at the back of the house, away from the road, or hanging dark curtains to block out a streetlight.

❏ If your bedroom looks like it has more cords and electrical devices than a small recording studio, get them out of the bedroom. There is some evidence that simply being around electrical fields can disturb the body's normal circadian rhythms. This means no TV in the bedroom.

❏ Relax for an hour before retiring. Listen to relaxing music, read (avoid the murder and horror genre), or watch television (not the news or high drama; stick to self-help or reruns of the soaps). Do not work or study.

❏ Herb pillows made from an assortment of dried herbs including hops, lavender, and chamomile placed under your pillow can be helpful, or place a few drops of the essential oils on your pillowcase each night.

❏ If you feel your insomnia may be due to a past traumatic episode, hypnotherapy or kinesiology may help break its hold over you.

❏ Avoid or limit daytime naps to half an hour.

❏ Keep calm colors in your bedroom such as dark blue, violet, and indigo. Lime green, bright yellow, and orange are considered mentally stimulating colors.

❏ Shift workers who suffer from insomnia may need to consider their line of work—is this job really worth the effect on your health?

❏ Sleeping tablets are among the most commonly prescribed drugs. They are often addictive and many also affect sleep quality, so you may get to sleep but wake up feeling like you haven't. However, sleeping tablets have their place; some sleep can be better than none. Talk to your doctor if you wish to wean yourself off these drugs, as rebound insomnia may occur if you cut them out too quickly.

❏ Poor sleep often becomes a habitual problem. Like all habits, you need to repeat the behavior consistently to change the habit. This is true with insomnia. When you find something that works, don't stop after one or two good nights. Keep up the "habit" or supplement for a few weeks until the body is used to the new routine.

AROMATHERAPY

Blend the following essential oils in 120 ml of orange blossom water, or lavender hydrosol, or an essential oil solubilizer, and shake well. Spray on your bed linen, pajamas, and/or pillowcase before sleep, and dream well! Alternatively, for a relaxing bath soak, blend with 200 grams of Epsom salts and 50 grams of bicarb soda, and halve the amount of drops of essential oils.

❏ 4 drops of vetiver oil—nervine, sedative

❏ 10 drops of chamomile oil (Roman or German)—sedative, insomnia, nervous tension

❏ 6 drops of neroli—anxiety, depression, nervous tension

❏ 10 drops of lavender oil—antidepressant, sedative, nervine

❏ 5 drops of sandalwood oil—sedative, nervous tension, stress-related complaints

AT A GLANCE

DIET

➠ Eat a light supper containing a little protein and carbohydrate before going to bed. This will keep your blood sugar levels steady.

➠ Avoid eating a large meal within three hours of bedtime.

➠ Alcohol may make you sleepy, but it can interfere with your sleeping patterns and leave you feeling unrefreshed in the morning.

REMEDIES

➠ If you have trouble falling asleep, take a dose of sleeping herbs at dinnertime (see above for suggestions). If you have problems staying asleep, take another dose at bedtime. These herbs can also be taken during the day as they can calm the nervous system.

➠ Calcium and magnesium are soothing minerals. Taken at night, they can help you sleep.

➠ Bach flower remedies are particularly helpful if stress and anxiety are the cause of your insomnia.

OTHER

➠ Exercise is important to tire the physical body. Try to get into a morning routine of gym, walking, swimming—whatever rocks your boat.

➠ A hot bath or shower last thing at night heats up the body. As the body starts to cool down, this will send sleepy-time messages to the brain.

➠ Belly breathing (see above) switches on the parasympathetic, or calming, nervous system—just what you need as you head into the land of Nod.

➠ If your insomnia is due to past stressful events, hypnotherapy and kinesiology can help.

➠ Once you have a set of routines and remedies that work, don't stop. Insomnia is a pattern, as is good sleep. Keep up the good routine, and happy dreams!

IRRITABLE BOWEL SYNDROME (IBS)

WHAT IS IT?

Irritable bowel syndrome (IBS) affects around one in six people. About half the people who visit a gastroenterologist (bowel specialist) leave with a diagnosis of IBS. A diagnosis of IBS is based on a group of symptoms known as the Rome III criteria. Rome, huh? It makes IBS sound rather romantic. Criterion I, you have a Botticelli bottom. Tick. Criterion II, the tinkling sounds in your belly remind one of the Trevi Fountain. Tick. And Criterion III, your bowel movements resemble a perfectly filled cannelloni. Err, tick. Actually, the Rome criteria for IBS state a diagnosis depends on your having abdominal pain or discomfort for at least three days a month for the last three months, associated with two or more of the following symptoms: a change in the frequency of bowel movements, a change in the appearance of bowel movements, and your symptoms improve with a bowel movement. On second thought, Venice sounds nice.

SYMPTOMS

- ☑ Diarrhea
- ☑ Constipation
- ☑ Alternating diarrhea and constipation
- ☑ Abdominal pain
- ☑ A feeling of fullness
- ☑ Bloating
- ☑ Flatulence
- ☑ Symptoms improve with bowel movement
- ☑ Lack of appetite

WHAT CAUSES IT?

- ❏ Some people carry their stress in their neck, some suffer headaches, while others feel tight knots in the muscles of their shoulders. People with IBS experience stress in their bowels. Worry is the enemy of the intestine. Irritable bowel syndrome is very often a visceral sign of stress. The physiological explanation of this process is the close connection between the nervous system, the digestive system, and the brain. When you experience stress of any kind, it causes a commotion in the nervous system, and this hubbub is then relayed to the bowel. Around 95 percent of the body's "happy" neurotransmitters, serotonin, are located in the digestive system. Stress causes a decrease in serotonin. Alterations in serotonin affect the movement of the bowel, and vice versa.

- ❏ Food sensitivity may cause or trigger IBS. Wheat, dairy, fructose, alcohol, and spicy food are some common culprits.

- ❏ Infection. One interesting theory is that IBS is initiated by a bacterial or viral infection. Although the infective agent may have left the building, its presence caused major disruption to the microflora within the bowel, and in the ensuing months or years can result in the presentation of IBS symptoms. It's the same sad lament one hears with so many conditions. Unhappy microflora; unhappy bowel; unhappy you.

- ❏ Hormones may not be the cause, but many women suffer an increase in IBS symptoms prior to menstruation.

WHAT TO DO

Diet

❑ IBS responds well to good eating habits. So, sit down to eat. Don't eat standing up. Don't eat working at your desk. Don't watch TV at dinnertime. Eat meals at regular times and don't miss any. Like small children, bowels respond best to routine. Chew each mouthful well. Peristalsis begins the moment you start to chew, so wolfing down your food sends a similarly rushed message to the bowel.

❑ Eat lightly when stressed. Keep to soups, steamed vegetables, chicken breast, or white fish.

❑ Avoid foods that trigger your IBS (which may include wheat, dairy, onions, brassicas, legumes, sugar, coffee, and alcohol).

❑ Avoid artificial sweeteners, particularly sorbitol, which interferes with peristalsis.

❑ Stick to a low-fat diet. Avoid deep-fried foods.

❑ Don't chew gum. It is one of the worst things you can do to your digestive system. When you start chewing anything, hormonal and nerve messages are swiftly sent to other parts of the digestive system to prepare for food. When no food arrives, there is understandable confusion.

If you have to, chew gum immediately after a meal to clean your teeth, but not at any other time.

❑ Prebiotic and probiotic foods can help restore and maintain healthy bowel flora. Prebiotic foods include asparagus, Jerusalem artichokes, leeks and onions, and legumes such as baked beans, chickpeas, and lentils. Probiotic foods include yogurt, miso, sauerkraut, kefir, natto, tempeh, and kimchi.

❑ Fructose malabsorption is the most recent food sensitivity on the nutritional scene. Pioneered (and marketed) by Australian dietician Sue Shepherd, fructose malabsorption is where you have difficulty in digesting fructose, a sugar found in fruits and vegetables. If not adequately digested, fructose (and fructose-like molecules) travel down the intestine where they ferment, releasing gas and creating havoc with peristalsis. Many people with IBS respond well by decreasing fructose foods from their diet. Fructose malabsorption can be detected by a hydrogen breath test. High-fructose foods include fruit juice, tinned and dried fruit, grapes, guava, apple, coconut milk and cream, honeydew melon, mango, nashi fruit, papaya, pear, quince, star fruit, tomato, watermelon, Lebanese cucumber, sweet potato, tomato

---

BEHIND THE SCENES: IN DEPTH

IBS is known as a "functional disorder" rather than the other option, an "organic disease." The difference is that an organic disease is where there is damage or change to an organ or body part, whereas with a functional disorder, a change has occurred to the normal functioning of a body process. This means that when IBS is investigated via a colonoscopy (a scope up the rear), there is no discernible damage to the bowel wall, unlike ulcerative colitis or Crohn's disease (both organic diseases), where there is often inflammation and ulceration to be seen. With IBS, it is thought that peristalsis (the wave-like movement which occurs throughout the bowel) is disrupted, which causes the symptoms of IBS that include abdominal pain, diarrhea, constipation, abdominal pain, flatulence, and lack of appetite.

paste, relish, sweet and sour sauce, BBQ sauce, fructose corn syrup, fructose, honey, fortified wines, globe artichokes, asparagus, garlic, green beans, onions, leek, shallots, and wheat.

Remedies

❑ Effective in tablet or extract form, ginger, lemon balm, chamomile, valerian, aniseed, peppermint, and fennel are excellent for treating the symptoms of IBS. Also, try one or more as a herbal tea, sipped throughout the day.

❑ Very often bowel flora is disturbed. Take probiotics including a single or variety of *lactobacillus fermentum, lactobacillus plantarum, lactobacillus acidophilus,* and *bifidus.* Take one teaspoon or three capsules every morning before breakfast.

❑ Take a large tablespoon of psyllium along with a glass of water each evening. Psyllium is a prebiotic as well as being helpful for both diarrhea and constipation.

❑ Magnesium helps muscle spasm, including the muscle of the bowel.

❑ If bloating is a major symptom of your IBS, take a digestive enzyme tablet before or with each meal.

❑ Enteric-coated peppermint oil capsules ease many IBS symptoms. "Enteric-coated" means that the medicine is coated with a substance that allows it to pass through the stomach and into the intestines where it is needed. Many substances are changed by stomach acid.

Other

❑ Stress is almost always a trigger with IBS, and IBS symptoms can be a sign that you are internalizing your stress. Learning relaxation techniques and how to manage your stress is paramount to controlling this uncomfortable condition. Meditation, yoga, counseling, whatever rocks your boat—and bowel.

❑ The Bach flower that helps stop incessant thoughts is White Chestnut; Pine is for those who feel guilty and never good enough; and Vervain is for those who have too much on the go at the one time.

❑ Buteyko breathing (see Appendix F) is the perfect remedy for IBS. This type of breathing relaxes smooth muscle (which lines the bowel), and switches on the relaxing parasympathetic nervous system. Exactly what is required. Get to it.

❑ Regular exercise is important. Swimming in particular can be helpful for IBS, perhaps due to the stretching of the abdominal muscles particularly from overarm and breaststroke.

AROMATHERAPY

Blend the following oils into a 20 ml base oil. Use in a soothing clockwise abdominal massage or as a warm compress on the abdomen and lower back. Mixed with some Epsom salts, it can also be used as a bath soak.

❑ 4 drops of sweet marjoram oil—soothing on the digestive system, can relieve cramps, indigestion, and constipation, and cleanse the gut

❑ 4 drops of black pepper oil—strengthening effect on the stomach, aids with flatulence, and calms in cases of nausea; tonifying to the smooth muscles of the colon

❑ 2 drops of peppermint oil—soothing, antispasmodic effect on the smooth muscles of the stomach helping to alleviate pain, colic, diarrhea, indigestion, and nausea

DIET

➡ Focus on acquiring and maintaining good eating habits. Chew each mouthful well. Don't rush your meals, and sit down to eat.

➡ Avoid foods that trigger IBS. Common offenders include wheat, dairy, onions, brassicas, legumes, sugar, coffee, and alcohol.

➡ Eat more prebiotic and probiotic foods. Improving your microbiome, or bowel bugs, often sorts out IBS.

➡ If you suspect that fructose malabsorption is behind your IBS, decrease high-fructose foods and see if it makes a difference.

REMEDIES

➡ A probiotic supplement can be helpful to overcome IBS. Take one daily. The strains of bacteria shown to be of most help include *Lactobacillus fermentum, Lactobacillus plantarum, Lactobacillus acidophilus,* and *bifidus.*

➡ Herbs such as ginger, lemon balm, chamomile, valerian, aniseed, peppermint, and fennel are good friends to the bowel.

OTHER

➡ As stress is a major factor in most cases of IBS, it will serve you well to attend to reducing and learning techniques to cope with your stress.

➡ The Buteyko style of breathing (see Appendix F) reduces anxiety and relaxes the bowel. Why not give it a whirl?

JET LAG

WHAT IS IT?

It's hard to scoot around Macy's trying to look glam when all you want to do is go to bed in your jammies. Jet lag can do this to you. Although humans have always been travelers, we never suffered from boat lag, car lag, or horse lag. It's only since planes have allowed us to move so fast that our brain might know we are in London during the day, but our body feels like it is nighttime in LA. Jet lag occurs when your body clock "lags" behind (or in front) of local time.

SYMPTOMS

☑ Fatigue

☑ Sleepiness in the daytime

☑ Insomnia

☑ Irritability

☑ Clumsiness

☑ Impaired judgment

WHAT CAUSES IT?

❏ Jet lag occurs when you cross time zones. Journeys going east are more difficult to adjust to than westward journeys. You can avoid jet lag completely if you only travel north to south, up and down along the same time zone—although this does limit your holiday choices and business destinations! The reason for the lag is that our body follows a twenty-four-hour routine, known as the circadian rhythm. Body temperature drops at night, which is when we prefer to sleep. We urinate more during the day, and hormones fluctuate according to the time within the twenty-four-hour cycle. This all gets thrown out the window when you cross several time zones in just a few hours. With jet lag, your body clock doesn't know whether it's day or night, whether it's coming or going.

❏ Jet lag is made worse by travel fatigue. Sitting down for many hours in seats designed by Lego, squished side-by-side like a can of sardines, your muscles are bound to cramp and tire. Even sardines get to lie down.

❏ Reduced oxygen in the aircraft cabin can also play havoc with your well-being.

WHAT TO DO

Jet lag remedies are like bad jokes: everyone has one. The following have proved helpful to frequent travellers and airline staff.

Diet

❏ Eat lightly. Choose salads and vegetables. Avoid heavy meals and creamy, spicy, and rich food.

❏ Eat meals according to your destination's time zone. Most airlines adjust the meals to reflect this, which is why you might find yourself eating breakfast at a very odd time.

❏ If you're not hungry, don't eat. There is no rule that says you have to eat every meal that is served. Often it's due to boredom rather than hunger.

❏ The air circulating in planes is as dry as a chip. Dehydration can increase jet lag, so ensure that you drink plenty of water—200 ml (around 7 ounces) per hour at least.

❏ Drink no more than a glass of wine with dinner—except French champagne, see below—as alcohol is a diuretic, causing you to become even more dehydrated. It can also disrupt sleeping patterns.

❏ Drink coffee only when it is morning time at your destination.

Remedies

❏ To help you sleep at night, try a herbal tablet, tincture, or tea containing valerian, passionflower, hops, Californian poppy, and/or chamomile.

❏ To help you stay alert in the morning, try a herbal preparation containing Siberian or Korean ginseng, gotu kola, and/or damiana.

❏ Melatonin, a hormone produced by the pineal gland in the brain, helps to balance out our circadian rhythms. Take a tablet an hour before you wish to sleep. You may need to see your doctor for a prescription in some countries. Homoeopathic melatonin also be helpful.

❏ The homoeopathic remedy arnica is terrific for jet lag—take a dose every couple of hours.

❏ If you suffer from anxiety when flying, take some Bach Rescue Remedy as well as the herb kava.

❏ If you are prone to water retention, take a 100 mg tablet of vitamin B_6 with each meal.

❏ Deep vein thrombosis (DVT) is a very real threat for those who take long-haul flights. A blood clot can form, usually in the calf, which may result in a potentially fatal pulmonary embolism. Vitamin E, gingko biloba, butcher's broom, and a remedy made from Japanese natto miso, nattokinase, can help. Take singly or in combination for a few days before and after your journey.

❏ Sitting in a crowded plane increases your chance of catching a cold. To prevent this from happening, take echinacea for a week before, as well as during, your flight.

Other

❏ The trick is to set your watch to the time of your destination as soon as you embark. This means that you try and sleep when it is nighttime at your destination, and eat at your destination's meal times.

❏ The downside to drinking water is the need to urinate, which can be inconvenient when you are in the middle seat. However, the trip to the toilet can double as "exercise."

❏ For flights over six to seven hours, you will need to exercise to prevent swelling of the ankles and legs and prevent "economyclassitis" (also known as deep vein thrombosis, a potentially fatal condition that comes from being cramped in a confined space for hours). Most airlines offer a set of exercises on information sheets or via their onboard entertainment system. At the very least, wear comfortable shoes and every hour or so stretch and scrunch your toes. In addition, rotate your ankles clockwise and counterclockwise hourly, as well as standing and walking when you are able.

❏ If it is sunny when you arrive, stay outside for an hour or so, without sunglasses. This is to allow the sunlight to hit the retina, be registered by the pineal gland, and promote the production of natural melatonin.

❏ Gentle exercise, moving your legs, and compression stockings can all help prevent DVT.

❏ When you arrive, if it is nighttime, take a hot bath with lavender oil.

❏ If you have the time, try to break up your journey with overnight stops. This will greatly relieve jet lag and your bank balance.

❏ Travel first class. French champagne is known to prevent jet lag and travel fatigue. Dosage: one glass per hour. When sleepy, snuggle in between those crisp white sheets, and remember your earplugs to block out unwanted sounds.

❏ Exercise for twenty to forty minutes as soon as you can after arriving at your destination. Swimming is the best exercise, preferably in the sunshine. Shopping is not exercise.

❏ Meditate regularly during the flight. Many people swear that meditating banishes jet lag.

❏ Sitting for hours and hours can lead to water retention and bloating. Don't wear tight-fitting clothes or shoes, walk around, and if possible put your feet up.

◼ AROMATHERAPY

To deter jet lag, the goal is to promote alertness, energy, strength, stamina, and balance within the nervous system. Blend the following essential oils with 10 ml of jojoba oil or 10 ml of coconut oil. Use as needed throughout and after the journey.

Alternatively, this blend can be combined with purified water and an essential oil solubilizer and used as a personal spritzer.

❏ 7 drops of peppermint oil—alertness, strength

❏ 6 drops of rosemary CT Cineole oil—mental fatigue, balance, strength

❏ 4 drops of black pepper oil—focus, strength, and stamina

❏ 3 drops of geranium oil—balance, uplifting, energizing

At a Glance

Diet

➠ Avoid large, rich, and spicy meals, sticking to salads and lighter snacks.

➠ Eat according to your destination's time zone. Breakfast at their breakfast time.

➠ If you are not hungry, miss a meal.

➠ Drink 200 ml (about 7 ounces) of water every hour to avoid dehydration.

Remedies

➠ An hour before bedtime—remember this is the bedtime of your destination—take sleeping herbs such as valerian, passionflower, hops, Californian poppy, and chamomile.

➠ The natural hormone melatonin can be helpful; take an hour before bedtime.

➠ In the morning, take some energy herbs including Siberian or Korean ginseng, gotu kola, and/or damiana.

➠ To avoid deep vein thrombosis (DVT), take vitamin E, ginkgo biloba, butcher's broom, and/or nattokinase a few days before, during, and after your flight.

➠ If you are an anxious flyer, take kava and some Bach Rescue Remedy.

➠ To avoid getting a cold, take some echinacea before and during your flight.

Other

➠ As soon as you embark, adjust your watch to the time of your destination. This will give your brain, at least, the heads up about the new time zones, allowing your body to catch up a little quicker.

➠ Wear comfortable shoes and loose-fitting clothes that allow you to stretch, and exercise can help prevent DVT.

➠ When you arrive at your destination in the daytime, exercise for twenty to forty minutes, preferably in the sunshine.

➠ If it's nighttime when you arrive, take a warm bath with lavender oil.

➠ Meditation reduces the effect of jet lag.

➠ See also Motion Sickness on page 236.

KIDNEY STONES

WHAT IS IT?

Kidney stones, also known as renal calculi, are formed from small crystals that grow over weeks or months to form stones. It is when these stones decide to move out of the kidneys and down to the bladder (via the ureters) and then urinated out (via the urethra), that you know you have a problem. A very painful problem.

The initial crystals are formed when calcium combines with other substances to form stones (calcium oxalate makes up 60 percent of all kidney stones). Very small grain-sized stones can pass through the bladder and out with the urine. It is the larger stones (up to the size of a golf ball) that cause the problems. Apart from the sidesplitting pain, complications from kidney stones include irreparable damage to delicate kidney tissue, increased risk of infection, blockage of the ureter, and loss of function of the affected kidney.

If you have had a bout of kidney stones, there is a 75 percent chance that you will form more. In short, it is best to prevent the formation of kidney stones if possible.

SYMPTOMS

☑ Pain that comes as suddenly as it goes. Pain may be felt in the abdomen, back, and groin area.

☑ Blood in the urine

☑ Chills and fever

☑ Nausea and vomiting

WHAT CAUSES IT?

❏ Men are more likely to form kidney stones than women.

❏ Kidney stones are often hereditary.

❏ Not drinking enough fluids. Kidney stones are more likely to form if you drink less than a liter of fluid a day.

❏ Certain medications can increase your tendency to form stones including chemotherapy drugs, diuretics, aspirin, and acyclovir.

❏ Struvite stones are caused by recurrent urinary tract infections. This type of stone affects more women than men.

WHAT TO DO?

Diet

❏ It is important to know which stone variety you are dealing with (your doctor will be able to let you know). For instance, if your stones are made from calcium oxalate, you will need to avoid foods high in oxalates. If your stones are made from uric acid, you will need to decrease purines in your diet and follow the principles outlined for gout. (See Gout, page 172.)

❏ The most important thing you need to do to prevent a recurrence of kidney stones is to increase your fluids. Water is best, closely followed by kidney-friendly herbal teas (see Remedies, below). Drink 2 to 3 liters of fluid a day.

❏ For calcium-oxalate stones, avoid high-oxalate foods such as coffee (including decaf), tea, chocolate, cola, nuts, spinach, strawberries, rhubarb, and beetroot.

❏ For uric-acid stones, avoid high-purine foods including offal or organ meats (liver, heart, spleen, intestines) and sweetbreads (thymus, pancreas), red meat, poultry, deli meats, shellfish, crustaceans, yeast, herring, sardines, mackerel, anchovies, asparagus, mushrooms, and spinach.

❏ Although excess calcium may increase your risk of calcium-oxalate stones, this is not a reason to reduce dairy or calcium-rich foods from your diet as calcium plays an important role in the body. Instead, eat in moderation.

❏ Decrease salt (sodium chloride) in your diet. This means not adding salt to your cooking and meals, as well as getting serious about reducing packaged, processed, and takeout foods that hide horrific amounts of salt. Sodium increases the levels of calcium in urine, and increases the crystallization of this mineral. Decreasing salt is also a good strategy for decreasing blood pressure, an extra burden on the kidneys. Happy kidneys are healthy kidneys.

❏ Normalize blood sugar levels. High-circulating glucose (blood sugar) places a strain on the kidneys and is an early sign of diabetes. Avoid sugar, eat frequent meals to keep blood sugar steady, and follow the recommendations for diabetes.

❏ Magnesium can help prevent kidney stones and facilitate an easier passing of them. Foods with a good magnesium-to-calcium ratio include barley, corn, buckwheat, rye, oats, brown rice, avocado, bananas, lima beans, and potato.

❏ Reduce protein in your diet. The breakdown products of protein create more work for the kidneys. Red meat in particular increases the urinary excretion of calcium, phosphate, oxalate, and uric acid—the entire mineral repertoire of the kidney stone. Reduce animal protein and incorporate more vegetarian protein sources including legumes, nuts, and seeds.

❏ Kidney-friendly foods include watermelon, citrus fruits, pumpkin seeds, and cranberries.

❏ Citrate is a molecule that binds to calcium in the urine, preventing the formation of stones. Citrate is found in citrus fruits (lemons, oranges, mandarins, tangerines, and grapefruit).

❏ Drink the juice of half a lemon in hot water first thing in the morning. Good for your kidneys, liver, and bowel.

Remedies

❏ Herbs that act as a kidney tonic include crataeva (a key herb), shatavari, uvaursi, dandelion leaf, couch grass, marshmallow, and corn silk. Take them in tablet or tincture form, or better still as a herbal tea. Double the action of great herbs for the kidneys and increase your fluid intake at the same time. You're in luck, as kidney herbs taste pretty good. Well, compared to sleep herbs or liver herbs.

❏ Viamin B_6 can help reduce the production of calcium oxalate and prevent the formation of stones of this nature.

❏ Magnesium relaxes smooth muscle, allowing small stones to pass through more easily. It can also increase the solubility of calcium, reducing stone formation.

❏ Don't take calcium supplements if you are prone to kidney stones, as most stones contain calcium. If, however, you have been advised to take extra calcium, choose a calcium citrate supplement that has less chance of stone formation.

❏ There has been torrid controversy in nutritional circles over whether vitamin C supplements can increase calcium oxalate stone formation. The final word is that taking vitamin C is absolutely fine, and will not increase your risk of stone formation. It is actually good for dissolving calcium phosphate stones and the less common magnesium ammonium phosphate stones (struvite).

Other

❑ Weight-bearing exercise such as walking, jogging, and gym work can help keep more calcium in the bones rather then being excreted in the urine.

❑ Kidneys are the organs of fear. Have you anything to fear or do you live your life fearfully? If you identify with feeling fearful, there are two Bach flowers that may assist. Mimulus is the one for known fears (e.g., fear of flying, fear of spiders) whereas Aspen is for generalized apprehension and anxiety.

AT A GLANCE

DIET

➩ Water is your friend. Keeping the kidneys flushed with fluid can help prevent crystals forming into stones. Drink at least 2 liters a day.

➩ Reduce salt (sodium) in your diet. Sodium increases the chance of calcium crystallizing to form stones. Sodium also has the potential to increase blood pressure, which adds stress to the kidneys. Avoid adding salt to your meal and also be careful of processed, packaged, and takeout foods.

➩ Citrus fruits contain citrate that can help prevent the formation of stones.

➩ Eat more vegetarian protein foods such as legumes, nuts, and seeds. A diet high in animal protein increases your risk of kidney stones.

➩ If your stones are calcium oxalate, reduce high oxalate foods such as coffee (including decaf), tea, chocolate, cola, nuts, spinach, strawberries, rhubarb, and beetroot.

REMEDIES

➩ Crataeva is the pick of the herbs that act as a kidney tonic, but take one or all of the herbs mentioned above as a tea or in tablets or tincture.

➩ B_6 and magnesium can help reduce stone formation.

OTHER

➩ Kidneys are the organs related to fear—is there anything in your life that is frightening you?

MEMORY AND CONCENTRATION

WHAT IS IT?

Is your mind as sharp as a tack? Remembering names and numbers no problem? Ideas flow as swift and strong as the Mississippi? Do you breeze through your working day clearheaded and efficient? You do? How nice. Unfortunately, there are many people for whom a clear and focused mind is a rare pleasure.

Poor memory, also known as CRAFT disease (Can't Remember a Freaking Thing), and poor concentration are common complaints, even for people in their thirties and forties. There is only so much one little mind can deal with, which can mean less important facts, like your daughter's boyfriend's name, can escape you. As long as you remember to feed the dog.

HERBS AND MEMORY

Gotu kola combines the ability to relax the body and still the mind, which is why for centuries, it has helped Indian meditators to meditate. It is said to strengthen the crown chakra: the energy center at the top of the head, which is closest to heaven. Indian elephants love gotu kola leaves, and as everyone knows, elephants never forget. Rosemary, a beloved herb of the Mediterranean, stimulates clear thoughts: "There's rosemary, that's for remembrance. Pray you, love, remember." (Shakespeare) Brahmi is another ancient herb in the Ayurvedic tradition. Not only is it good for improving memory and acquiring and retaining information, brahmi can help regenerate nerves that have been damaged, making it a particularly good herb for recovering from a stroke. A study showed that brahmi reversed memory loss in aged rats. Now, where did I leave my cheese?

WHAT CAUSES IT?

- ❏ Stress. Lapses of memory and poor concentration are often the result of an overcrowded and stressful life. The hormone cortisol, which literally floods the body during times of stress, can cloud the mind.

- ❏ Alcohol. Although you might be the life of the party after a few drinks, alcohol is actually a depressant, sedating the nervous system and reducing the normal amount of stimuli the brain receives.

- ❏ Avoid or reduce recreational drugs such as ecstasy, alcohol, cocaine, and marijuana. To get the most out of your brain cells, it's best not to harm them.

- ❏ Dementia is where there are changes to the brain. The most common kind of dementia is Alzheimer's disease. Symptoms may include changes to language, personality, cognitive skills, and memory.

- ❏ Age is not a cause of poor memory or concentration, although dementia is more common among the elderly.

- ❏ Poor circulation. The brain keeps all the body's systems shipshape—from maintaining body temperature to releasing hormones and controlling organs—and requires a steady supply of oxygen. Poor circulation can be due to insufficient exercise, cigarettes, low thyroid activity, or atherosclerosis.

- ❏ Blood glucose. The one fuel all nervous tissue requires, including the brain, is glucose. This requirement for glucose does not mean you should munch candies all day long, but eat a low-glycemic diet that releases a steady flow of glucose.

- Depression and anxiety can increase cortisol and affect neurotransmitters and brain function. As a result, this can be a common cause of lapses in memory and concentration.

- Food sensitivity. Poor memory and concentration can result from a reaction to a food or chemical to which you are sensitive.

- Prescription medications such as antidepressants, tranquilizers, and blood pressure medication may be the cause of your mental fogginess. Do not reduce or discontinue your medication without talking to your doctor first.

- A few days of brain fog and confusion, or "chemobrain," after chemotherapy treatment can be common.

- Nerve or brain diseases (such as Parkinson's or multiple sclerosis), or a trauma to the head, can all affect memory and concentration.

- PMS, menopause, and pregnancy are times of surging hormones. For some women this can affect their concentration levels.

- Insufficient sleep. If you are an insomniac or burn the candle at both ends, this can have a negative impact on your ability to think clearly. See Insomnia on page 206.

WHAT TO DO?

Diet

- The brain relies on a steady flow of blood glucose. Symptoms resulting from a less than continuous supply of glucose may include poor concentration and memory, fatigue, irritability, hunger or nausea, and dizziness. The trick is to keep your blood glucose levels constant by eating a small meal every two to three hours that contains a little protein. Breakfast is particularly important, something along the lines of an omelet, baked beans or feta, and avocado on toast. Studies performed on school children that missed breakfast showed that they had poor concentration and lowered academic performance.

- A dehydrated brain is a sluggish brain. Make sure you are drinking at least 2 liters of fluid a day, including lots of fresh water.

- Avoid sugar. It won't make you smarter. Even though you'll feel a buzz for a short while, the resulting crash can affect your mental processes. Don't be dopey; give sugar a miss. This includes sugar found in packaged and processed foods.

- Many people drink coffee to keep them alert. And that is exactly what it does. A cup of coffee or more can increase your capacity for intellectual work, decrease drowsiness, and promote a more rapid and clear flow of thought. However, keep it to just a couple of cups a day.

- Tea contains a little caffeine that can help keep you on your mental toes, as well as theanine, a compound that can be calming and improve mind function. Theanine is found in all tea: green, black, oolong, and white.

- The omega-3 fatty acid DHA (docosahexaenoic acid) can help cognition, memory, and concentration. It is found in fish (which is why fish used to be called brain food), and can be converted in the body from all omega-3 fatty acids as found in chia seeds, linseeds, and walnuts.

- If you notice that your concentration falters after eating some foods, try to nail down if you might have a food sensitivity by avoiding that food for a month. Possibilities include wheat, diary, chocolate, eggs, and soy. Also look at preservatives and colorings.

Remedies

❏ Ginkgo biloba can help with difficulties in concentration and memory, absentmindedness, and mental fatigue, and has a reputation for treating cerebral insufficiency. (Don't we all feel cerebrally insufficient at some time or another?)

❏ Many herbs sharpen the mind. Other herbs that have been used over the centuries to improve memory and concentration include brahmi, gotu kola, rosemary, sage, lemon balm, and rhodiola. Sage was revered by the ancient Greeks, and in 1597, John Gerard, botanist and herbalist, wrote in the widely read herbal *Generall Historie of Plantes* that sage "is singularly good for the head and brain, and quickeneth the nerves and memory." Even more recently, in the twenty-first-century, sage has been found to facilitate the action of the important neurotransmitter acetylcholine, which helps with memory and cognition. There are some studies showing that sage may slow the progression of Alzheimer's disease.

❏ Stress can play mind games. Or rather, it plays with the mind. The stress hormone cortisol dulls concentration and affects memory. The adaptogen group of herbs (see page 92) can help clear the mind and reduce stress. These herbs include Siberian ginseng, licorice, Korean ginseng, schizandra, astragalus, gotu kola, tulsi, rhodiola, and withania.

❏ The amino acid, glutamine, plays a key role as a neurotransmitter in memory and concentration. For best effects, take between meals.

❏ DHA found in fish oil can help improve cognition. Take a fish oil that contains a fair proportion of DHA to EPA.

BEHIND THE SCENES

Memory is either immediate (covering the past few seconds); intermediate (up until the past few days); or long-term (extending back to childhood). The immense amount of information that humans are able to process is staggering, and memory plays an indispensable part in that process. We take our ability to remember things for granted—until we start to lose it.

From time to time, everyone forgets names and appointments—either from being too tired or too busy, or because facts just slip the mind. However, sometimes there is an underlying physical reason for your poor memory. Answer yes or no to the following questions.

❏ Are you experiencing an increased difficulty in learning new tasks?

❏ Do you frequently forget material you have just read?

❏ Are you forgetting people's names or appointments?

❏ Are you forgetting where you've placed your keys?

❏ Have you been told you are repeating yourself?

❏ Are concentrating and focusing becoming more difficult?

❏ Are everyday tasks like sending emails, making calculations, or recording TV shows becoming more difficult?

Responding yes to three of these questions is normal, but if you said yes to four or more, you may be experiencing memory problems. If the suggestions in this chapter don't help, and your memory keeps deteriorating, check with your doctor to rule out dementia.

Other

❏ Meditation. The Dalai Lama was once heard to say, "I have a busy day ahead. I must meditate twice as long." Although it's tempting to keep thinking of all the things you have to do, it is more helpful to clear the mind of clutter for at least a few minutes every day. Regular meditators know that meditation makes them more focused and mentally efficient.

❏ Buteyko breathing (see Appendix F) can help the mind in two ways. Firstly, by switching on the relaxing nervous system, it can reduce the stress hormones that so affect concentration, and secondly, it improves circulation to the brain, allowing more oxygen and glucose to nourish those lagging brain cells.

❏ Music can influence the mind. Studies published in *Nature* showed first-grade students who participated in special music classes saw their reading and math skills increase dramatically. Other studies have shown an increase in learning by 24 percent and memory by 26 percent after listening to appropriate music. Music that has a rhythm of 60 to 80 beats a minute is calming and relaxing. Coincidentally (or not) the resting human heart has precisely the same rhythm. Baroque music composed mainly in the seventeenth and eighteenth centuries has such a soothing beat. Composers of mind-empowering music include Pachelbel, Debussy, and Bach.

❏ Use it or lose it. Whether it is Sudoku, crosswords, bridge, or studying for your master's degree, use the mind you have been blessed with.

❏ The Bach flower Clematis is good for the absentminded.

❏ Use it or lose it, but don't abuse it. Be selective in what you want to remember or devote your mind to. Unless you want to "zone out" (and that's okay too), choose quality reading material and TV that will enhance your life.

❏ Heard a good joke lately? Psychologist Daniel Goleman in his book *Emotional Intelligence* said that "laughter helps people think more broadly and associate more freely."

❏ Aromatherapy has a lot to offer the befuddled mind. Smell goes straight to the emotional part of the brain, bypassing thought processes. If our emotions are centered, it is likely that the mind will be too. Burn some aromatherapy oils (rosemary, sage, and peppermint) in the room where you need to focus.

AROMATHERAPY

Blend these three essential oils into a base of 10 ml of brahmi oil. Massage into the scalp and temples.

❏ 1 drop of basil oil—cephalic

❏ 3 drops of lemon oil—known for lifting mental fatigue

❏ 2 drops of rosemary oil—known for remembrance

DIET

➡ Drink plenty of water. Dehydration dumbs you down.

➡ Although the brain relies on a steady flow of blood glucose, this does not mean a diet of gummy bears and chocolate will improve your mental prowess. Quite the opposite. Eat regular meals comprising low-glycemic food, and avoid sugar.

➡ Tea and coffee can help you concentrate, but don't go overboard.

➡ Fish is brain food. Containing the omega-3 fatty acid DHA, fish helps memory and concentration.

REMEDIES

➡ Stress increases cortisol. Cortisol decreases brain function. The adaptogen group of herbs helps the body cope with stress.

➡ Other herbs such as brahmi, ginkgo biloba, gotu kola, rosemary, sage, and rhodiola have been used for centuries to help hone the mind.

➡ The amino acid glutamine is used by the brain as a smart neurotransmitter.

OTHER

➡ Meditation calms the mind, reduces stress hormones, and allows nerves and neurotransmitters to work their thoughtful magic.

➡ Buteyko breathing (see Appendix F) increases the transport of oxygen and glucose to the brain, reducing stress.

➡ Aromatherapy oils can help concentration and memory. Try burning aromatherapy oils or massaging them onto your scalp and temples.

➡ Laughter and music are good medicine for the mind.

MENOPAUSE

WHAT IS IT?

At menopause, after thirty to forty years of active service doggedly slaving away month after month, producing eggs and estrogen, a woman's ovaries submit their letter of resignation in the hope of a quiet retirement. Menopause signals the end of a woman's reproductive years, and officially occurs at the end of the last menstrual period. The transition to menopause, known as perimenopause, takes from two to five years and can affect each woman differently. Some women breeze through symptom free, while others suffer a mixed bag of distressing symptoms. Studies have shown that women who have a healthier lifestyle, eat a good diet, and exercise regularly, suffer less symptoms of menopause.

The average age of menopause is fifty. Between the ages of forty-five and fifty-five is considered normal. Premature menopause is before forty, and an early menopause is before forty-five years of age. After menopause, women are more at risk of heart disease and osteoporosis, as estrogen has a protective effect on these conditions.

SYMPTOMS OF PERIMENOPAUSE AND MENOPAUSE

☑ Hot flashes (night and day)

☑ Night sweats

☑ Dry vagina

☑ Insomnia

☑ Forgetfulness

☑ Poor concentration

☑ Itchy skin

☑ Mood swings

☑ Depression

☑ Irritability

☑ Anxiety

☑ Palpitations

☑ Joint aches

☑ Low libido

☑ Prolapse of bladder, uterus, or bowel

☑ Increased bladder and vaginal infections

☑ Decreased bladder control

SYMPTOMS OF PERIMENOPAUSE

☑ Heavy bleeding.

☑ Painful periods.

☑ PMS symptoms.

WHAT CAUSES IT?

❏ Menopause is a natural event in a woman's life.

❏ On average, women who smoke experience menopause five years earlier than women who don't.

❏ Thin women suffer more menopausal symptoms than their curvaceous sisters. This is because fat cells produce a small amount of estrogen that can help reduce menopausal symptoms.

❏ Stress increases menopausal symptoms. Adrenal glands can produce some estrogen after menopause, but they are also responsible for producing the stress hormone cortisol. If the adrenal glands are preoccupied with the production of cortisol, this will negatively impact on estrogen production.

❏ Premature menopause may be caused by removal of the ovaries, surgery, medication, radiation, and chemotherapy.

WHAT TO DO

Hormone replacement therapy (HRT) is the conventional medical solution for menopause. HRT involves taking synthetic hormones, usually in tablet form. Some women find HRT an answer to their prayers, some experience side effects, while others prefer to enter this phase of their lives without chemical interference.

Following are some natural remedies that may help reduce the symptoms of menopause—they can be taken in conjunction with HRT.

Diet

❏ Avoid sugar and reduce caffeine and alcohol. The healthier your diet, the fewer your symptoms.

❏ Reduce packaged and processed foods.

❏ If you experience hot flashes, avoid triggers such as spicy foods, alcohol, and hot drinks.

❏ Introduce and increase phytoestrogen-rich foods such as soya sprouts, alfalfa, green beans, split peas, olives, soya beans, miso, tempeh, parsley, chickpeas, cherries, corn, oats, barley, rye, wheat, rice, pomegranate, hops, sesame seeds, linseed, buckwheat, millet, sage, fennel, celery, carrots, cabbage, rhubarb, and garlic.

Remedies

❏ Chop six to seven fresh sage leaves and soak overnight in lemon juice. In the morning, strain and drink the juice, diluting with water if preferred. After a week or so this mixture can help control hot flashes with the added benefit of improving digestion.

❏ Phytoestrogen herbs and other tonic herbs are excellent for the treatment of menopause. There are dozens to choose from, but the most helpful include black cohosh, red clover, dong quai, wild yam, soy, sage, and hops. (Note: if you are perimenopausal and still menstruating, these herbs may not be as helpful as for when you are actually menopausal. In this case, use the remedies mentioned below.)

❏ Vitex agnus-castus is such a lovely herb. Useful for virtually all occasions of hormonal misbehavior, it is excellent at both perimenopause and menopause itself.

❏ Evening primrose oil is also a good remedy during the perimenopausal time. Especially good for tender breasts and mood swings. Take at least 6 grams daily. Vitamin B_6 is indicated here also.

❏ Herbs to help with sleep problems include passionflower, Californian poppy, St. John's wort, valerian, lavender, and kava. Zizyphus can also help with sleep and hot flashes.

❏ Herbs that support the nervous system, adrenal glands, and hormones are indicated now. Choose from St. John's wort, withania, verbena, rhodiola, rehmannia, zizyphus, and kava.

❏ For low libido, choose from tribulus, shatavari, and/or panax ginseng.

❏ A reduction in estrogen creates a thinning of the vaginal wall. If you suffer from vaginal dryness, squeeze the contents of a 500 IU vitamin E capsule into the vagina each night. A dry vagina is one of the more stubborn symptoms of menopause. If the natural remedies are not effective, try estrogen cream prescribed by your doctor. The amount of hormone absorbed from the cream into the body is minimal.

❏ Depression descends on many women during

BEHIND THE SCENES

Phytoestrogens are natural chemicals present in certain plants. They exert a very weak hormonal influence, much weaker than that of the real hormone produced by the ovaries. Throughout the body, on most cells are receptor sites capable of being activated by certain substances. In the case of the hormone estrogen, there are thousands of receptor sites that are coded only for estrogen. At the time of menopause, these receptor sites are "hungry" for estrogen, and menopausal symptoms occur at this time. Eventually, after a time without estrogen, the receptor sites get sick of waiting and close up shop. End of story. No more menopausal symptoms. How the phytoestrogens work is that they look enough like estrogen to keep the receptor sites happy, although they are in no way as strong as the real-deal hormone. You keep taking the phytoestrogens as long as you experience symptoms. One day they will stop. Promise. If you are in perimenopause and are experiencing heavy bleeding, hold off on the phytoestrogens for a while, and take vitex agnus-castus instead. You can also try the recommendations for heavy periods on page 141.

menopause. St. John's wort is the best herbal medicine for you at this time.

❑ The Bach flower remedy Walnut is recommended during times of change, helping you to traverse this hormonal crossroad with grace.

Other

❑ Hop to it. Regular exercise can reduce all symptoms of menopause.

❑ If irritability and stress are part of the picture, incorporate relaxation techniques such as yoga and meditation.

❑ If you suffer from hot flashes, wear cotton clothes in layers that you can easily remove.

❑ A cool(ish) bath or footbath with 20 drops of peppermint oil in the evening can help reduce hot flashes and aid sleep. During the day, soak a washcloth in cool water and add a few drops of peppermint oil.

❑ The Bach flower Walnut is perfect for this time of transition and change.

❑ Menopause, a time of change in a woman's hormones, can often coincide with a time of change in other areas of life. If you had chil-

dren, they may be leaving home, or parents may be aging or have passed away. You no longer need to put others' needs ahead of your own. It's decision time—decisions made by you, for you. Go for it, girlfriend.

AROMATHERAPY

Use this blend in 20 ml of sweet almond oil mixed with 10 ml of borage-infused oil. Use as a body massage oil or in the bath. If using as a personal perfume, halve the blend of essential oils and blend in jojoba oil.

❑ 8 drops of bergamot oil—a wonderful uterine cleanser; excellent for anxiety and depression while possessing sedative properties, and yet at the same time being rather uplifting

❑ 3 drops of sweet fennel oil—a great body cleanser; said to mimic the hormone estrogen; good in cases of fluid retention; may help with low libido

❑ 4 drops of cypress oil—great for treating heavy bleeding and edemas of any kind; can be calming on the mind while putting a lid on anger and frustration; excellent for excessive sweating too!

CONTROVERSY CORNER

Over the last couple of decades, treating menopause has become mired in controversy—not only with prescription HRT, which may or may not be linked with an increased risk of breast cancer, but also with natural remedies including black cohosh and soy. Some time ago, a few cases of liver damage were reported in people after taking black cohosh. When this was investigated further, it was unclear whether black cohosh was actually taken, and whether or not the people had pre-existing liver disease. The only known side effects of black cohosh—reported by herbalists over hundreds of years—is a skin rash and diarrhea affecting a small percentage of patients. Even though there is no proven link between black cohosh and liver damage, due to government regulation, labels have a warning to this effect. No wonder confusion abounds. With regard to soy as a supplement or food, there is no evidence that it increases a woman's risk of breast (or any other cancer), and in fact, there is some evidence that it may reduce the risk of breast cancer.

DIET

→ The healthier your diet, the fewer menopausal symptoms you will have. So, avoid sugar and reduce caffeine and alcohol. Reduce packaged and processed foods, and eat plenty of fresh fruit and vegetables.

→ Add some phytoestrogen foods to your diet (see above).

REMEDIES

→ To control hot flashes, try fresh sage leaves soaked overnight in lemon juice (see above).

→ Herbs containing phytoestrogens are useful for reducing symptoms from hot flashes to faltering memory (see above).

→ Vitex agnus-castus is good for regulating hormones throughout perimenopause and menopause.

→ If you have mood swings, either up or down, St. John's wort, verbena, withania, rhodiola, rehmannia, and/or zizyphus can help.

OTHER

→ Exercise can help reduce all symptoms of menopause.

→ Wear layers of cotton clothing to add and remove as the hot flashes dictate.

→ A time of change in hormones and often life circumstances, menopause is a time to make big decisions and take charge of your life's direction from now on.

MOUTH ULCER

WHAT IS IT?

Only those who have had them can understand the exquisitely tender pain caused by a coven of mouth ulcers. Mouth ulcers, canker sores, or if you're in the mood for ancient Greek, "aphthous stomatitis" affects around 20 percent of the population. They are generally less than a centimeter in diameter, and start life as little red craters that soon fill with pus from white blood cells and bacteria. Mouth ulcers tend to recur, with each episode lasting from five to seven days.

SYMPTOMS

☑ Painful sores on the lining of the mouth

☑ Pain and irritation inside the mouth

WHAT CAUSES IT?

❑ Mouth ulcers are reliable signposts of stress— exams, overwork, overtraining, being overwrought, late nights, or personal dramas.

❑ They can pop up during fevers.

❑ Mouth ulcers can indicate a gluten or fluoride intolerance.

❑ Mouth ulcers may result from trauma to the inside of the mouth (e.g., from braces, hard-bristled toothbrushes, or chewing the inside of the cheek).

❑ Many women find that an outbreak will occur just prior to menstruation when immune levels are at their low point.

❏ Mouth ulcers can appear alongside an outbreak of cold sores or oral thrush—both signs that your immune system is below par.

WHAT TO DO

Diet

❏ When you have a mouth ulcer, eating a bland diet can help prevent the ouch factor. Although it's really a case of "taste it and see," in general avoid pepper, chili, tomatoes, vinegar, lemon, pineapple, mustard, cherries, plums, and citrus. Try cooling foods like watermelon, pear, cucumber, acidophilus yogurt, and lettuce. Bland foods include white rice, steamed chicken breast, and white fish.

❏ If the ulcers are really bad, live on smoothies for a few days to avoid chewing. Try a banana, raw egg, unsweetened yogurt, milk (cow, almond, soy, or rice), chia seeds, and honey, if desired.

❏ If you constantly get mouth ulcers and are not under a lot of stress and/or can't think of any other obvious cause, avoid gluten for a month. If your ulcers disappear in that time, you may be intolerant to gluten.

❏ If your immune system is struggling, give it a boost by avoiding sugar, processed carbohydrates, coffee, and alcohol.

Remedies

❏ Suck on a combined zinc and vitamin C lozenge every couple of hours.

❏ Make a mouthwash using a combination of echinacea, thyme, goldenseal, and/or calendula. Dilute if using a tincture, or if using herbal tea, make it strong. Swill and swallow three times a day.

❏ Slippery elm is healing for mucous membranes.

There are lozenges available containing slippery elm and other healing compounds such as zinc. Suck on these throughout the day.

❏ The bee product propolis is healing for ulcers. Dab a little on the ulcers several times a day.

❏ Aloe vera gel is healing and blessedly cooling. Apply several times a day.

❏ A less acidic environment will temporarily ease the pain, so suck an antacid tablet (from the drugstore), or pack your ulcer with paste made from the very alkaline bicarbonate of soda mixed with a little water.

❏ Rinse your mouth with acidophilus powder in water each morning to reduce sensitivity and restore healthy microflora to the area.

❏ If your ulcers are due to stress, take a strong B-group vitamin each day.

❏ If your ulcers are a sign that your immune system is under par, try a course of vitamin C and zinc as well as andrographis, echinacea, and/or cat's claw.

Other

❏ Although not an allergy, fluoride intolerance may manifest as mouth ulcers. Try a fluoride-free toothpaste for a couple of months to test this theory.

❏ If you insist on being heavy-handed with your toothbrush, change to softer bristles or an electric brush, and ask your dentist to teach you a gentler brushing technique.

❏ Avoid chewing gum; you are tempting fate.

❏ Rather than despair over an outbreak, be grateful to your mouth ulcers for showing you that all is not well. Learn to manage your stress before your immune system crumbles further. Try meditation, counseling or belly breathing. See Stress on page 276.

DIET

➡ If your ulcers are severe, drink smoothies for a few days.

➡ During an outbreak, stick to foods that are bland and cooling.

➡ Try a gluten-free diet for a month to test whether your ulcers are the result of a gluten intolerance.

REMEDIES

➡ Every few hours, suck on a combined zinc and vitamin C lozenge; if you find one with slippery elm in it too, all the better.

➡ Create a herbal mouthwash (see above). Swill and swallow three times a day.

➡ If your mouth ulcers are due to stress, take a B-group vitamin twice daily.

OTHER

➡ See your dentist if braces or harsh-brushing technique are the cause of your ulcers.

➡ If stress is behind your symptoms, treat the cause. Learn to meditate, go to counseling, or try belly breathing (see Appendix F). Find out how to manage your stress and enjoy an ulcer-free mouth.

MULTIPLE SCLEROSIS

WHAT IS IT?

Multiple sclerosis (MS) is an autoimmune condition whereby cells from the body's own immune system damage patches of the myelin sheath (the protective sleeve around nerves). This leaves the nerve beneath exposed and vulnerable while causing an alarming array of symptoms. Multiple sclerosis affects twice as many women as men, usually striking those between twenty and fifty years of age. The severity of symptoms can range from temporary and trivial to causing permanent and serious disability. Onset can be sudden and severe or insidious and mild. There can be times with total remission.

SYMPTOMS

☑ Muscles—weakness and/or spasms in the muscles of one or more limbs

☑ Senses—tingling, pins and needles, burning, numbness, feeling that the body is tightly wrapped

☑ Pain can occur anywhere on the body at random times.

☑ Vision—blurring, loss of vision, double vision

☑ Fatigue is a common symptom regardless of the severity of other symptoms.

☑ Depression is experienced by around 60 percent of those affected with MS.

☑ Advanced symptoms may include loss of bladder and bowel control, cognitive decline, and memory loss.

WHAT CAUSES IT?

❑ MS is one of a mysterious group of autoimmune conditions that, as yet, no one has found a definitive cause.

❑ The closer you live (or spent the first fifteen years of life) to the equator, the less your chance of being diagnosed with MS, which explains why more Scots and Scandinavians are affected than Maoris and indigenous Australians.

❑ Low levels of vitamin D might put you more at risk of MS.

❑ There is possibly a viral link, where a virus such as Epstein-Barr may be the trigger for unlocking the genetic susceptibility for MS.

❑ Stress is nearly always involved in exacerbating the symptoms of MS.

WHAT TO DO

Diet

❑ Avoid animal fats. It was first suggested as far back as 1950 that there may be a relationship between the consumption of animal-derived (saturated) fats and MS. Numerous studies since then have shown that patients on a low-saturated-fat diet had fewer episodes and less severe symptoms. Restrict foods containing animal and other saturated fats including butter, full-cream milk, cheese, cream, ice cream, red meat, pork, and coconut and palm oil products. In addition, avoid the highly processed oils that occur in margarine and some cooking oils, keeping to cold-pressed vegetable oils such as olive oil.

❑ Taken to its ultimate conclusion, avoiding animal fats completely would transform your diet into that of a vegan. Why not try a vegan diet for a month and see how you feel and if your symptoms respond positively? The long-term vegan needs to keep an eye on their B_{12} and iron levels. Also eat plenty of nuts and seeds to ensure enough of the right kind of fats.

❑ Avoid sugar, coffee, and alcohol. They are all draining on the immune and nervous system.

❑ Eat fish three to four times a week. The omega-3 fatty acid EPA, found in fish, is anti-inflammatory. Fish containing the most EPA are the fattier fish such as sardines, salmon, mullet, halibut, trout, and tuna.

❑ Cook with ginger and turmeric for their anti-inflammatory properties. They taste good, too.

❑ Various natural substances have the potential to stop the expression of certain genes. If MS (along with many other conditions) is the expression of a gene you don't want expressed, then taking these substances in food or supplements may prove helpful. These substances include the micronutrients such as zinc and folic acid, as well as phytochemicals such as EGCG (found in green tea), curcumin (found in turmeric), resveratrol (found in red grapes, peanuts, pistachios, pomegranates, and berries), and oligomeric proanthocyanidin complexes (OPCs) from grapeseed and maritime pine bark.

Remedies

❑ Evening primrose oil (EPO) has anti-inflammatory properties. In addition, GLA, the active constituent in EPO, is incorporated in the myelin sheath. Take 10 ml daily.

❑ Fish oil is also anti-inflammatory, and may be taken in combination with or instead of EPO.

❑ Check your vitamin D levels, and if they are on the low side, sunshine is not enough; you need to supplement with this vitamin.

- Find an antioxidant tablet that includes folic acid and zinc, as well as one or more of EGCG, resveratrol, or OPCs.

- MS episodes are often triggered by stress. Calming herbs for the nervous system include kava, St. John's wort, passionflower, zizyphus, and vervain.

- B complex vitamins can help your nervous system.

- The herbs used for autoimmune conditions, including MS, serve to modulate and regulate immune function, rather than to rev up and stimulate. Herbs include echinacea, rehmannia, bupleurum, cat's claw, and astragalus.

Other

- Stress is the wild card for MS. Learn to calm your nervous system with meditation, belly breathing (see Appendix F) or yoga. If you are finding life and your situation difficult, do not hesitate to seek the help of a good counselor.

- Keep cool. MS symptoms are worse for the heat.

At a Glance

Diet

- Avoid animal fats. There may be a link between saturated fats (particularly animal fats) and MS. Avoid red meat and milk products.

- Avoid sugar, caffeine, and alcohol.

- Cook with ginger and turmeric for their anti-inflammatory properties.

Remedies

- Take 10 ml of evening primrose oil for its anti-inflammatory properties, and a B complex each morning.

- If your vitamin D levels are low, top them up with a D supplement.

- Herbs that can help modulate and regulate immune function include echinacea, rehmannia, bupleurum, cat's claw, and astragalus.

Other

- Learn to avoid or deal with stress, and learn to calm your nervous system.

- Keep your cool. MS symptoms are worse for the heat.

NAUSEA AND VOMITING

WHAT IS IT?

Vomiting is the forcing of the contents of the stomach up into the esophagus and out of the mouth. It is one of the body's more ostentatious methods of elimination. Nausea is the stomach-churning sensation that usually precedes retching or vomiting.

SYMPTOMS

☑ To feel nauseous or queasy is to have sense of unease or discomfort in the upper abdomen.

☑ You feel like vomiting, although this may not occur.

WHAT CAUSES IT?

Nausea is an unpleasant symptom of various conditions (see below).

FOOD POISONING

WHAT IS IT?

Food poisoning occurs when you have eaten contaminated food. Vomiting is nature's way of promptly ridding the body of toxic pathogens before they are absorbed. The contaminant may be bacterial, viral, or the toxins made from these pathogens. Food poisoning can occur immediately after eating the contaminated food, or up to twelve hours afterward. Symptoms usually resolve within twenty-four hours, but can continue for three to four days. Common pathogens include salmonella, E. coli, enteritis, and campylobacter.

WHAT CAUSES IT?

❏ Food poisoning is most often caused by poor hygiene practices such as not washing hands after going to the toilet.

❏ Poor food hygiene: cross-contamination from raw meat to vegetables; not washing vegetables; not allowing food to defrost at the correct temperature; undercooking food.

❏ Traveling: food poisoning is more frequent when traveling to countries with less stringent food hygiene laws.

OTHER SYMPTOMS

❏ Abdominal cramps.

❏ Diarrhea.

❏ Fever.

❏ Headaches.

❏ Weakness.

WHAT TO DO

Diet

❏ Generally, you won't be able to keep any food down; however, try to eat a little dry toast, white rice, banana, or a cracker.

❏ Dehydration is the greatest risk with food poisoning. Sip warm ginger tea with honey, peppermint tea with honey, ginger ale, lemonade, black tea with honey, and/or diluted sports electrolyte replacement drinks.

Remedies

❏ Symptoms should resolve within a day. The offending pathogen is better outside your body than within so best to allow nature to take her course, and keep hydrated.

❏ After the storm has passed, take a good quality probiotic to restore microbial harmony. Take for at a least a week.

❏ The homoeopathic remedy arsenicum album can be useful in food poisoning.

Other

❏ Avoid dodgy restaurants and food outlets.

❏ Take a prophylactic probiotic before and during travel.

❏ Soak a hand towel in cold water with about 5 drops of spearmint oil or a cup of cold spearmint tea. Wring out the cloth and place it on your upper abdomen. If you don't have spearmint, use peppermint instead.

❏ Place an ice pack (or unopened pack of frozen peas) on the back of your neck.

❏ Press the acupuncture point *He-Gu* or "Joining of the Valleys," which is situated at the vortex between the thumb and first finger. Dig deep into this spot with the opposite thumb and massage in a tight circle for about a minute. Then for another minute, massage the scalp deeply as a good hairdresser does when shampooing you.

❏ Food poisoning can be very severe. If it continues more than twenty-four hours, seek medical help.

CHEMOTHERAPY

WHAT IS IT?

The drugs used for chemotherapy in cancer treatment commonly cause nausea and vomiting. Very often, antiemetic—or antivomiting—drugs are given concurrently with the medication.

SYMPTOMS

☑ Lack of appetite.

☑ Nausea and vomiting.

WHAT TO DO

Diet

❏ Even though you may not be hungry, try to eat small meals frequently, such as a boiled egg on a cracker, steamed chicken breast and a salad, or a few nuts. Each meal needs to contain a little protein, which has been shown to reduce the feelings of nausea during chemotherapy.

❏ Avoid sugar.

Remedies

❏ Ginger tablets have been shown to reduce nausea in addition to nausea medication.

❏ Sip on warm ginger or peppermint tea.

❏ The homoeopathic remedies nux vomica, arsenicum album, or ipecacuanha can be helpful. They will not interact with your other medications.

Other

❏ Speak to your doctor or cancer nurse if nausea is affecting you severely. An adjustment in dosage or an alternative medicine may be needed.

❏ A spearmint or peppermint hand towel on your upper abdomen, an ice pack on the back of your neck or pressing the acupuncture point *He-Gu* ('Joining of the Valleys') can also be helpful (see above).

❏ Marijuana is illegal in many states; however, THC (found in marijuana) can be helpful in relieving nausea and pain.

MORNING SICKNESS

WHAT IS IT?

Morning sickness occurs during pregnancy. It usually reaches its peak by week nine, but for some women, the nausea may extend to week twenty or more. Unfortunately, it can occur at any time of the day. Take solace in the knowledge that morning sickness coincides with a lower rate of miscarriage.

SYMPTOMS

☑ Nausea at the smell of certain foods

☑ Nausea and vomiting

☑ Nausea is often felt more at the beginning of the day.

WHAT TO DO

Diet

❏ Keeping blood sugar levels steady is one of the most important factors in reducing morning sickness. Eat small meals frequently. Even before you get out of bed, eat something. A dry cracker or a piece of toast. Each meal should contain a little protein.

❏ Avoid food and drink with strong smells.

❏ Avoid sugar.

❏ Keep your fluids up but avoid drinking more than a glass of fluid with meals.

Remedies

❏ Vitamin B_6 is excellent for reducing morning sickness. Take in combination with ginger.

❏ Ginger, cinnamon, chamomile, peppermint, black horehound, and chen pi can all be safely taken during pregnancy to reduce nausea.

❏ Homeopathic remedies that may help morning sickness include sepia and pulsatilla.

Other

❏ Rest up.

❏ Acupuncture and acupressure can be very helpful for reducing the symptoms of morning sickness.

❏ A spearmint- or peppermint-moistened hand towel on your upper abdomen, an ice pack on the back of your neck, or pressing the acupuncture point *He-Gu* ("Joining of the Valleys") can also be helpful (see above).

MOTION SICKNESS

WHAT IS IT?

Motion sickness can occur in boats, cars, trains, and planes, as well as on the big dipper and crazy mouse.

WHAT CAUSES IT?

Motion sickness is caused by mixed messages to the brain. Your sense of equilibrium is sensed via fluid in the inner ear and by sight. The brain takes in both messages and then judges one's position in space. If, for example, you are looking at the horizon while sailing, your eyes are resting on a still point, while your body is lurching from the swell of the sea. Vomitsville. Just why the mixed message to the brain should involve the stomach at all is open to speculation. One theory is that the brain decides one of the senses is hallucinating due to a toxin and orders the stomach to eject the poisonous substance.

SYMPTOMS

☑ Nausea and vomiting

☑ Sweating

☑ Hyperventilating

WHAT TO DO

Diet

❏ If you are particularly prone to travel sickness, don't eat before the journey, and if it is a short trip, avoid eating at all. Try small meals that are not fatty, spicy, or strongly flavored.

❏ Avoid alcohol before and during travel.

Remedies

❏ Feeling sick and the process of vomiting are intrinsically frightening. Vomiting can make even the strongest person feel vulnerable. A few drops of Bach Rescue Remedy will take the edge off fearfulness.

❏ Sip sweetened ginger tea or suck on crystallized ginger.

❏ The homoeopathic remedy ipecacuahna is good for motion sickness.

Other

❏ Can you not walk there instead?

❏ Open the window and grab some fresh air (not recommended on planes).

❏ Sit where there is least movement in the craft. Over the wings in a plane, midship on a boat.

❏ Drive rather than be a passenger. If this is not possible, bag the front seat, and keep your eyes on the road and scenery.

❏ A spearmint- or peppermint-moistened hand towel on your upper abdomen, an ice pack on the back of your neck, or pressing the acupuncture point *He-Gu* ("Joining of the Valleys") can also be helpful (see above).

❏ When going to an amusement park, avoid the Rotor ride. If you ignore this advice in addition to eating a corn dog, you will garner no sympathy from this quarter.

GALLSTONES

WHAT IS IT?

Rich foods such as creamy sauces or a roast dinner may trigger a gall-bladder attack, with nausea and vomiting a common symptom. If a stone is lodged in the bile duct, the pain is acute, and surgery to remove the gall bladder is often indicated.

WHAT CAUSES IT?

A stone lodged in the bile duct.

SYMPTOMS

☑ Upper abdominal pain

☑ Diarrhea

☑ Jaundice

☑ Fever and chills

WHAT TO DO

Diet

❏ Drink plenty of water, at least 2 liters daily. This is most important to keep the bile from becoming too concentrated.

❏ First thing each morning, drink a cup of hot water with the juice of half a lemon squeezed in it. Good for liver; good for gall bladder; good for you.

❏ Eat plenty of high-fiber foods including vegetables, legumes, and whole grains.

❏ Avoid fatty food.

Remedies

❏ Take a teaspoon of herbal bitters in some water before each meal.

❏ St. Mary's thistle, globe artichoke, turmeric, chelidonium, calendula, ginger, and peppermint can all help the gallbladder and liver. Take a tincture or tablet of one or more of these herbs once or twice a day.

Other

❑ To treat the painful abdominal symptoms, apply a heat pack to the area. A ginger or castor oil compress will add to the soothing effect.

❑ Acupuncture is an effective treatment for gallbladder disease.

❑ A spearmint- or peppermint-moistened hand towel on your upper abdomen, an ice pack on the back of your neck, or pressing the acupuncture point *He-Gu* ("Joining of the Valleys") can also be helpful (see above).

OTHER CAUSES FOR NAUSEA

❑ Helicobacter pylorus. Nausea is a common symptom of peptic ulcers and gastritis, and a symptom of the presence of helicobacter pylorus, the bacteria that is a major cause of these conditions (see peptic ulcer and gastritis).

❑ Low blood-sugar levels. If you feel nauseous, ask yourself when last you ate. If it was more than four hours ago, your blood sugar levels may be low.

❑ Migraines (see page 181).

❑ Hangover.

❑ Food allergies (see page 152).

❑ Swallowing mucus from a cold (see page 97) or sinusitis (see page 271).

❑ The presence of gallstones may cause nausea, particularly in response to a fatty meal (see page 163).

❑ Anything that ticks off the liver. Overburdening the liver with too much fatty food or alcohol can often cause nausea. The remedies for this are similar to those recommended for gallstones. (See page 164).

❑ Stress affects everyone differently. Some people respond to stress by feeling nauseous (see page 276).

❑ Overeating. Simply overfilling the confines of the stomach may make you vomit. Two thousand years ago, the Romans had specially built vomitariums so that they could more conveniently empty their stomachs to keep on eating.

❑ Annoying people—as in, "You make me sick."

❑ From an esoteric view, vomiting might be viewed as a resounding rejection of an idea or an experience.

AROMATHERAPY

This calming antinausea blend can be used as a dry inhalation and sniffed as needed. Simply sprinkle the drops onto a tissue and smell deeply. Alternatively, you can blend into 5 ml of sweet almond oil and gently rub on to the abdomen.

❑ 1 drop of ginger oil—analgesic, antispasmodic, digestive

❑ 1 drop of peppermint oil—analgesic, cephalic, nervine, vasoconstrictor

❑ 1 drop of cardamom oil—antispasmodic, cephalic, digestive

❑ 2 drops of mandarin oil—antispasmodic, sedative, calmative, digestive

DIET

➠ If your nausea is a passing phase, then it is best to eat nothing for a day or so, until you feel hungry.

➠ Avoid fatty foods—they will only make matters worse. Keep to bland, nonsmelly foods.

➠ Eat a little food every two to three hours; whatever you can stomach.

➠ Drink. Vomiting frequently can cause you to become dehydrated very quickly without realizing it. Some rehydrating fluids to sip slowly include plain, room-temperature water, as well as the old faithful flat lemonade or ginger ale, Chinese green tea, black tea, ginger or mint tea, or soda water. Diluted sports drinks can also replace lost electrolytes.

REMEDIES

➠ Ginger is an excellent herb for nausea for all reasons. Take as a tablet, tea, tincture, crystallized, or in a syrup.

➠ Homoeopathic remedies such as the following can work very quickly for nausea and are safe in pregnancy:

• nux vomica—nausea that is worse in the morning, irritability.

• sepia—nausea that is worse for thinking about or smelling food.

• pulsatilla—nausea worse for a stuffy room or fatty foods.

• arsenicum album—vomiting and diarrhea, food poisoning.

• ipecacuanha—motion sickness.

OTHER

➠ A spearmint- or peppermint-moistened hand towel on your upper abdomen, an ice pack on the back of your neck, or pressing the acupuncture point *He-Gu* ("Joining of the Valleys") can also be helpful (see above).

➠ Feeling sick and the process of vomiting are intrinsically frightening. Vomiting can make even the strongest person feel vulnerable. A few drops of Bach Rescue Remedy can take the edge off your fearfulness.

OSTEOPOROSIS

WHAT IS IT?

Bone mass peaks in late adolescence. This makes living into your nineties a downhill spiral unless you take particularly good care of dem bones. Osteoporosis is a condition where the density of the bone, particularly of the hip and spine, reduces to such a degree that fractures and falls are likely. Breaking a bone when you're a kid means having a cool plaster cast, which your pals can pen jokes on, and within six weeks, you're back on your bike with the broken bone long forgotten. However, a fracture in your seventies onward is a different kettle of fish, resulting in a much-diminished life often dependent on others, or even the cause of your demise. Osteoporosis affects one in two women and one in three men over the age of sixty. Osteopenia is a reduction of bone density, which is not as severe as osteoporosis, but is still heading down that path.

SYMPTOMS

☑ Osteoporosis is named the "silent killer," as very often the first symptom you experience is a fall or fracture.

☑ Compression of the spine can result in a dowager's hump or stooped upper back, and is thought to be the cause of Quasimodo's hunched back in *The Hunchback of Notre Dame.*

☑ Pain can result from the compression of the vertebrae.

WHAT CAUSES IT?

❏ After menopause, with a sharp decline in estrogen, bone density loss is at its most rapid.

❏ A family history of osteoporosis can increase your risk of osteoporosis.

❏ A sedentary lifestyle. Nowadays, there is not much physical work in the course of everyday life. Over the years, life has become easier on the body. Compare today's computerized washing machines to those twin-tub contraptions that required hauling loads of wet sheets from tub to tub, followed by a tug-of-war with towels through the wringer.

❏ Heavy metals from the environment such as lead, cadmium, and aluminum contribute to osteoporosis as they compete with calcium to be absorbed into bone, making bone less strong. Unfortunately, once these bad metals are incorporated into bone they are unlikely to leave.

❏ People with fair skin have a greater risk of osteoporosis than those of a darker hue.

❏ Illnesses including inflammatory bowel disease, celiac disease, and chronic diarrhea usually result in malabsorption of minerals, and can therefore result in osteoporosis.

❏ A history of anorexia nervosa will increase your risk of osteoporosis. Anorexia combines a limited nutrient intake together with lowered estrogen (often menstruation ceases during anorexia).

❏ Smoking decreases estrogen production and increases calcium excretion.

❏ Certain medications, including cortisone, can increase bone loss.

WHAT TO DO

Prevention is key. Once your bones are osteoporotic, it is much more difficult to treat. In fact, diet and supplements will, at best, keep levels the same. It is virtually impossible to reclaim bone unless you take medicine, which may have side effects. If you feel you might be at risk of osteo-porosis, have a DEXA scan (a dual energy x-ray absorptiometry scan) sooner than later. Reduced bone density, when diagnosed early enough, can be redressed by diet, exercise, and supplements.

Diet

❑ Increase calcium-rich foods including spinach, broccoli, bok choy, cheese, milk, yogurt, canned fish with edible bones, sardines, salmon, white-bait, tofu, almonds, tahini, sesame seeds, pars-ley, sprouts, and dried figs.

❑ Decrease coffee and tea, avoid sugar, and reduce salt as they all increase calcium excre-tion. Reducing salt not only means minimiz-ing the amount you add to your meals, but also reducing packaged, processed, and takeout food, which are often studded with sodium.

❑ Animal protein decreases bone mineralization. However, insufficient protein in the diet also decreases bone density. The answer is to in-crease plant proteins at the expense of animal protein. Plant protein can be found in legumes such as soy and lentils, as well as nuts and seeds.

BEHIND THE SCENES

We tend to think of bones as inert still-life structures propping up the body. However, bones are constantly in micromotion. Bone is made up of a protein lattice made from col-lagen. It is speckled with various minerals, including calcium and silicon, which serve to increase the bones' load-bearing capability. Bones hold 99 percent of the body's calcium, and act as a calcium storage facility, allowing calcium to freely move from bone to blood and vice versa, facilitating calcium to perform its other duties in the body including muscle contraction and nerve transmission.

❑ Dietary phytoestrogens may increase bone den-sity, particularly after menopause. Such foods include soya sprouts, alfalfa, green beans, split peas, olives, soya beans, miso, tempeh, parsley, chickpeas, cherries, corn, oats, barley, rye, wheat, rice, pomegranate, hops, sesame seeds, linseed, buckwheat, millet, sage, fennel, celery, carrots, cabbage, rhubarb, and garlic.

❑ Drink in moderation. A glass of alcohol a day decreases your risk of osteoporosis; more than two drinks increases your risk.

❑ An acid-forming diet can increase your risk of osteoporosis (see Appendix E: Acid-Forming Food).

Remedies

❑ A calcium supplement is helpful, particularly if you are in the osteopenic range of bone den-sity. Osteopenia is a condition of lowered bone density, a step on the way to osteoporosis if preventative measures are not adopted. A dose taken twice a day can optimize absorption. Make sure your supplement contains a range of calcium-enhancing minerals including mag-nesium boron, zinc, manganese, silicon, stron-tium, and copper as well as vitamins K and D.

❑ Vitamin D is crucial for calcium absorption. It has been shown to decrease your risk of frac-ture. If your blood levels of vitamin D are low (as found in a blood test), take a supplement until they are above midrange.

Other

❑ Enjoy regular weight-bearing and resistance exercise. With exercise, muscle pulls on the bone, causing them to become stronger. Try weightlifting, balancing (as in strong yoga poses), tai chi, jogging, dancing, cross-country skiing, and gym work. The aim is to strength-en bone as well as improve muscle tone and balance to help prevent falls.

- Enjoy some sunshine (out of the midday sun) to help maintain your vitamin D levels.

- Don't smoke.

- If you believe you may have been exposed to heavy-metal toxicity in your life, for instance from pollution, mining, or agricultural practices, a hair mineral analysis can be done to diagnose which minerals are involved. A process known as chelation can then be undertaken, which draws the toxic minerals from your bone. Certain environmental doctors and some naturopaths specialize in this area.

CALCIUM AND DAIRY

Dairy products are often recommended for their high calcium levels. And indeed, they do contain admirable amounts of calcium. However, milk products are not the only source of calcium in food. Nuts and seeds, leafy green vegetables, and legumes all contain calcium. Osteoporosis is less common in Asian countries where diets are traditionally dairy free. Magnesium is important for calcium absorption and utilization. They need to be in a certain ratio for this to be optimized: that is, 2 parts calcium to 1 part magnesium. In the case of milk, the ratio is 10 parts calcium to 1 part magnesium. Enjoy good quality milk products such as unsweetened yogurt and whole milk cheese as part of a good diet, but don't be bullied by the media into thinking you "have" to eat milk products in order to prevent osteoporosis. If you are not fond of dairy products, or have a dairy sensitivity, then ensure you are eating an array of other calcium-rich foods.

AT A GLANCE

DIET

- Increase calcium-rich foods. (See Appendix D, Food Sources.)

- Reduce coffee, tea, sugar, and salt as they all increase calcium excretion.

- Decrease animal protein in your diet and increase plant protein. Down with meat, up with legumes, seeds, and nuts.

REMEDIES

- Take a calcium supplement if you are at risk of osteoporosis or a scan has shown that your bone density is less than ideal.

- If your vitamin-D levels are low, take a supplement until your blood tests show levels above the midrange.

OTHER

- Exercise is vital to prevent osteoporosis. Weight-bearing and balance exercises are best.

- Don't leave it too late. Get a DEXA scan if you think you might be at risk of osteoporosis. Prevention is far better than cure.

- Enjoy some sunshine.

OVERWEIGHT

Overweight is a large (sorry!) subject about which gazillions of words are written and squillions of diet books have been sold. The following are my thoughts on the topic and what has worked well for my patients over the years.

If you are overweight, you have two issues to deal with. Firstly, being overweight puts you at risk of heart disease (stroke, heart attack), diabetes, and some cancers—all the common killers of today. The second issue is that you are under constant societal pressure to look differently (i.e., thin) from what you are (i.e., fat). Generally, it's the second issue people are motivated by, rather than the patently more important first issue, which explains why fad diets are so popular. Losing weight to conform to society's narrow view of attractiveness takes up enormous amounts of emotional energy, time, and money—and only confirms that we humans are queer creatures (except thee and me). What sane animal would obsess about this issue?

WHAT IS IT?

Two simple ways to determine if you are overweight is by taking your body mass index (BMI), and measuring your waist.

BMI

The body mass index is a measure of a human's body shape based on weight and height.

Underweight: less than 18.4
Overweight: 25–29.9

Healthy weight: 18.5–24.9
Obese: 30+

To get to these figures, you will need to put your math head on, but it's not too difficult to calculate. Your BMI is measured by dividing your weight in pounds by your height in inches^2 and multiplying that result by a conversion factor of 703. For example, if you are a 180-pound woman measuring 70 inches (5 feet, 10 inches), your BMI would be 180/(70 x 70) = 180/4900 x 703 = 25.82, which is slightly over ideal, but not too bad. (If math is not your bag, there are plenty of online calculators that make it easy.)

There are limitations to this one-size-fits-all BMI calculation. Athletes, for example, may be very heavy for their height, but much of their weight is in muscle mass, which is a good health look, whereas some elderly or sedentary folk may weigh less, but have a bigger fat to muscle ratio. BMI is also unsuitable for children under eighteen and pregnant women. And some people really do have big bones.

Waist Measurements

The other determinant to being overweight is to measure your waist. A tape measure sounds very old-fashioned, but this simple technique compares favorably with the more modern, fancy-pants, high-tech medical equipment when it comes to assessing your risk of heart disease and diabetes.

Women

Increased risk: more than 31 inches

Substantially increased risk: more than 34.6 inches

Men

Increased risk: more than 37 inches

Substantially increased risk: more than 40 inches

WHAT CAUSES IT?

❑ Very often, overweight is caused by the simple mathematical equation of too many calories in, and not enough calories out, so the excess calories are stored as fat.

❑ A sedentary lifestyle. Humans were apparently designed to walk over 25 miles a day. We do much less with our bodies and eat more ice cream than our ancestors ever did.

❑ Genes do play a role. If you come from a family who are overweight, it is likely you will have more difficulty losing weight than some skinny mini.

❑ After menopause, a woman's metabolic rate drops, causing weight gain.

❑ Polycystic ovarian syndrome (PCOS) interferes with insulin resistance, and often has weight gain as part of its symptom profile.

❑ Certain conditions including hypothyroidism (low thyroid function) can increase weight.

❑ Various medications, including cortisone and some antipsychotic medicines, can increase weight.

❑ Lack of sleep is known to pile on the pounds.

❑ Stress, particularly ongoing stress, can increase weight. This is due to the diabolical stress hormone, cortisol, which is chemically identical to cortisone.

❑ One diet too many. If you have been a yo-yo dieter, trying many diets over your life, particularly low-calorie diets, you will probably be heavier than people who have never dieted.

❑ Emotional eating. Overeating is an addiction to food that should be given the same consideration as any other addiction, including alcohol and heroin. The problem with food addiction is that you can't go cold turkey. When you were a baby and terribly vulnerable, an important source of comfort and nourishment was mother's milk (or formula). When you were afraid or tired or angry and cried, you were given the breast or bottle. As an adult, when you are upset or stressed, it is common to crave food to feel comforted, just as you did as a baby. Trouble is, eating more than your body needs is a fleeting comfort and probably a source of your distress.

❑ The more you watch TV the more likely you are to be overweight.

WHAT TO DO

Losing weight isn't easy, but it doesn't have to be difficult. Once you get your head around a few simple rules, you are set for life. Quick-fix diets don't work. Studies have found that over 95 percent of dieters who lose weight on stringent diets will regain the lost pounds plus extra within a year. I have developed an eating plan with a few simple rules that allows you to eat healthily while losing or maintaining your ideal body weight. Most people feel more energy, notice better concentration, and improved general health. You can live a normal life, go out to restaurants, and not rely on "special" foods. This diet is not only good if you want to lose weight, but it can also help prevent diabetes, some cancers, and heart disease. A good choice for a healthy, lifelong way of eating.

❑ The Beaming with Health eating plan works well for children and teenagers; however, they need to eat more starches as energy requirements are proportionately higher. The best starches would be whole grains and potatoes with skins, rather than processed products.

The Low-Starch Eating Plan
(or the Beaming With Health Eating Plan)

❏ Avoid sugar. Absolutely no refined sugar added to or within your diet. Any packaged or processed food that has over 5 grams of sugar per 100 grams of food has sugar added. (Be aware of all the different names for sugar on labels. Google this if necessary or out of interest.)

❏ Eat protein with each meal. For main meals, this means about the size of your palm and as thick as a pack of cards. For snacks or smaller meals, halve this amount. Protein foods include lean meat, chicken, fish, eggs, nuts, seeds, and legumes.

❏ Reduce starchy carbohydrates. If you want to kick start your diet, avoid them completely for one month. For a slower weight loss and maintenance, include two to three starches in your diet a day. Choose from the list on the next page. Starchy foods generally have a high-glycemic index (GI). High-GI foods cause a rapid increase in blood sugar levels, which in turn causes an increase in the amount of insulin. High amounts of insulin in the blood-stream increase fat storage.

❏ Don't go hungry. Eagerly anticipating a meal is a good thing, but when you are very hungry it indicates your blood sugar levels have dropped too low—and you are likely to eat something that you will later regret.

❏ There are two types of people. Those who do best by grazing and those who thrive on three square meals a day. You know who you are. Grazers are known to quiver and feel faint and queasy if they don't eat lunch on the dot of 12, while the three-square-meal types can more easily miss a meal. Grazers need to ensure they eat a small meal every two to three hours. The three-square-meal individuals must make sure that they don't miss meals, especially breakfast, as this will lower your metabolism.

❏ Don't go low fat, but don't go crazy. If you like yogurt, choose full cream (unsweetened of course), good quality probiotic yogurt, and have a small serving. Same goes for cheese and milk.

❏ Don't eat food containing artificial sweeteners. Not only will they keep your sweet tooth ignited, they do not supply you with any nutritional goodness—the overwhelming characteristic of any good food. Studies have shown that people who drink diet sodas are heavier than people who drink the normal fizzy drinks—with their nine teaspoons of sugar!) Avoid both kinds, please.

❏ Eat no more than three pieces of fruit daily, and although not "starchy," also avoid the fruits with higher sugar levels such as melons, grapes, and dried fruits.

❏ Most people feel fantastic eating this way. However, by removing breads, pasta, and cereals, inadvertently you are also removing a certain amount of fiber, which may result in constipation. So it's important to ensure that you drink plenty of water (1.5 to 2 liters a day) and eat a wide variety of vegetables, nuts, seeds, and legumes to increase fiber. If this is still not enough, supplement with two tablespoons of psyllium husks daily.

❏ The low-starch eating plan is designed as a life-long diet. You do not need to buy special foods or supplements, and you can still go out to restaurants with your family and friends. For instance, if you love spaghetti marinara, you can still enjoy eating it, but it means you forego toast for breakfast and a sandwich for lunch.

Starchy Foods

One serving of the following is equivalent to one serving of starch.

Grains

Bread	one slice
Rice	³/₄ cup (cooked)
Pasta	³/₄ cup (cooked)
Oats	³/₄ cup (cooked)
Quinoa	³/₄ cup (cooked)
Crackers (e.g.,Vita-Wheat, rice cakes)	two pieces

Fruit

Banana	one average

Vegetables

Potatoes	3 small; 1 medium
Pumpkin	1 small piece
Peas	¹/₂ cup
Corn	¹/₂ cup
Parsnip	1 average

Other

❑ All fruit except bananas, melons, grapes, and dried fruit. (You can eat these, but they will take up one of your starch options.)

❑ All vegetables except peas, potatoes, corn, parsnip, pumpkin. (Again, be aware that these will take up one of your starch options.)

❑ All protein foods: meat, chicken, fish, eggs, nuts, seeds, cheese, legumes, and tofu.

❑ Protein powders: pea protein, soy protein, rice protein, and whey protein.

❑ Fats and oils: walnut oil, sesame oil, cold-pressed olive oil, macadamia oil, flaxseed oil, and coconut oil.

❑ All spices and herbs; soy sauce.

❑ Alcohol. If you like to drink alcohol, you can enjoy one or two glasses of dry white or red wine, spirits or champagne daily. Avoid beer, liqueurs, and sweet wines.

❑ Juice. Avoid fruit juices; they are high in sugar. Better to eat the whole fruit rather than its juice. But if you want to, dilute a little with water. Vegetable juice once a day is okay.

Meal Suggestions

Breakfast

❑ Scrambled, poached, or boiled eggs on a bed of spinach and/or mushrooms and/or tomato.

❑ A smoothie made from soymilk, cow's milk, juice from an orange or other fruit and/or yogurt. Add an egg for protein or LSA, a mixture of ground linseeds, sunflower seeds, and almonds. You can buy this blend readymade from health food shops or supermarkets.

❑ Try a combination of chopped almonds, walnuts, and/or cashews together with sunflower seeds, sesame seeds, linseeds, and/or pumpkin seeds. Have as much as you like mixed with a spoonful of milk or yogurt.

❑ A cup of ricotta mixed with fruit such as apricots, kiwifruit, or berries.

❑ If you wish to have starch at this meal, try toast, oatmeal, baked beans, or a banana.

Lunch/dinner

❑ Meat or chicken casserole and vegetables.

❑ Fish, meat, or chicken, and salad.

❑ Meat, chicken, or tofu, and vegetable soup.

❑ Stir-fry vegetables with meat, chicken, fish, or tofu.

❑ Fish (canned or fresh), and salad (e.g., canned tuna with grated beetroot and carrot).

❑ If you wish to have starch at this meal try bread, rice, or pasta.

Snacks

❏ Meat, chicken, or tofu, and vegetable soup.

❏ Almonds, walnuts, and so on.

❏ A boiled egg.

❏ Small can of tuna with lettuce or salad.

❏ Small can of baked beans.

❏ Fruit and cheese.

❏ If you wish to have starch at this meal, try crackers, baked beans, bread, or a banana.

Remedies

❏ Health foods shops, pharmacies, and online superstores are heaving with weight-loss potions. The bottom line is that they don't work. Better not to waste your money. Sorry. My rationale for not recommending supplements for weight loss is that it takes the onus off the individual to do the hard work and take responsibility for their own health. Maintaining weight is a lifestyle choice, not something to fix with a pill. What a nag I am. Having said that, there are a few situations where supplementation will assist in weight loss, in addition to exercise and the low-starch plan.

❏ If you have low thyroid function, supplementation will assist your weight loss. Take rehmannia, iodine, or kelp.

❏ Likewise, if you have polycystic ovary syndrome (PCOS), try the herbs and supplements listed here to help you lose weight. The low-starch diet mentioned in this chapter is also perfect for this condition as it helps those with insulin resistance, which is part of PCOS.

❏ If your excess weight is due to stress and the effect that cortisol has had on your body, take a B complex each morning and the adaptogen herbs (see page 92), including Siberian ginseng, schizandra, licorice, withania, and rhodiola.

❏ The Bach remedies may help if emotions are getting in the way of weight loss. Crab Apple is the one for feeling ashamed of the way you look. Chestnut Bud hits the spot if you tend to repeat the same pattern of sabotaging your diet.

Following is a list of foods and supplements that have been shown in some studies to assist in weight loss.

❏ Tyrosine—can possibly suppress appetite; stimulate brown fat cell metabolism; precursor to thyroid hormones.

❏ Carnitine—an amino acid that facilitates the breakdown of fats.

❏ Damiana—a good herb for energy; sometimes promoted as a weight-loss agent.

❏ Fish oil—some evidence that EPA reduces insulin resistance, thus improving weight loss (see Diabetes on page 123).

❏ Ginger—a few studies have shown that ginger helps in weight loss, for reasons unknown.

❏ Green tea—studies have shown green tea reduces food consumption by possibly decreasing the appetite hormone, leptin. Green tea may also increase your metabolic rate. These studies have been done on animals, however, not humans.

❏ Guarana—decreases appetite and increases metabolic rate, working very similarly to caffeine.

❏ Gymnema—this herb is interesting as it decreases your desire for sweet food, decreases appetite, and improves insulin resistance.

❏ Licorice—one study showed licorice reduced thigh fat! One thing licorice is very helpful for is to decrease the effect of cortisol, the stress hormone.

- Oranges—a chemical found in oranges, synephrine, can increase fat breakdown.

- Psyllium—this soluble fiber taken before meals will increase your sense of fullness, reducing the temptation to overeat.

Other

- Exercise is the other essential ingredient to losing weight. There are three reasons why exercise helps to lose weight, and these reasons will inform which exercise you choose. The first reason is that when you exercise aerobically, where your heart and lungs are working hard and you are increasing your heart rate, this will burn calorie and more importantly, boost your metabolic rate for up to forty-eight hours after the activity. The second reason is that when you exercise to increase muscle mass, such as cycling or lifting weights, you burn calories again, but more importantly, you increase the number of your muscle cells. Muscle cells, even at rest, burn considerably more calories than fat cells. And thirdly, exercise helps reduce stress levels. Stress is associated with weight gain via an increase in cortisol. If you are an emotional eater, exercising will reduce the triggers for overeating.

- Which exercise to choose? Luckily many exercises and sports incorporate both aerobic and muscle building—jogging, hill walking, cycling, gym classes, flowing yoga, skiing.

- Meditation is one of the most effective activities to reduce stress hormones. Learning this skill will markedly improve your health—and help you lose those excess pounds.

- If you find that you are sabotaging your diet, or know that you eat for emotional reasons,

---

RATIONALE BEHIND THE LOW-STARCH DIET

EVOLUTION

Our body (and digestive tract) has remained essentially unchanged for hundreds of thousands of years—yet the food we eat has changed substantially. Grains (including rice, rye, wheat, barley, and corn) have only been cultivated for the last ten thousand years—the beginning of agriculture and civilization—long after our digestive systems were up and running. In the modern diet, there is an overemphasis on grains such as wheat, which appears in bread, pasta, biscuits, and most breakfast cereals. This is not to suggest that we go back to prehistoric times and eat cockroaches and dinosaur dung, but return to the kind of foods our bodies were evolved to thrive on: leaves, seeds, nuts, fruits, meat, eggs, vegetables, fish, and the occasional flower.

RECENT HISTORY

Over forty years ago, the Western world was swept up by Pritikin fever. The U.S.-based Nathan Pritikin wowed the experts with evidence that fat was a major cause of heart disease, then the number-one killer of Americans. Pritikin recommended a diet severely restricted in all kinds of fat. Chips and chops were out, boiled potatoes and pasta were in. Lots of people lost weight, and lots of people avoided heart disease. However, the news wasn't all good. By focusing on processed carbohydrate foods (at the expense of "good" fat and protein), this ultimately causes a shift in the way the body deals with glucose, encouraging weight gain and even a tendency toward diabetes and obesity—diseases that are now epidemic.

then why not seek counseling? The therapist you choose does not need to specialize in eating problems—your emotional eating is only a symptom, and you need to address the originating cause or find ways to handle your day-to-day stress. Once you understand what drives you, your desire to overeat or eat foods that undermine you, will be much diminished.

AT A GLANCE

THE LOW-STARCH EATING PLAN

➠ Avoid sugar. Sugar is only going to add calories with no nutritional benefit. Ditch the poison. Read labels carefully as any food that has over 5 grams of sugar per 100 grams of food has been sweetened. Be aware that sugar goes by other names.

➠ Eat some protein with each meal.

➠ A key to this diet is to reduce starchy carbohydrates. Depending on your requirements, having none to three starches a day will have you losing weight and maintaining a healthy weight for the rest of your life.

➠ Stick to two standard units of alcohol a day.

➠ Stick to two to four pieces of fruit daily (but not grapes, melons, or dried fruit).

REMEDIES

➠ If you have low thyroid function, this will affect your weight. See hypothyroidism on page 284.

➠ If you have PCOS this will often affect your glucose metabolism, in addition to the diet take a supplement containing zinc, chromium, and B vitamins.

➠ Reduce the stress in your life if this is affecting your weight, and try some herbal supplements.

OTHER

➠ In addition to the low-starch eating plan, regular exercise is important for weight loss and good health. Combine aerobic exercise with muscle-increasing exercise so as to burn calories.

➠ If you choose the wrong foods or eat more when you are stressed or upset, try counseling and take up meditation to reduce the triggers that may sabotage your good diet.

PEPTIC ULCER

WHAT IS IT?

Peptic ulcers are not only the domain of power-breakfasting type A personalities. Even school-children are capable of growing their own. A peptic ulcer occurs when the protective lining of the stomach is damaged. If this happens within the stomach itself, it's called a gastric ulcer. If this happens just outside the stomach in the first part of the small intestine, it's called a duodenal ulcer. They have similar symptoms and are treated in the same way. Once the thick lining of mucus coating the stomach is disturbed, hydrochloric acid and pepsin (a protein-digesting enzyme) eat away at the tissue beneath, causing an ulcer. Some people think a peptic ulcer is caused by an excess of stomach acid. This is not the case. Stomach acid needs to be ruggedly acidic in order to do its best work. Rather, it is when the lining has been damaged and acid is able to reach unprotected tissue that problems arise. Gastritis, an inflammation of the stomach lining, is but a skip and a jump along the path to an ulcer.

SYMPTOMS

☑ Pain in the upper abdomen and chest, variously described as burning or gnawing

☑ Pain occurs when the stomach is empty or within one to three hours after eating.

☑ Upper abdominal pain that wakes you up at night

☑ Loss of appetite

☑ Nausea and vomiting

☑ Black, tarry stool. This is a sign the ulcer may have perforated. See your doctor immediately.

WHAT CAUSES IT?

❏ The bacteria *Helicobacter pylorus* (known as *H. pylorus* to its friends and researchers, and *H. pylori* when there is a gathering of *H. pyloruses*) is implicated in 95 percent of all peptic ulcers. Since triple therapy (two antibiotics with an acid-inhibiting drug) has been introduced, the recurrence of stomach ulcers has been reduced by 90 percent.

❏ Excess alcohol can cause peptic ulcers. Alcohol irritates the lining of the stomach. In addition, a certain percentage of alcohol is absorbed directly from the stomach, which explains why you can feel tipsy within minutes after your first sip of champers. Most foods are absorbed after leaving the stomach, in the small intestine. Presumably, some acid is drawn along with the alcohol, creating or exacerbating damage to the stomach lining. Drinking on an empty stomach is particularly harmful.

❏ Nonsteroidal anti-inflammatory drugs (NSAIDS), including aspirin, are another common cause and trigger in peptic ulcers. They irritate the lining of the stomach and inhibit the repair of tissue.

❏ Although most cigarette smoke goes to the lungs, some ends up in the stomach, where it is an irritant. Cigarette smoke also decreases bicarbonate production from the pancreas into the small intestine. Bicarbonate is important for buffering or reducing the acidic contents after their release from the stomach. As you can imagine, if the acid contents are not quickly alkalized, they are likely to damage any area not protected. Passive smokers may also be at risk.

- Formerly thought to be the major cause of peptic ulcers, stress is still considered an exacerbating factor.

WHAT TO DO

While the dietary suggestions and remedies mentioned below are very effective, sometimes it will be necessary to complete a course of triple therapy as peptic ulcers are not to be trifled with—they can perforate and cause internal bleeding.

Diet

- Avoid alcohol and any foods that aggravate your ulcer. Common aggravators include curry, pepper, chilies, coffee (even decaf), black tea, orange juice, and tomatoes. You know your own ulcer—if a food not on this list causes you curry-like aggravation, even if it's not curry, avoid it until your ulcer has healed.

- For breakfast (or any time), you might like to try this therapeutic "soothie": blend milk (cow, goat, soy, rice, or almond), yogurt (sheep, goat, or cow), a teaspoon of probiotic powder or the contents of three capsules, a teaspoon or two of slippery elm, a small banana, manuka honey, and cinnamon to taste.

- Avoid sugar. Bacteria thrive on it, including *H. pylorus.*

- The humble cabbage contains S-methyl methionine that stimulates the healing of cells and speeds up the production of the protective mucus lining. The best way to enjoy the healing power of cabbage is to juice it. Blend two cups of sliced cabbage (green or red), two sticks of celery, and two carrots. Drink this through the day, every day, for seven days.

- To prevent *H. pylorus* from gaining a foothold and to restore microbial balance (especially after antibiotic therapy), eat plenty of probiotic foods such as yogurt made with acidophilus or bifidus, miso, leben, and sauerkraut. If you can cultivate a taste for sauerkraut it would be splendid, because it offers both the cabbage and the probiotics.

- Manuka honey contains a substance that inhibits the growth of *H. pylorus.*

- A little plain acidophilus yogurt is soothing and not a strain on your digestion.

- Adopting good eating habits is important. Eat your food slowly. Don't eat lunch at your desk while working. Eat your meals at the same time each day. Don't miss meals. Don't chew gum between meals, and eat small meals that create less work for the digestive system.

- Avoid red meat as digesting it is asking way too much from a stressed-out stomach.

- Mucopolysaccharides help to heal an ulcer. Try foods such as oysters, tripe, shellfish, oatmeal, aloe vera, slippery elm, pig's feet, okra, and cactus (peeled).

- If your ulcer is giving you a lot of pain, try pureed soup or baby food until you can take more demanding meals.

Remedies

- Drink 50 ml (less for children) of aloe vera juice, morning and night. Aloe contains mucopolysaccharides, and will soothe and heal an angry ulcer or inflamed stomach wall.

- Slippery elm cannot be surpassed. Its gentle slipperiness is just the thing for healing. Slippery elm doesn't linger, so take a teaspoon three times a day before meals. When things have calmed down, take once daily. (Powder is best here, rather than tablets.)

- Take a good probiotic each morning. This will help reduce the *H. pylori* population and is absolutely vital to take after any antibiotics to restore harmony to the microbial population of your stomach. The bugs that have thus far been proven to be helpful against Mr. *H. pylorus* are *L. rhamnosus GG, lactobacillus casei,* and *Johnsonii La1*. No doubt as research continues, more probiotics will be added to this list, but in the meantime, take a supplement containing at least one of these guys in addition to including probiotic food in your diet.

❑ Traditional herbal formulations for peptic ulcers contain antibiotic herbs such as goldenseal and calendula, as well as soothing and other healing herbs like licorice, chickweed, chamomile, meadowsweet, and marshmallow root.

❑ Vitamin A and zinc will help heal the damaged mucous membranes.

❑ The amino acid glutamine increases cell replication and aids healing, particularly of the mucous membrane lining of the digestive tract.

Other

❑ Stop smoking.

❑ Stop stress. Or at least find ways to manage your stress levels. Meditation, scrabble, quitting the job you hate, making a tree change.

AT A GLANCE

Depending on the severity of your condition, it might be necessary to take a course of triple-therapy medicine. The following suggestions can help relieve symptoms, assist healing, and prevent a recurrence.

DIET

➨ Avoid alcohol. It irritates the lining of the stomach.

➨ Avoid any food that causes you pain.

➨ Try a soothie (see above).

➨ Avoid sugar.

➨ Cabbage contains S-methyl methionine that stimulates healing to the stomach lining.

➨ Eat probiotic foods to restore microbial harmony in your stomach.

REMEDIES

➨ Aloe vera juice will soothe and heal inflamed and ulcerated tissue.

➨ Slippery elm is superb for any digestive inflammation.

➨ To reduce *H. pyloruses* and hold and restore microbial harmony, take a good probiotic each morning.

➨ Herbs are excellent for healing inflamed and distressed mucous membranes: Goldenseal, calendula, licorice, chickweed, chamomile, meadowsweet, and marshmallow.

➨ The amino acid glutamine increases cell replication and aids healing.

OTHER

➨ Stop smoking.

➨ Deploy all your stress-management tools.

PREGNANCY

A good diet and healthy lifestyle before and during pregnancy is all you need to make a healthy baby. However, some people like to tick every box, and then some. If you have the luxury of time, start implementing positive health changes three months before you plan to conceive. Following are some tips to help baby and mom during these interesting and exciting months of pregnancy, and also some advice on preconception care for Dad. The herbs and supplements recommended below are safe to take during pregnancy.

WHAT TO DO

Diet

❏ Even before your baby is a glint in anyone's eye, antioxidants can help improve the health of both sperm and egg. Antioxidants are found in good food. Naturally colored fruit and vegetables are best. Employ the old adage "eat like a rainbow," ensuring a broad range of antioxidants as each of the different colors bring their own addition to the table, literally. Think broccoli, beetroot, pumpkin, carrots, kale, Asian greens, rocket, berries, red grapes (including the seed), turmeric, and green tea.

❏ Fish and seafood. An excellent source of omega-3 fatty acids and protein, but also one of the few reliable sources of iodine.

❏ One for the guys. Omega-3 fatty acids, especially EPA and DHA, are especially needed for the healthy development of the nervous system, as well as cognition and eyesight in babies. They also increase movement and flexibility of the sperm, which makes swimming to their destination easier. Sources high in omega-3 include chia seeds, walnuts, and fish. Avoid fish that may contain high levels of mercury, such as swordfish, shark, and bluefin tuna. (Most tuna sold in tins and in general is yellowfin, and is not a great mercury risk.) This warning applies to men as well as women.

If either parent is allergic to fish or does not like it, or are vegetarian, then omega-3-rich algae supplementation is recommended.

Alcohol

The general recommendation prior to pregnancy (for women) is a maximum of one to two glasses a day and none during pregnancy. The time of most risk to the baby is the first few weeks after conception, which is often the time many women don't even realize they may be pregnant. For this reason, it is best to go easy if you are planning to have a baby.

Fetal alcohol syndrome is one of the potential risks for the baby, but this mainly occurs when the mother drinks a large amount of alcohol, not a glass or two, so don't beat yourself up if you find out you are pregnant after drinking a glass of champers. After all, women in Italy and France routinely have a glass or two of wine with meals throughout their pregnancies, and there is no evidence that their babies have suffered.

Remedies

❏ Folic acid (also known as folate) is often recommended as a preconception vitamin, as if it is deficient in the diet, the baby has a slightly higher risk of having spina bifida (a condition where the spinal column does not fully develop). Although this deficiency has been well researched, it makes sense that all the essential vitamins and minerals are necessary for the health of the unborn baby.

❏ For women, I recommend taking a good multivitamin before pregnancy, during, and while breast-feeding. Look for one that contains at least 400 micrograms (mcg) or 400 mcg folic acid, iodine, and zinc. In addition, take extra fish oil and calcium later in the pregnancy.

❏ Mom needs magnesium, especially in the last trimester when leg and back aches are worse. It can also make for an easier birth.

❏ Both parents need to check their vitamin D status, and take this vitamin if deficient or on the low side of normal.

❏ For fathers, take a male multivitamin daily with added fish oil and zinc as you need these in greater amounts than can be supplied by the multi.

❏ Iodine is required by the thyroid glands to produce thyroid hormones. A deficiency of iodine during pregnancy may result in poor physical and mental development of the baby, and worst-case scenario is cretinism. If the soil is deficient in iodine, so will the food that is grown in it. Government public policy has been to add iodine to salt; however, with the rise of gourmet salts, which do not contain iodine, iodine deficiency has become more common. Seaweed, seafood, and eggs contain iodine. Try 220 mcg during pregnancy, and 270 mcg while breast-feeding.

❏ Iron is necessary for hemoglobin to carry oxygen around the body and to the unborn baby. Iron is not necessary to take *unless* a blood test has shown that you are low. However, if you are low in iron, a supplement is a must. If you become constipated taking regular iron tablets, the herbal iron tonics are good and do not cause this side effect.

❏ The omega-3 fatty acids EPA and DHA are pretty much only found in seafood. They are required for a healthy nervous system, cogni-

tion, and eyesight. If you don't plan on eating three servings of fish each week, it is a good idea to take a supplement containing these nutrients. Try 1 to 2 grams daily.

Men

❏ For years, it has been an assumption that a woman's health is the only focus for the health of a baby. However, recent research has shown that the father's health, or at least the health of his sperm, is at least as important as mom's. Testes produce sperm at a rate of 100 million per day in a healthy male, with 85 million sperm per ml of semen. The process from go to "whoa there" takes approximately 75 days. If you are not as healthy as you could be, and you are planning a baby, this gives you around three months to clean up your act.

❏ There are many male multivitamin tablets available that contain all the nutrients mentioned below. The well-known preconception vitamin for women, folate, which is responsible for cell division, is also essential for sperm development.

❏ Zinc is vital for sperm production and the creation of testosterone.

❏ Ever since the late 1970s, vitamin C has been known and recommended to improve sperm formation and viability.

❏ Selenium, a mineral and antioxidant in short supply in many soils, has been found in several studies to increase sperm motility and protect sperm from free-radical damage.

❏ L-carnitine can also be useful, especially for healthy fatty-acid production that can help create healthy sperm.

❏ Omega-3 fatty acids are important for sperm health. If you don't eat a lot of fish, it is worth taking a supplement of 2 to 3 grams of fish oil daily. A multivitamin cannot supply this quantity without the tablet becoming humungous.

Women

❏ A good female multivitamin containing folic acid, zinc, and iodine in addition to 2 to 3 grams of fish oil is recommended, as is 1,000 mg of calcium in the last trimester and during breast-feeding.

SOME COMMON CONDITIONS DURING PREGNANCY

Reflux

❏ Reflux is a common symptom of pregnancy, particularly as the baby grows and presses on the stomach. Eat smaller meals and take a teaspoon of slippery elm powder before each meal.

❏ The herbs meadowsweet, peppermint, chamomile, and ginger are also helpful for reflux and are absolutely fine to be taken during pregnancy. Take a few drops of tincture in water before meals or drink in a cup of herbal tea after each meal.

Constipation

❏ The hormone progesterone increases during pregnancy and has the effect of slowing down the movement of the bowel. This explains why many women experience constipation even quite early in their pregnancy. The upside of this slower movement is the increased absorption of minerals such as zinc and iron.

❏ Take 2 to 3 tablespoons of psyllium husks daily and increase water consumption to 2 liters daily.

Hemorrhoids and varicose veins

❏ Piles and varicose veins are basically the same thing, just located in different parts of the body. They occur when veins become distended and engorged. There is nearly always a genetic tendency, and being pregnant can force the issue.

❏ Hemorrhoids may occur during and often after a natural delivery. Take a teaspoon of slippery elm powder twice a day. It can help heal the area. The gentle fiber slippery elm comes into its own in the treatment of piles. Take three tablets or a teaspoonful of the powder each night. If you have a stubborn case of piles, slippery elm powder should become part of your life.

❏ Psyllium husks are a soluble fiber supplement that will keep the stool soft and easy to pass, without aggravating the pile. Take two tablespoons daily, along with a large glass of water.

❏ For varicose veins in particular, if possible, avoid standing for extended periods of time. Don't cross your legs. Exercise regularly; swimming is particularly good. At some time each day, but best at the end of the day, lie with your legs elevated, up the wall if you are able, allowing blood to circulate back to the heart.

❏ Eat foods containing the bioflavoids including the pith of citrus fruits, cherries, berries, rye, rosehip tea, and buckwheat.

❏ Quercetin and rutin are bioflavonoids, both excellent for healing and repairing veins. Quercetin relieves inflammation, while rutin acts to strengthen blood vessel walls.

❏ Calcium fluoride (calc. fluor.) and silicea are tissue salts that are good for strengthening vein walls. Take before and during pregnancy.

Morning sickness

❏ Morning sickness may occur at any time of the day, and although it usually abates by the end of the first trimester, it can last the full term. Take heart—there is some evidence to suggest that morning sickness means a healthy baby and less likelihood of miscarriage.

❏ Eat small meals regularly, including *before* you get out of bed in the morning. Try a plain arrowroot biscuit or a slice of dry toast on your bedside table to nibble before you get up.

❏ Ginger is very effective. Take as a tea or tablets every day.

❏ Raspberry leaf tea or in tablet form is often recommended later in the pregnancy, but is also effective for morning sickness.

Other

❏ Lose excess pounds before becoming pregnant. Apart from the fact that being overweight makes it more difficult to conceive (for men and women), many women put on more than the recommended 26 pounds per pregnancy. Overweight can increase risk of high blood pressure and diabetes during pregnancy.

❏ Quit smoking.

❏ For optimal sperm motility and production, testicular temperature should be somewhat lower than body temperature. For this reason (and to be fashion-forward) ditch those tight-fitting pants and underwear.

AT A GLANCE

Good Food

➟ Eat plenty of vegetables, fruit, and protein.

➟ Avoid alcohol.

Remedies

➟ Lose weight.

➟ Stop smoking.

➟ Stress less, and guys, loosen those pants!

➟ Don't rush this stage of your life. It is a time to enjoy.

PREMENSTRUAL SYNDROME (PMS)

WHAT IS IT?

"It must be that time of the month" is the derisive comment offered by some men in response to a woman who is teary or irritable. Perhaps she is just teary or irritable, but the truth is, it could actually be that time of the month when a woman's hormones are in flux. Nevertheless, he is a thoughtless fool for saying so, and deserves that dirty look.

For some women, the premenstrual time sees them change from feeling in control and calm, to being strapped in the front seat of an emotional rollercoaster. Of course this does not mean that women are less able to achieve tasks or make important decisions, it's just a tad more difficult when you are managing hormonal hijinks as well.

The premenstrual body is a vulnerable body. Your pain threshold is lower—don't get your legs waxed. Your immune system is under par—the perfect time to catch a cold. Your vaginal pH changes—thrush is more likely to appear. It is not only the physical body that is more vulnerable; your emotions are also tested at this time.

Premenstrual syndrome (PMS) occurs in the second half of the menstrual cycle, during the luteal phase, anywhere from two weeks to the day before your period. Symptoms of PMS were first described in the medical literature in 1931, and for many years, the diagnosis was scoffed at by the medical fraternity.

A woman's menstrual cycle averages 29.5 days—a lunar month. If you are not sure how long your cycle is, keep a track of dates in your diary. Officially, the day your period starts is day 1. Midway through, ovulation occurs, and the last day of the cycle is day 29. This is "average," but it is perfectly normal to have a cycle slightly longer or shorter than this. PMS is the collective name for the 200 symptoms that may occur in any combination, the most common mentioned below. Premenstrual symptoms resolve during the first couple of days of your period.

SYMPTOMS

- ☑ Swollen breasts
- ☑ Pelvic discomfort, a dragging or cramping pain
- ☑ Change in bowel habits, often a looser bowel movement
- ☑ Headaches
- ☑ Weight gain
- ☑ Pimples
- ☑ Swelling of hands, ankles, and feet
- ☑ Back and leg pain
- ☑ Food cravings, often for chocolate or starches
- ☑ Fatigue
- ☑ Insomnia
- ☑ Anxiety
- ☑ Mood swings
- ☑ Depression
- ☑ Irritability
- ☑ Lack of concentration
- ☑ A subgroup of PMS is premenstrual dysphoric disorder, or PMDD. For up to 8 percent of women, their PMS time is characterized by very severe mood changes including depression, anger, and anxiety.
- ☑ The PMS time often sees a worsening of already existing conditions such as IBS, headaches, and herpes (cold sores and genital herpes).

WHAT CAUSES IT?

Up to 90 percent of women experience one or more symptoms of PMS. The actual cause is unknown, but an imbalance between estrogen and progesterone is a likely hypothesis.

WHAT TO DO

❏ PMS responds very well to natural remedies. It may take a couple of cycles for symptoms to respond, and up to four cycles for significant improvements.

Diet

❏ Women who eat a plant-based diet suffer less from PMS than meat-eating women do. So eat plenty of fruits, vegetables, whole grains, and legumes.

❏ Reduce dairy.

❏ Increase foods containing soluble fiber including legumes, vegetables, and chia seeds. Soluble fiber can stop excess estrogen from recirculating.

❏ Eat fish four times a week to provide the omega-3 fatty acid EPA that will help ease the inflammatory symptoms of PMS.

❏ Cut out all sugar, salt, and white flour products. A study revealed that women with PMS consumed 75 percent more refined sugar, and 62 percent more white flour products than did women without PMS. It also found that women with PMS consume 79 percent more sodium.

❏ Reduce caffeine (including coffee, cola, chocolate, guarana) all month, and cut it out midway through your cycle. The xanthines in coffee and chocolate have an effect on estrogen receptors in the breasts, contributing to breast tenderness and enlargement. Caffeine also increases PMS irritability.

❏ Drink dandelion root coffee instead. Dandelion root is good for the liver, which helps excrete excess hormones.

❏ If your PMS symptoms include cravings for sweet foods, mood changes, or forgetfulness, eat small meals frequently to steady blood sugar levels. Each meal should contain a little protein.

Remedies

❏ Vitex agnus-castus is a natural for PMS as it helps smooth hormonal regularities. Take a dose every morning throughout the month.

❏ Other herbs helpful for normalizing hormones include paeonia, dong quai, and false unicorn root.

❏ If you suffer an angsty time premenstrually, St. John's wort, passionflower, kava, and pulsatilla can prove useful.

❏ There are several good "women's formulation" multivitamin and mineral supplement tablets available specifically for PMS. They have higher amounts of B_6, magnesium, and zinc. Take a tablet daily until ovulation, then double the dose until your period arrives.

❏ Magnesium helps relieve breast tenderness, weight gain, fatigue, anxiety, cramping, and nervous tension. Take extra magnesium, twice a day for two weeks prior to your period.

❏ If you crave chocolate and starches, take a supplement containing chromium, gymnema, zinc, and B vitamins.

❏ Take vitamin E every day throughout the month. Vitamin E will relieve breast tenderness and normalize hormones.

❏ Evening primrose oil (EPO) can be very successful in relieving many of the symptoms of PMS. It contains gamma-linoleic acid (GLA) that is converted in the body into hormone-regulating prostaglandins. In order to be effective, GLA needs to be incorporated into every cell, which is why you need to take EPO for several months.

❑ If you suffer from premenstrual fluid retention, vitamin B_6, dandelion leaf, and the tissue salt natrum sulphate (nat. sulph.) can be helpful.

Other

❑ Women who partake of regular aerobic exercise have less PMS symptoms than women who don't. However, ease up the intensity a couple of days before and during your period.

❑ Massage can help relieve fluid retention and premenstrual pain.

❑ There is often no smoke without fire. In the time before the period everything in the body is more vulnerable. Whatever the emotions you feel in the PMS days, whether it be sadness, irritability, or murderous rage, they are magnified versions of what is happening the rest of the month, only you are no longer able to keep these feelings under wraps. Rather than ignoring these "out of control" feelings, try to figure out what might be happening for you. In the cold light of day (after your period), perhaps you could analyze whether there is any substance to your feelings, instead of brushing them off as PMS dramatics. Counseling can also be helpful.

❑ The Bach flower Walnut may be helpful at this time as it protects against outside influences, just the thing if you are feeling vulnerable. Mustard can help if you feel more depressed at this time, and Willow or Holly may fit the bill if you feel resentful and angry.

❑ For many women with busy work and family commitments, it is difficult to tune in to your body's rhythms. However, the premenstrual time can be quite rewarding if you can manage to slow down, listen, and feel. As your feelings are heightened, so too is your awareness, and we can be more sensitive to deeper insights, both emotionally and spiritually. It is a time of reflection. Don't push yourself. Now is not the time for hard physical exercise; stay with stretching and walking.

❑ PMS is an opportunity for some "gentling" activities like meditating, soaking in a hot lavender bath with candlelight, or writing in your diary.

AROMATHERAPY

The following blend can be used for a full body massage when blended in 20 ml of almond oil. Try an abdominal massage beginning up to a week before the onset of menstruation, or in a bath combined with Epsom salts, or as a personal perfume in jojoba oil.

❑ 3 drops of clary sage oil—excellent uterine tonic, regulator of irregular menstruation, easer of painful cramping in the lower abdominal area; it's great for easing tension and anxiety while uplifting in cases of depression

❑ 3 drops of geranium oil—helps in the balancing of hormones; it can also help in cases of menstruation-related depression and decongestion of the breasts by utilizing its diuretic properties along with its ability in relieving inflammation

❑ 2 drops of rose otto—warming, comforting, and uplifting on the emotions enabling stress relief; it is a stimulating tonic for the uterus with calming and regulating properties

❑ 2 drops of neroli oil—wonderfully uplifting to the mood, tonifying on the nervous system, and an antispasmodic aiding in uterine discomfort

AT A GLANCE

Diet

⟹ Avoid red meat and dairy foods (except plain yogurt), and eat more fruit and vegetables, whole grains, and legumes.

⟹ Cut out all sugar, salt, and white flour products. They add to your premenstrual distress by increasing fluid retention.

⟹ Reduce caffeine (including coffee, cola, chocolate, guarana) as it has an effect on estrogen receptors in the breasts, contributing to breast tenderness and enlargement.

⟹ To reduce premenstrual craving of chocolate and carbohydrates, eat a small meal or snack that contains some protein every two to three hours.

Remedies

⟹ The best herb for PMS is vitex agnus-castus as it helps to regulate hormones.

⟹ If you find yourself depressed or anxious at this time, take St. John's wort, passionflower, kava, and/or pulsatilla.

⟹ Take a multivitamin specially formulated for PMS that contains B$_6$, magnesium, and zinc.

⟹ If you experience cramping, headaches, and backache, take extra magnesium.

⟹ Evening primrose oil (EPO) helps with many of the symptoms of PMS. You need to take it consistently for best results.

Other

⟹ Regular aerobic exercise reduces all symptoms of PMS. Take out a gym membership, jog in the park or join a sports team.

⟹ If you find yourself more angry, irritable or depressed at this time, it could be worthwhile to book a few sessions with a counselor to see if there are any underlying issues that bubble up at this time.

⟹ Your body is more vulnerable too. Treat yourself gently and try having long soaks in the bath or watching soppy DVDs.

PROSTATE ISSUES

WHAT IS IT?

The prostate, a small organ about the size of a walnut that snugly fits at the base of a man's bladder, is involved in providing and storing 70 percent of the fluid that makes up semen. A large proportion of men over sixty years of age develop benign prostatic hyperplasia (BPH), an enlargement of this gland. When the prostate reaches a certain size, it may partly or completely block the outlet from the bladder, causing untold problems in the plumbing department. Benign prostatic hyperplasia does not cause prostate cancer, but men at risk of BPH are also at risk of this common cancer. The treatments offered below will reduce your risk of both conditions and are also helpful for inflammation of the prostate, prostatitis.

SYMPTOMS

✓ Interrupted flow and force of urination

✓ Getting up to urinate during the night

✓ Urgent need to urinate

✓ Incomplete voiding of the bladder

✓ Dripping after urination

WHAT CAUSES IT?

❑ It is not certain why this enlargement happens, although it seems likely that there are hormonal influences, possibly an increase in estrogen. (Men have some estrogen, just as women have some testosterone.)

❑ You have an increased risk of developing BPH if you also have diabetes type 2, or increased insulin levels.

❑ High blood pressure also increases your risk of BPH.

❑ BPH is associated with being exposed to heavy-metal toxicity such as chromium, pesticides, and other chemicals.

❑ There is some evidence that BPH is an autoimmune condition.

WHAT TO DO

Diet

❑ The two groups of men with the lowest incidence of BPH are the Japanese who eat a traditional diet, and vegetarian men. Clearly you are on a lucky streak if you are a vegetarian Japanese male.

❑ A diet high in animal fats increases your risk, so decrease red meat, deli meats, and high-fat dairy such as cream, ice cream, camembert, and yellow cheeses.

❑ Caffeine is a urinary system irritant. Decrease or avoid all caffeine including coffee, cola, chocolate, guarana, and tea (except some green tea).

❑ Decrease sugar and refined carbohydrates to decrease your risk of diabetes, itself a risk factor for BPH.

❑ Eat some baked tomatoes with your scrambled eggs. Lycopene, an antioxidant found in tomatoes, helps prevent BPH. Lycopene levels increase when the tomatoes are cooked, so tomato paste is also on the menu. Fancy some spaghetti Napolitana?

❑ Increase zinc-rich foods including oysters, seafood, pumpkin seeds, sunflower seeds, leafy green vegetables, and barley.

❑ Even though you might be tripping to the toilet more often, don't let this stop you drinking sufficient water (2 liters of fluids daily).

❑ Eat tofu and tempeh as they contain daidzein

and genistein, substances that can help decrease the risk of prostate (and breast) cancer.

❑ Green tea offers protective properties against BPH.

❑ Avoid beer. It contains hops, which have an estrogenic effect. Australia is an enthusiastic beer-drinking country—and has one of the highest rates of prostate disease.

Remedies

❑ Herbal remedies are very effective for BPH. Old herbal texts refer to saw palmetto as the "old man's friend," and it is the star herb when it comes to treating and preventing BPH. Other herbs good for prostate health and prevention of BPH are pygeum, nettle root, and epilobium. Crataeva is an excellent herb for bladder irritation, which is often affected due to the proximity of the prostate gland.

❑ Zinc supplementation is recommended to help reduce the size of the prostate gland.

❑ The amino acids L-glycine, L-alanine, and glutamine have shown in scientific studies to reduce the feelings of urgency to urinate as well as frequency of urination.

❑ Selenium and the B group vitamins are also helpful in reducing BPH.

Other

❑ Men who exercise regularly have less risk of BPH. Additionally, exercise decreases the other risk factors for BPH, diabetes and high blood pressure.

❑ Regular ejaculation is important for prostate health.

❑ A yoga posture that encourages circulation to the prostate is to lie flat on your back, bring your knees in, and put the soles of your feet together. Hold on to each shin with your hands and pull your heels towards your stomach. You may look like a recently sprayed cockroach, but don't let this dissuade you.

AT A GLANCE

DIET

➡ Eat less red meat and animal fats. That will leave you with more vegetables, whole grains, and legumes.

➡ Caffeine is an irritant to the urinary system, so reduce your intake of coffee, tea, cola, and chocolate.

➡ Reduce sugar and refined flour products; this will decrease your risk of diabetes, which in turn decreases your risk of BPD.

➡ Increase zinc-rich foods including oysters, seafood, pumpkin seeds, sunflower seeds, leafy green vegetables, and barley.

REMEDIES

➡ Saw palmetto is an important herb when it comes to preventing and treating BPH. Other good choices include pygeum, nettle root, and epilobium.

➡ Take a daily zinc tablet.

➡ Selenium and the B group vitamins are also helpful in reducing BPH.

OTHER

➡ Regular exercise reduces your risk of prostate problems.

PSORIASIS

WHAT IS IT?

Psoriasis is a common skin condition that affects two to three in every 100 people. It is an autoimmune condition whereby the skin cells divide faster than normal, resulting in a thickening of the skin and silvery scales. Some people may have a little patch that appears only when they are stressed, whereas other poor souls may be covered from top to toe with itchy, white scales. Eczema and psoriasis are often confused; however, psoriasis usually visits the knobby bits of elbows and knees, whereas eczema is more likely to affect the inner bends. Psoriasis also often visits the scalp and shins. Psoriatic arthritis can appear along with psoriasis. Treating the psoriasis can also help the arthritis.

SYMPTOMS

- ☑ Thickened salmon-pink to red skin

- ☑ Flaky, silver-white scales

- ☑ Itchy and irritated patches of skin

- ☑ Areas often affected include the scalp, elbows, knees, shins, torso.

- ☑ Nail changes can include thickened nails, nails with yellow-brown discoloration, and pitting of the nails that looks like pinpricks.

- ☑ Can be associated with psoriatic arthritis

WHAT CAUSES IT?

- ❏ In around 50 percent of cases, there is a family history of psoriasis.

- ❏ Psoriasis is often triggered by stress. Other triggers include trauma to the skin including cuts, burns, sunburn, and insect bites.

- ❏ Allergies may be a factor. Gluten is the first food to suspect.

- ❏ One naturopathic view is that psoriasis is due to a "leaky gut." A "leaky" gut or bowel is when toxic substances are absorbed into the bloodstream from the bowel. Leaky gut is also thought to be a major cause of food allergy.

- ❏ In addition to a leaky gut, it is likely that you have a dodgy liver too. Although this sounds dire, a "naturopathically dodgy" liver is nothing to be too alarmed by. We like our livers to be squeaky clean. Just treating your liver with TLC can likely result in improvement for your psoriasis. Avoiding alcohol, reducing fatty foods, and drinking lemon juice each morning is plenty of TLC.

- ❏ There is nearly always a candida overgrowth in those with psoriasis. Possibly due to the leaky gut scenario.

WHAT TO DO

Diet

- ❏ The forbidden foursome: sugar, alcohol, coffee, and red meat. Avoiding them entirely is very important as well as very effective. The foursome are generally enough to bid psoriasis adieu, but sometimes dairy avoidance will do the trick. So make that a fivesome.

- ❏ As the yeast *Candida albicans* often cohabits with psoriasis, in addition to avoiding sugar and alcohol as recommended above, reduce yeasted foods such as Vegemite, Marmite, bread, and yellow and blue cheese. (See Candida on page 73.)

- ❏ A plant-based diet will serve you well. However, if you don't want to go the whole hog (or in this case the whole hazelnut), adding fish to your diet will provide the anti-inflammatory omega-3 fatty acids your skin will love.

- A diet high in soluble fiber, including legumes, whole grains, fruit, and vegetables, can improve intestinal flora and reduce bowel toxins.

- Drink the juice of half a lemon in hot water first thing each morning to aid the bowel and liver.

- Drink at least 2 liters of pure water daily. It is always recommended to drink plenty of water with any skin condition as the skin is the largest organ of elimination.

- Reduce animal fats and deep-fried foods.

Remedies

- Herbs work particularly well in the treatment of psoriasis, especially St. Mary's thistle, sarsaparilla, coleus, Oregon grape, gotu kola, burdock, red clover, and fumitory. These herbs are generally good for the skin and liver. Take one or a combination of these herbs in tea, tablet, or tincture form three times a day.

- Cod-liver oil combines vitamins A and D. Both vitamins are necessary for normal cell growth, which isn't happening in the case of psoriasis where cells are growing in a topsy-turvy fashion.

- Evening primrose oil is an excellent supplement for psoriasis. It is anti-inflammatory, and so good for skin conditions. Heavy-handed dosages work best.

- B_{12} and folate can also help in cell differentiation and growth. They are also methyl donors, which are recommended in any autoimmune condition as they help "turn off" the genetic switch that codes for this disease.

- The minerals zinc and selenium can help in the treatment of psoriasis.

- The topical application of creams containing selenium, B_{12}, vitamin D, gotu kola, lavender oil, aloe vera, and/or evening primrose oil can be helpful.

- A good daily probiotic will help restore microbial balance and treat your leaky gut.

- Check your vitamin D levels. If they are low, catch some rays and take a supplement.

- If psoriasis is in your scalp, wash your hair with an antidandruff shampoo that contains selenium.

Other

- Sunshine is an effective and inexpensive treatment for psoriasis, particularly so when combined with seawater. If you are lucky enough to live near the ocean, take a walk in the sun by the seaside several times a week. Make sure you splash seawater on your skin. It is the UVB rays that are so healing. No need to get sunburnt, just reveal your skin to the gentle rays of the sun as often as you can. There are also UVB sunlamps available.

- Magic psoriasis cure stories abound from people who have swum in the Dead Sea in Israel. If Israel is not on your travel plans, there are products made from the salts derived from there.

- Dry skin is an invitation for a visitation from any skin condition you are predisposed to. Keep your skin well moisturized even when you are not suffering an outbreak of psoriasis.

- Avoid soap and wash with a stocking filled with oats.

- As stress is a major trigger, deal with it.

AROMATHERAPY

Mix 5 ml of cold-pressed avocado oil and 5 ml of borage oil with 20 grams of unscented vitamin E cream, and massage into the affected area at least twice daily then use as needed. The following blend can also be used with Dead Sea salts in a full bath as an allover general method.

❏ 5 drops of lavender oil—antimicrobial, antiseptic, nervine, immune defense, and vulnerary

❏ 3 drops of tea tree oil—antiseptic, anti-inflammatory, and vulnerary

❏ 4 drops of cajeput oil—antimicrobial, carminative, and antineuralgic

❏ 2 drops of Virginian cedar wood oil—antiseborrheic, antiseptic, balsamic, and astringent

AT A GLANCE

Diet

➺ Avoid sugar, alcohol, coffee, and red meat. Do this, and you will be a long way down the path to being psoriasis-free. If your psoriasis does not completely clear with this combination, add dairy to the mix.

➺ Drink the juice of half a lemon in hot water first thing each morning to aid the bowel and liver.

➺ Avoid fatty and deep-fried foods.

Remedies

➺ Vitamins A and D are required for normal cell growth. Cod liver oil combines both of these vitamins.

➺ If you are low in vitamin D, take a supplement. The amount present in cod liver oil is insufficient to boost low levels.

➺ Evening primrose oil has anti-inflammatory properties that are particularly effective in skin complaints such as psoriasis.

➺ Zinc and selenium can help.

➺ Keep the skin well moisturized. After each shower, apply a cream containing selenium, B_{12}, vitamin D, gotu kola, lavender oil, aloe vera, and/or evening primrose oil.

➺ Take a good probiotic each day.

Other

➺ Sunshine and seawater are a lovely combination at any time, and just happen to help psoriasis. UVB sunlamps are available if sunshine is in short supply.

➺ If you find stress a trigger, as many do, find some solace in meditation, counseling, or belly breathing (see Stress, page 276).

REFLUX

WHAT IS IT?

Reflux, commonly known as heartburn, strikes in the chest, and can feel frighteningly like a heart attack. Known medically as gastroesophageal disease (GORD, or Oh Gawd), it occurs when the stomach contents (both food and liquid) leak out of the stomach and up into the esophagus. The issue is not an excess of stomach acid, although it may feel that way, but with a defect in the closing of the esophageal sphincter that separates the stomach from the esophagus. By design, the sphincter should keep a tight seal, only allowing food and drink to travel in a downward direction, not the reverse.

SYMPTOMS

☑ A feeling of food being stuck or a lump behind the sternum (breastbone)

☑ A burning or acidic sensation in the sternum and up into the throat

☑ Symptoms are usually worse after meals, particularly large ones, when leaning forward or lying down, and late at night.

☑ Unexplained cough

☑ Hoarseness of the voice

☑ Sore throat

☑ When the reflux is asymptomatic, or you are unaware of its occurrence (i.e., there are no symptoms), it is called silent reflux. Although you may feel no discomfort, this condition needs to be resolved as constant erosion of the tender mucous membrane cells lining the esophagus, known as Barrett's esophagitis, increases one's risk of cancer in this part of the body.

WHAT CAUSES IT?

❑ Many women experience reflux during pregnancy. This is due in part to the hormones that relax smooth muscle (in this case the esophageal sphincter), and also later in the pregnancy due to the upward pressure from baby on the stomach.

❑ A hiatus hernia can often cause reflux. A hiatus hernia is when part of the stomach is forced through a small opening (a hiatus) in the diaphragm into the chest.

❑ Reflux is a common symptom of that old friend, stress.

❑ Food triggers include alcohol, chocolate, coffee, spicy foods, tomatoes, capsicums, cucumbers, and citrus fruits.

❑ Smoking.

❑ Obesity.

❑ Peppermint is usually the recipient of rave reviews for any digestive disorder; however, for some people, peppermint can relax the esophageal sphincter and trigger reflux. It's moments like these when you don't need a mint.

❑ The bacteria often responsible for stomach ulcers, *Helicobacter pylorus* (*H. pylorus*), may also be responsible for reflux.

❑ Some medications have reflux as a side effect. Check with your doctor.

❑ Gluten sensitivity may be the cause.

WHAT TO DO

Diet

❏ Become acquainted with your triggers and avoid them.

❏ While you're off your coffee and alcohol, why not drink herbal teas that help reflux instead, like licorice, chamomile, meadowsweet, and lemon balm. Ginger is excellent for reflux, helping the stomach to empty downward, the correct direction. Add ginger to your meals or drink as a tea.

❏ Eat small meals; large meals can be a common trigger for reflux.

❏ Eating when stressed or in a hurry increases the chance of reflux. Take your time over your meal and chew each mouthful well.

❏ Avoid drinking more than a glass of fluids during, half an hour before, and an hour after larger meals.

❏ If there does not appear to be any other good reason for your reflux, avoid gluten for four weeks, and see if this improves symptoms.

Remedies

❏ Slippery elm is an absolute must when treating reflux. It soothes and heals. Take a teaspoon of slippery elm powder before or with each meal, mashed with a little yogurt or banana or in hot water. Slippery elm powder is better for this condition than slippery elm capsules or tablets as the medicine needs to come into direct contact with the inflamed mucous membranes.

❏ The herbal teas mentioned above are terrific remedies for relieving the symptoms of reflux and soothing the mucous membranes of the esophagus. In addition, calendula and goldenseal are excellent healers of inflammation.

❏ Glutamine is an amino acid that has an excellent reputation for preventing damage to and repairing cells lining the intestine, including the esophagus.

❏ Aloe vera is anti-inflammatory and helps heal ulcerations. Take 10 ml of aloe juice before each meal.

❏ Zinc is a mineral necessary for healing. Combine it with vitamin A for healing mucous membranes.

❏ The tissue salt, calcium fluoride (calc. fluor.), taken twice daily can, after some months, strengthen the esophageal sphincter. This is particularly helpful for hiatus hernia.

❏ If your reflux is caused by *H. pylorus,* a good probiotic supplement taken each morning can help. Also, get this checked out and treated by your doctor, with triple therapy if necessary, as infection by *H. pylorus* may result in a peptic ulcer (see Peptic Ulcer, page 250).

Other

❏ To stop reflux from troubling you at night, elevate the head of the bed six inches or so. Try a couple of books under each bed leg. Some people find that sleeping on their left side helps.

❏ If stress is a trigger for your reflux, learn to manage your stress levels.

❏ Lose weight if necessary.

❏ Stop smoking.

DIET

⇒ Avoid foods that may trigger reflux such as alcohol, chocolate, coffee, spicy foods, tomatoes, capsicum, cucumbers, peppermint, and citrus fruits.

⇒ Certain herbal teas can be very calming for reflux, such as licorice, ginger, chamomile, meadowsweet, and lemon balm.

⇒ Tidy up your eating habits. Eat smaller meals, chew your food well, and avoid eating when stressed or too late at night.

⇒ Gluten sensitivity may be the cause of your reflux. Avoid gluten for four weeks and see if symptoms improve.

REMEDIES

⇒ The soothing and healing qualities of slippery elm powder makes this remedy a priority when treating reflux. Take a teaspoon of slippery elm powder before or with each meal, mashed with a little yogurt or banana or in hot water.

⇒ Herbal remedies for relief of reflux symptoms include lemon balm, licorice, chamomile, meadowsweet, ginger, and chamomile. Herbs for the healing of mucous membranes are calendula and goldenseal.

⇒ The amino acid glutamine is very good at repairing cell damage to the esophagus.

⇒ Aloe vera can help heal and calm inflamed mucous membranes. Take 10 ml aloe juice before each meal.

OTHER

⇒ Lose weight if necessary.

⇒ Stop smoking.

⇒ Stop stressing.

ROSACEA

WHAT IS IT?

Rosacea, from the Latin word *rosaceus,* meaning "rose-colored," describes the main feature of rosacea: rosy red skin. Sometimes known as acne rosacea or adult acne, rosacea is not related to pimples (acne vulgaris) even though there can be red bumps and lumps that may look a little similar. Rosacea becomes noticeable as small blood vessels (capillaries) become dilated and eventually burst, resulting in a constant state of redness.

Rosacea affects mainly light-skinned folk of Celtic and northern European origin, occurring mainly between the ages of thirty and fifty. It occurs more frequently in women but more severely in men. The redness can present as an attractive blush of the cheeks, but for some people, over time, the skin thickens, and small bumps and fluid-filled cysts can erupt. In extreme cases, the nose itself enlarges, creating the bulbous schnoz of a chronic boozer—without the years of drinking.

Although not a threat to health, rosacea can be an embarrassing condition causing some to avoid social situations, and may even lead to depression.

SYMPTOMS

☑ Redness affecting the central region of the face, most commonly cheeks, forehead, and lower half of the nose

☑ Bumps and thickening of skin, mainly over nose and cheeks

☑ On occasion, rosacea may affect the eyelids and eyes, causing inflammation, itching, and dryness.

☑ A tendency to blush or flush easily

WHAT CAUSES IT?

❏ Rosacea is a baffling condition. No one knows the cause; however, there is often a genetic link, with cases flaring up among various family members.

❏ There appears to be a connection between a small mite (*Demodex folliculorum*) that is commonly found in the hair follicles of rosacea sufferers. There are two possible scenarios. Firstly, the activity of the mites set up an inflammatory response in surrounding blood vessels, or the mites might convene after the skin is already inflamed.

❏ Another theory is that rosacea occurs due to an underfunctioning digestive system. In particular, hypochlorhydria, or low stomach acid. If you burp, bloat, and fart, improving your digestion may also improve your rosacea. A win–win situation.

❏ Although not causative, the following factors are common triggers of rosacea: strong sunlight, wind, cold, heat, humidity, hot drinks, alcohol, caffeine, spicy food, and stress.

WHAT TO DO

Diet

❏ Reduce dietary triggers such as spicy foods (especially chilies), caffeine, and alcohol.

❏ Drink your beverages warm rather than piping hot.

❏ Increase foods containing proanthocyanins, the type of bioflavonoids that strengthen capillary and other blood vessel walls. This will serve to reduce the progression of the condition and improve the appearance of your skin. Proanthocyanins are found in many foods but particularly apples, pears, red grapes (particularly skin and seeds), nuts, cocoa, green tea (drunk warm), cherries, and all berries.

❏ If you burp and bloat (signs of low stomach acid), eat bitter foods including cress, endives, radicchio, olives, and grapefruit.

❏ Try two teaspoons of apple cider vinegar (the best ones are with the "mother"—i.e., traditionally fermented vinegar that has not been filtered) with honey in warm water each morning. This is an excellent way to start the day, especially if your digestive system is under par.

Remedies

❏ One thing is clear: those fragile little blood vessels bear the brunt of rosacea, becoming irreparably broken after repeated dilation. The following supplements all serve to strengthen capillaries: quercetin, vitamin C, rutin, resveratrol, pine bark, and grapeseed extract.

❏ Herbs that help treat and prevent capillary fragility include horse chestnut, ginkgo biloba, bilberry, grapeseed, butcher's broom, and gotu kola, the great repairer of tissue.

❏ A combination of digestive enzymes and hydrochloric acid will assist a feeble digestive system. There are tablets that combine both. Take one before each meal.

❏ Another digestive remedy to boost stomach-acid production is old-fashioned herbal (or Swedish) bitters. Take one teaspoon of bitters in a small glass of water before dinner.

Remedies

❏ Avoid overheating the body as it will dilate the blood vessels and trigger rosacea. Choose gentle rather than vigorous exercise. Swimming is perfect.

❏ Saunas and steam rooms are no-go zones.

❏ The topical application of creams can address the problem externally. You also need to combat the condition by using natural antibiotic remedies to decimate the mites, as well as strengthen the integrity of capillary walls. Cal-endula, tea tree, and colloidal silver are antibiotic for mite control, while green tea, grapeseed, resveratrol, coenzyme Q_{10}, and gotu kola are capillary strengtheners. Search for face creams containing these ingredients. Or you may wish to use diluted colloidal silver as a toner between cleansing and moisturizing.

❏ Wear a hat in sunny weather, and try to protect your face from harsh cold and winds.

❏ If stress triggers rosacea, look at remedies and techniques to help, including meditation (see Stress, page 276).

❏ Rosacea sufferers often tend to be shy. If this describes you, and it affects your self-confidence, would you consider some counseling?

❏ If you are a shy person who easily blushes, the Bach flower Mimulus is for you.

At a Glance

Diet

➡ Reduce foods and dietary triggers that may set off an episode of rosacea.

➡ Proanthocyanins are bioflavonoids that strengthen capillary walls, thereby reducing the appearance and slowing down the progression of rosacea. Proanthocyanins are found in apples, pears, red grapes (particularly the skin and seeds), nuts, cocoa, green tea (drunk warm), cherries, and all berries.

Remedies

➡ Try supplements and herbs to strengthen capillaries (see above).

➡ Bloating and burping may be signs of low stomach acid. Take a combination of digestive enzymes and hydrochloric acid before each meal.

Other

➡ Avoid overheating the body with vigorous exercise, saunas, steam rooms, or going out in the noonday sun.

➡ Use facial creams that have an antibiotic action to control the mites, as well as creams that include capillary-strengthening substances.

➡ If you are shy and retiring and would prefer to be more extroverted, why not enroll in some self-assertiveness training or seek counseling.

AROMATHERAPY

Use this calming, soothing, cleansing, and restorative blend mixed with 30 grams of aloe vera gel as needed on cleansed skin.

❏ 2 drops of German chamomile oil—antiallergenic, analgesic, antibacterial, tissue repairing

❏ 2 drops of yarrow oil—anti-inflammatory, astringent, promotes healing, anti-itch

❏ 3 drops everlasting oil—anti-inflammatory, antimicrobial, antiseptic, blood purifying

❏ 5 drops of lavender oil—analgesic, antimicrobial, antitoxic, antiseptic, tonifying, and tissue repairing

❏ 3 drops of palmarosa oil—antiseptic, hydrating, stimulates circulation

SINUSITIS

WHAT IS IT?

It is always difficult to ignore pain, and it is almost impossible to ignore when the pain is literally "in your face." Which is why sinusitis is so horrible. The sinuses are hollow bones, as narrow as a pencil lead, situated within the skull. Lined with sensitive mucous membranes, the sinuses become swollen and secrete mucus in response to a trigger such as an allergy or a head cold. Since the sinus cavities are tiny, any buildup is bound to increase pressure and block fluid from draining away, causing the pain of sinusitis. What's worse is that these tiny stagnant rivers of mucus are begging to be sites of infection.

SYMPTOMS

✓ Headache, usually painful and often throbbing, behind and above the eyes. If you are unsure whether your headache is due to congested sinuses, press firmly with your fingertips on the eyebrows and cheekbones. If you squeak with pain at either location, your sinuses are most likely inflamed. The other giveaway is the headache is worse when you bend forward.

✓ Eyestrain and eye pain

✓ Swelling and puffiness under the eyes

✓ A congested honker

✓ Postnasal drip; mucus dripping down the back of throat

✓ Sore throat

✓ Bad breath

✓ Fatigue

✓ Loss of smell

WHAT CAUSES IT?

❏ A head cold is a common precursor to sinusitis. First the cold virus creates inflammation, and the subsequent mucus production creates an open invitation for bacteria to swan in and form a secondary bacterial infection.

❏ A mechanical deficiency in the nasal department such as a deviated septum means the sinuses are unable to drain adequately. Combine this with an allergic disposition, and you are bound to suffer from sinusitis. Surgery may be the best solution if bony bits are behind the blockage.

❏ Nasal polyps will also block the way for sinuses to drain. However, nasal polyps are as much a symptom of inflammation as a cause of sinusitis. If they are surgically removed, odds on, they will grow back. The treatment options below should sort it out.

❏ Some people are born with extra-narrow sinuses that clog easily when an allergy or cold occurs. If this is you, you need to always be mindful of this proclivity, and use some options below as preventative measures.

❏ Your chronically inflamed sinuses could be due to a fungal overgrowth. Quite probably in your home or environment, and possibly in your very person.

WHAT TO DO

Diet

❏ During a sinus attack, give alcohol a miss as it further swells mucous membranes.

❏ Drink at least 3 liters of clear fluids daily. This will help stop the mucus from becoming too thick, which is when it tends to become infected.

❏ Eat copious amounts of garlic and onions as they are mucolytic (they can break up mucus) and antibiotic (they can kill microbes).

❏ Other good foods include horseradish, chili, ginger, fenugreek, wasabi (Japanese green mustard), and nasturtiums (put the peppery leaves and pretty flowers in salads).

❏ Avoid dairy products and sugar for the duration of the attack; they both can increase mucus production.

❏ Your sinusitis might be due to a food allergy. First foods to suspect are dairy and wheat.

❏ If you suspect your sinusitis might be due to a fungal overgrowth, check this by having a look

at Candida on page 73. Following the candida diet may give you permanent relief.

❏ Increase foods high in vitamin C, a natural antihistamine, such as citrus, papaya, kiwifruit, strawberries, pineapple, guava, rock melon, broccoli, cauliflower, Brussels sprouts, and capsicum.

❏ There may be a link between a high-salt diet and sinusitis, as there is with hay fever and asthma. Reduce added salt and packaged food, which often has high levels of salt.

Remedies

❏ As part of your 3 liters of fluid (less for children), enjoy two to three cups of this therapeutic brew. In your favorite teapot, plunger, or thermos, combine the juice of a lemon and add half of the lemon rind, chopped up, half a stick of cinnamon, a handful of fresh thyme crushed or chopped, about one inch of fresh ginger root thinly sliced or grated, and a good dollop of honey. Add boiling water and let stand for five minutes (or hours in the thermos).

❏ Sinus-beating herbs include elder, eyebright, goldenseal, echinacea, and goldenrod.

❏ Vitamin C will stem an infection and is an effective natural antihistamine.

❏ If you are sinus-prone, take horseradish, vitamin C, and garlic tablets throughout the year.

Other

❏ A Vicks inhalation before bed can help clear the sinuses, as will the steam from a hot shower.

❏ God's gift to sinus sufferers is the Neti pot (see page 179).

❏ Where possible, avoid or reduce known allergens such as chemicals, mold, and dust in your home and work environment.

❏ Allergy desensitization is a long-term commitment, but is very effective. Firstly, an allergy specialist will determine the exact nature of your allergens by pricking the skin of the forearms with tiny amounts of the offending substances. A welt may appear, the size of which will depend on the extent of your allergy. Depending on the ilk of your practitioner, either vaccine or homoeopathic dosages of the allergen will be dispensed—sometimes as drops, other times via regular injection.

❑ Buteyko breathing (see Appendix F) works well for sinusitis, and even better for preventing sinusitis if you are a regular sufferer. This technique raises CO_2 levels, which has the effect of increasing nitric oxide levels. Nitric oxide, a naturally produced compound, has anti-inflammatory and antibiotic properties. Perfect for shrinking the swollen mucous membranes lining the sinuses as well as helping to combat the infection.

AROMATHERAPY

The following essential oils once blended together may be used as a steam or dry inhalation. Sprinkle 8 drops onto a tissue or into a bowl of steaming water or into a room vaporizer. Mix with 20 grams of aloe vera gel and apply to the chest and neck area. Mix with 125 grams of Epsom salts and relax in a warm bath.

❑ 2 drops of everlasting oil—antitussive, expectorant, mucolytic, anti-inflammatory

❑ 3 drops of cajeput oil—analgesic, febrifuge, antiseptic, expectorant

❑ 3 drops of ravensara—antimicrobial, antiviral, antiseptic, immune stimulant, expectorant

❑ 2 drops of eucalyptus peppermint—decongestant, expectorant, mucolytic, balsamic

AT A GLANCE

DIET

➠ Avoid alcohol as it swells mucous membranes, the last thing you need.

➠ Drink at least 3 liters of clear fluids daily to thin the mucus and encourage drainage.

➠ Avoid dairy and sugar, increasing foods that improve sinusitis (see above).

REMEDIES

➠ Herbs are very effective for sinusitis (elder, eyebright, garlic, goldenseal, horseradish, echinacea, and goldenrod).

➠ Drink 2–3 cups of the lemon herbal tea daily (see above).

➠ Vitamin C has antihistamine properties that will reduce the swelling within the sinuses. If you are sinus prone, take a vitamin C tablet that is combined with garlic and/or horseradish throughout the year.

OTHER

➠ Unless you are very congested, use a Neti pot each morning. It works by improving drainage, as well as shrinking the swollen mucous membranes.

➠ Buteyko breathing can help cure and prevent sinusitis (see Appendix F). Buteyko breathing over time reduces your sensitivity to allergens.

SORE THROAT

WHAT IS IT?

Upon inspection, a sore throat looks red and irritated. If your sore throat is called tonsillitis, there may be white spots of infection. However, sometimes a sore throat just feels sore, and there is nothing to see at all.

SYMPTOMS

☑ Sore and irritated throat

☑ Difficulty swallowing

☑ If there is an infection present, swollen and tender lymph glands in jaw and neck

WHAT CAUSES IT?

❏ A sore and inflamed throat is one of the common symptoms of a cold or flu.

❏ Glandular fever nearly always presents with a sore throat.

❏ Tonsillitis is the mother of all sore throats. Tonsils are an aggregation of lymphatic nodules forming a ring around the back of the throat. Lymphatic nodules are also found in the armpits, groin, and abdomen. Their purpose is to act as a line of defense, the sentry stations of your immune system, filtering out bacteria and germs.

❏ If you wake with a sore throat every morning, it could be due to a dust-mite allergy, as dust mites lurk in mattresses and pillows. If you have a tendency to sneeze, have a dripping nose, and itchy eyes at the same time, these are also pointers to a dust-mite allergy.

❏ Actors, teachers, and singers often get a sore throat from overusing their voice.

❏ Breathing in pollution or smoky air can cause a sore throat.

❏ Stress. While everyone responds differently to stress, we all have our Achilles heel. For some people, they know they are stressed when their eczema reappears, for others it's a headache, for you it may be a sore throat.

❏ Snoring. If your mouth is dry and your throat is sore when you wake, you could be a snorer. Another clue is finding your bed companion on the couch in the living room.

❏ A sore throat may be a symptom of acid reflux (see page 266).

❏ A sore throat could be caused by a food allergy. Suspects include dairy, gluten, and eggs.

❏ Globus hystericus isn't hysterically funny. It is the feeling of a lump or something lodged in the throat. Globus hystericus is often a symptom of anxiety or stress.

WHAT TO DO

Diet

❏ Drink plenty of fluids including herbal teas, water, broths, and soups.

❏ If there is infection present, avoid sugar.

❏ Avoid alcohol as it can further swell the mucous membranes lining the throat. The exception to this rule is a therapeutic hot toddy. To a cup of hot water, add the juice of half a lemon, a teaspoon of honey, a clove, and a sprinkle of ground cinnamon. The final touch is the addition of a shot of brandy, whisky, or rum.

Remedies

❏ Gargling can help a sore throat. The old-fashioned and readily available salt and water gargle is effective. Add one-quarter to one-half teaspoon of salt to a cup of warm water. Dissolve the salt, and gargle several times. Spit out the water.

❏ Gargle with a teaspoon of colloidal silver to a cup of water. Spit out after gargling.

❏ If there is an infection present, a herbal gargle works like magic. Gargle strong herbal tea or a tincture diluted in water. Choose from sage, myrrh, echinacea, propolis, marshmallow, calendula, and/or poke root (particularly effective for tonsillitis). Swallow after gargling, as these herbs will help on the inside as well.

❏ For an infection, suck on lozenges containing zinc and vitamin C for rapid healing.

❏ Propolis lozenges are also very helpful for soothing and healing.

❏ If you are getting frequent infections, follow the advice for colds and flu on page 97.

Other

❏ If you rest in the early stages, there is a good chance that your sore throat will go away without doing anything else.

❏ Change your toothbrush every month, as an idle toothbrush may fester. Every couple of days, put a drop of tea tree oil on it to disinfect, then rinse the brush.

❏ If your sore throat is from teaching or singing, ask a voice coach for advice. You may need to follow a different breathing pattern, or you might need a microphone.

❏ If you have globus hystericus, Buteyko breathing can help (see Appendix F). This style of breathing helps anxiety and relaxes smooth muscle that lines the throat. A relaxed throat will melt away any hysterical lumps.

❏ If you have a dust-mite allergy, cover your mattress and pillows with cotton protectors. Wash often. Spray the mattress and pillows with weak black tea, diluted tea tree oil, or colloidal silver. Leave in sunlight if possible.

❏ Does your sore throat mean you are not speaking your truth? Try Cerato, a Bach Flower Remedy.

AROMATHERAPY

Blend the following oils into 10 grams of aloe vera gel, an unscented balm, or 10 ml of sweet almond oil/unscented cream. This blend can be rubbed on the throat and chest areas to remove those "razor blades." Use as needed.

❏ 4 drops of sandalwood oil—antiseptic, antispasmodic, bactericide, sedative

❏ 4 drops of eucalyptus or peppermint oil—antiseptic, antispasmodic, antiviral, analgesic

❏ 3 drops of thyme oil—antiseptic, bactericide

❏ 3 drops of geranium oil—antiseptic, antiinflammatory

DIET

⇨ Drink plenty of fluids: water, herbal tea, soups.

⇨ Generally avoid alcohol, with the exception of a hot toddy (see above).

REMEDIES

⇨ A salt-water gargle is a tried-and-true remedy for sore throats (see above).

⇨ Herbal remedies work well if there is an infec-tion present. Gargle a strong tea or diluted tincture of one or more of the herbs mentioned above.

OTHER

⇨ Your sore throat could be a sign of early infec-tion or stress. Take rest.

⇨ Does your sore throat mean you are not speak-ing your truth?

STRESS

WHAT IS IT?

Stress is the physical, emotional, and mental response to something you find stressful. The stres-sor can be as major as the death of someone you love or as trivial as missing the bus. Stress has an impact on the whole body, causing minute alter-ations in body chemistry, temperature, pH, and electrical charge. These tiny changes eventually converge into obvious physical and mental symp-toms such as recurrent colds, bowel problems, poor memory, and even serious illness including cancer. We tend to separate mind and body, but the distinction becomes meaningless when you contemplate that the body and brain share the same blood, nutrients, and oxygen. When the body and mind become so involved in dealing with stress, it is difficult to find happiness.

The main players in the body during stress are the stress hormones adrenaline and cortisol, and the nervous system, in particular the autonomic nervous system. The autonomic nervous system is beyond your conscious control, comprising the sympathetic (fight-or-flight) and the parasympa-thetic (relax and digest) systems. In response to stress, the sympathetic nerves send the message to the adrenal glands to release adrenaline.

SYMPTOMS

☑ Anxious thoughts

☑ Feelings of apprehension

☑ Avoidance of tasks

☑ Awareness of heartbeat

☑ Choking feeling

☑ Crying

☑ Depression

☑ Difficulty in completing tasks

☑ Difficulty in swallowing

☑ Fidgeting

☑ Lack of motivation

☑ Loss of interest in sex or increased, inappro-priate interest in sex

- ☑ Poor concentration
- ☑ Poor memory
- ☑ Getting impatient easily
- ☑ Restlessness
- ☑ Shakiness
- ☑ Sleep problems
- ☑ Strained facial muscles, for example, frowning, clenched jaw
- ☑ Tension headaches
- ☑ Waking feeling tired
- ☑ Clenching fists
- ☑ Grinding teeth
- ☑ Stiff or tense muscles
- ☑ Sore back or neck
- ☑ Nervous tic
- ☑ Finishing other people's sentences for them
- ☑ Feeling guilty if you relax
- ☑ Trying to fit too much into a day
- ☑ Assuming more and more responsibilities
- ☑ Finding it difficult to say no to more work
- ☑ Perspiring easily, particularly on the palms and underarms
- ☑ Becoming preoccupied with negative thoughts
- ☑ Finding it difficult to be alone
- ☑ Tending to be cynical
- ☑ Tending to be prone to outbursts of anger
- ☑ Finding yourself intolerant of people
- ☑ Increasing consumption of alcohol, recreational drugs, or cigarettes
- ☑ Under- or overeating
- ☑ Flatulence, burping, abdominal bloating, reflux, stomach ache
- ☑ Constipation or diarrhea
- ☑ Frequent urination
- ☑ Urgency to urinate
- ☑ More than three colds in a year

What Is This Thing Called Stress?

"I'm stressed" is a common refrain, and one that most of us can identify with. Stress as a common term really only came into being in the 1940s and hit its stride by the 1970s. Here in the twenty-first century, stress is still going strong. Although stress wasn't identified until around World War II, it did exist as a concept. Nervous breakdowns, men coming back from war shell-shocked, and homes for the bewildered give an inkling that stress existed, named or not.

In 1914, Harvard professor of physiology W. B. Cannon coined the term fight-or-flight syndrome. He observed physical changes in animals endangered by predators, such as increased heart rate and decreased digestion. These, and a whole range of other physical changes, also occur when a human perceives a threat. The fight-or-flight theory is helpful in understanding what happens to your body when you are stressed. A threat doesn't have to be physical—it can be a looming deadline or an argument with your spouse. However, the physical responses to stress evolved long ago to meet threats of a different kind, such as being trodden on by a mammoth or clubbed by a Neanderthal with a grudge. Our body responds just the same to a mammoth or a mammoth deadline.

The Three Phases of Stress

In the 1930s, Dr. Hans Selye, known as "the father of stress" (rather an unfortunate title), went further than Cannon and identified three stages in the body's response to stress.

Stage 1: Alarm Phase

The stress switch has been turned on; the trigger has been pulled. This is the fight-or-flight response—an immediate reaction to a threat, perceived or real. There is an instantaneous mobilizing of nerves and hormones. The body is abuzz with adrenaline. You are ready to rock and roll, fight or flee. Activation of the stress system heightens mental and physical arousal, accelerates reflexes, improves attention, decreases appetite, increases tolerance of pain. In small doses, adrenaline feels fabulous, and people can get addicted to these feelings. In fact, drugs such as cocaine, and to a smaller extent nicotine and caffeine, activate adrenaline.

Stage 2: Resistance Phase

If the alarm bells continue to ring, the body tries to adapt. You know how annoying a car alarm can be? The first time you hear it you look out the window, ready to apprehend a car thief. The fifth time the alarm goes off, you are looking for the numbnuts who owns the car. The resistance stage of stress is when you start to see some of the conditions associated with stress, including IBS, insomnia, and headaches.

Stage 3: Exhaustion Phase

You can only be on high alert for so long. The adrenal glands eventually become too pooped to pop. By this stage you will be experiencing a worsening of the symptoms that began in Stage 2, and are probably feeling very tired, depressed, and possibly showing early signs of heart disease, diabetes, and cancer.

Adrenaline and Cortisol— The Drama Queen and Cinderella

The adrenal glands deal with stress by pumping out another hormone in addition to adrenaline: cortisol. Adrenaline is the drama queen stress hormone for "right now" events (the fight-or-flight response), whereas cortisol is the resentful Cinderella who mops up the effects of adrenaline and deals with longer-term stress. If your body has suffered stress for a long period, it is a drain on your adrenal glands. Naturopaths call this adrenal exhaustion. If you are adrenally exhausted, you have few, if any, reserves left. Pushed beyond these reserves, you run the risk of falling seriously ill.

There are usually three indicators that you may be adrenally exhausted. Firstly, you have very low energy levels. Secondly, your pupils are unusually large. (When adrenaline is switched on, the pupils widen. Normally, after the adrenaline surge has gone, the pupils go back to their normal size, a third of the iris, but in the adrenally exhausted individual they stay dilated. This may be more apparent under the iridology torch, when the pupils fluctuate in and out in response to the light of the torch. Normally, the pupils will slightly constrict.) Thirdly, you find you are more tired after exercise. (Unless it's a marathon, exercise generally gives you energy, so if you are drained the afternoon or next day after a swim or fast walk, adrenal exhaustion is likely.)

Trigger-Happy

Adrenal exhaustion isn't the only effect of repeated exposure to stress. Every time you are exposed to stress it's as if a trigger has been pulled, causing your brain and adrenals to release hormones. Unfortunately, it takes less and less pressure on the trigger to create the stress cascade. The brain and adrenals become trigger-happy and hypersensitive. You may have noticed that if you've been under a lot of stress, you become stressed over the littlest things. You lose your cool over trivial stuff that has never bothered you before. Misplacing your keys becomes high drama instead of a small setback. You become startled and distressed by everyday noises such as barking dogs and slammed doors.

Cortisol's Effects

Although cortisol is the less dramatic of the stress hormones, it's the dark horse in the race as in the long term, excess cortisol poses a greater risk to your health than the occasional excess of adrenaline.

That is not to say that cortisol doesn't have its good points. It's more a question of quantity and the amount of time that high levels of cortisol are circulating in the body, rather than cortisol being "bad" per se. Cortisol has important anti-inflammatory properties. You may have heard of the drug cortisone—a man-made copy of the body's own cortisol—which is used medically to calm

ADRENALINE'S EFFECTS	
BODY SIGN	EVOLUTIONARY REASONS
PUPILS (dilate)	To enable you to see better running in twilight through deep jungle or stalking your prey.
SKIN (sweating increases, including palms and soles of the feet)	Sweating improves heat loss, all the better for keeping cool when fighting or running. Sweaty palms allow you to keep hold of your club when fighting, or swingfrom lianas when fleeing.
LUNGS (airways widen)	Adrenaline is given as emergency medicine for asthmatics to widen airways and for anaphylactic allergic reactions (as in an epi-pen). More air into the lungs makes it easier to breathe when running away from T. Rex or after your prehistoric adversary.
PENIS (engorges)	It's a guy thing. Spontaneous erection and ejaculation may (disconcertingly) occur. Perhaps it's to sire your progeny before you depart this mortal coil in combat.
BLOOD FLOW	Blood travels to the big muscle groups like the legs, arms, and heart that need to work hard, retreating from the less important areas such as the digestive tract and periphery (e.g., face and hands), leaving you looking pale and your fingers cold to touch.
BLOOD AND BLOOD VESSELS	Blood vessels constrict when bracing for an injury. Substances that increase clotting increase in the bloodstream, again just in case a tusk tears you apart. The downside in modern times is that these are also markers for a heart attack or stroke. Blood fats also increase, prehistorically to give you more energy to run further, but now just adding to the picture of stroke and diabetes.
MIND	Mental activity increases. You'd best have your wits about you in a fight to save your life. Anxiety levels go through the roof, but better to be scared and on guard rather than to be found lounging around the open fire, sucking on some fermented fruit.

down the inflammation of severe asthma, arthritis, and colitis. Cortisol's other role is to increase blood sugar levels. Back in the jungle, this was good news, allowing a constant stream of fuel to the brain and more energy for muscles. However, high-sugar levels on a day-to-day basis spells disaster.

Some of the types of stress that increase cortisol release include:

❏ Trauma to the body of almost any type, including bruises, cuts, and a fall.

❏ Infection.

❏ Intense heat or cold.

❏ Surge of adrenaline.

❏ Surgery.

❏ Illness.

❏ Lack of sleep.

❏ Emotional stress.

❏ Mental stress.

Following are some of the negative effects of higher than normal levels of cortisol.

Immune System
Acute stress of no more than three to five days' duration can increase immunity. In the middle of a crisis, you rarely get sick, but the minute the alarm bells have finished ringing, you are wide open to infection.

Long-term stress of more than five days or so and the associated higher cortisol output can decrease the number of immune cells in your blood and shrink the thymus gland and lymph tissue where immune cells mature.

Autoimmune conditions, such as ulcerative colitis, rheumatoid arthritis, and MS, are conditions where the body's immune system attacks certain cells in the body. A period of stress often precedes the onset and flare-up of an autoimmune disease.

Memory
High levels of cortisol interfere with memory. If stress exists for less than six months, the effect will not be permanent. However, repeated and longer-term stress can shrink the part of the brain where you store memories. A study reported in the *International Journal of Neuroscience* found that high stress levels could be linked with the onset of Alzheimer's disease. A low-stress life is looking more and more attractive.

Depression
Cortisol levels are elevated in people with depression. And vice versa, long-term stress can cause depression. The connection between stress and depression works like this. Stress causes a shift in brain biochemistry. The stress hormone cortisol decreases the availability of serotonin (the happy neurotransmitter). Low serotonin levels are linked to depression.

Muscle Loss and Weight Gain
Cortisol reduces protein synthesis and increases protein breakdown. High cortisol translates to loss of muscle tissue. Under lots of stress, our muscles get weak and lose tone. Due to its interaction with insulin, an excess of cortisol can lead to increased fat deposition. Life isn't fair.

High Cholesterol and Low Libido
Cholesterol is converted into cortisol in the adrenal glands. Cholesterol is also the "parent" molecule for other important molecules in the body, including testosterone, vitamin D, and the diuretic hormone. If you are exposed to a lot of stress, your adrenal glands are under pressure to produce loads of cortisol. This will cause high circulating levels of cholesterol to show up on your blood tests. The cholesterol is directed at making cortisol at the expense of the other molecules. With excess stress, testosterone levels decrease in both men and women, causing a decline in libido.

Fluid retention is also a common symptom found in the chronically stressed, and adds to the perception of weight gain.

Heart Disease

Cortisol increases circulating cholesterol and blood fats, both risk factors for heart disease. Combined with adrenaline's role of constricting blood vessels and increasing blood clotting, it's no wonder stress is so deadly.

WHAT TO DO

Diet

❏ With adrenaline and cortisol both having an effect on blood sugar levels and therefore influencing your mood, it's important you keep to a diet that minimizes rising and falling levels. Eat regular meals that include some protein such as eggs, fish, chicken, meat, legumes, nuts, and seeds.

❏ Avoid caffeine. The last thing you need when you are stressed is any stimulant. Caffeine increases adrenaline. Drink a maximum of two cups of tea and one cup of coffee, and make that *no* diet colas.

❏ Avoid sugar. The stress hormones are already doing their darnedest to disrupt your blood-sugar equilibrium, so don't make things worse. Eating protein with each meal will reduce your craving for sweet things.

❏ Reduce alcohol. Alcohol is a nervous-system depressant. If you enjoy a glass or two a day and it calms you down, go for it, but if you notice you are more stressed, anxious, or depressed the next day, or it interrupts your sleep, then best to cut alcohol out altogether.

❏ When you are stressed it is important that you eat well. Unfortunately, when you are stressed it is more likely you don't have the time or inclination to cook. On the weekend, or when you have some spare time, cook double or more of a nourishing casserole or wholesome soup, and freeze portions to use when you can't be bothered cooking.

❏ Keep hydrated. Drink at least 2 liters of fluid daily. Why not swap to some calming herbal teas such as licorice, chamomile, lemon balm, and/or ginger?

❏ Juices, particularly vegetable juices, are a good way to increase your vitamin and mineral content when your diet might be a bit dodgy. Base your juice on carrots, and add an assortment of beetroot, ginger, celery, parsley, and/or spinach. Drink your juice with a meal to ensure blood sugar levels don't spike.

Remedies

❏ Stress begins with the nervous system and the B complex vitamins can all be beneficial for a stressed nervous system. Take one with breakfast and another with lunch.

❏ Herbs to help calm an irritated nervous system include St. John's wort, kava, valerian, oats, passionflower, vervain, lemon balm, zizyphus, magnolia, and chamomile.

❏ If your shoulders are bunched up around your ears and your muscles tighten up when you are stressed, then magnesium is your friend. Take at night.

❏ For longer-term stress, and to avoid the health concerns that come with it, take several of the adaptogen herbs (see page 92) such as Siberian ginseng, licorice, Korean ginseng, schizandra, astragalus, gotu kola, tulsi, rhodiola, withania, and rehmannia.

❏ Bach flowers can be very helpful in stressful times. The classic is Rescue Remedy. Others that might appeal include Aspen for generalized anxiety, Mimulus for known fear, White Chestnut for thoughts that go round and round in the mind like a mouse on a wheel, Sweet Chestnut for appalling mental despair (the dark night of the soul stuff), and Star of Bethlehem for shock and the aftereffects of shock.

❏ Stress is the trigger behind many conditions from headaches to eczema. See each condition for more specific remedies.

Other

❏ When stressed, your breathing changes, becoming faster and more shallow. By focusing on breathing from your belly, you will feel calmer. Belly breathing switches on the parasympathetic nervous system (PNS), the part of the autonomic nervous system you want to dominate in preference to the sympathetic nervous system. (See Belly Breathing on page 319). Don't relegate belly breathing to practice at a particular time of day; make it your default breathing pattern. The more you belly breathe, the better you will feel—and the more natural it will become to breathe this way. Buteyko breathing also switches on the PNS. (See Appendix F, Buteyko Breathing.)

❏ Meditation is a winner when it comes to reducing the harmful effects of stress, lowering both adrenaline and cortisol levels. It doesn't matter which type of meditation you choose, just so long as you are able to reduce the "monkey mind" thoughts that will try and distract you. CDs and books are available, although it is often best to learn meditation in a group, on a course or meditation retreat. Countless studies have been done on the benefits of meditation for all sorts of conditions from heart disease, to cancer, to headaches.

❏ Last thing at night, take a long hot bath, with a handful of Epsom salts added to relieve muscle spasm and a few drops of lavender oil to ease your mind.

❏ Exercise helps reduce cortisol levels. It also uses up any spare adrenaline, making exercise an excellent stress management tool. Don't throw it away when the going gets tough. Even though you might have little spare time in the day, make some time for a twenty-minute walk or swim or some yoga stretches.

❏ How you handle stress is often how your parents handled stress. We learned before we could speak or properly understand family dynamics. If becoming angry or depressed was how members of your family handled stress, odds on that will be your default tendency. Understanding this is important, and then you can go on to changing your reactions so they are more helpful to the situation and less detrimental to your health. A good counselor can help with this.

❏ Counseling is useful during times of stress. Not only is it a supportive pair of ears, and a time devoted to you for you to unload, good counseling allows you to develop skills in order to cope with stressful situations, now and in the future. With counseling, it is important you find the right person for you; just because they have impressive qualifications doesn't mean they are good for you.

❏ Don't let stress destroy your happiness or your health.

AROMATHERAPY

Use this relaxing, calming, stress-relieving blend as needed. For a full body massage, dilute in 5 ml of arnica-infused oil with 25 ml of warm coconut oil. Or mix 10 drops with 125 grams of Epsom salts and relax back in a warm bath. Use 6 to 8 drops in a room vaporizer or blend with jojoba oil and use as a personal perfume. Mix with an essential oil solubilizer and use as a personal spritzer.

❑ 3 drops of lavender oil—carminative, hypotensive, nervine, sedative, antidepressant

❑ 3 drops of frankincense oil—sedative and calming

❑ 5 drops of bergamot oil—calming, uplifting, antidepressant, balancing, and stress relieving

❑ 4 drops of clary sage—antidepressant, hypotensive, nervine, stomachic, and sedative

At a Glance

Diet

➠ Under stress, your blood sugar levels will be all over the place. Eat regular meals every two to three hours that contain a little protein (eggs, fish, chicken, meat, legumes, nuts, and seeds).

➠ Avoid caffeine. Caffeine releases adrenaline, something you already have in excess.

➠ Avoid sugar. Sugary foods will only make things worse, I promise.

➠ When you are stressed, it's best to be well nourished. Freeze extra portions of nutritious casseroles and soups for when you don't feel up to making meals from scratch.

➠ Vegetable juices can add to your nutritional repertoire.

Remedies

➠ Take a strong B complex at breakfast and lunch. The B vitamins are good for your nervous system.

➠ Herbs for a stressed nervous system include St. John's wort, kava, valerian, oats, passionflower, vervain, lemon balm, zizyphus, magnolia, and chamomile.

➠ Herbs for the longer haul include Siberian ginseng, licorice, Korean ginseng, schizandra, astragalus, gotu kola, tulsi, rhodiola, withania, and rehmannia.

➠ Magnesium is relaxing for muscle spasms, a common symptom of stress.

Other

➠ Learn to belly breathe (see page 319). Stress makes breathing faster and more shallow. Belly breathing and Buteyko breathing (Appendix F) reverse this pattern and switch on the parasympathetic nervous system.

➠ Now is the time to bring out and dust your meditation stool or enroll in a meditation class. Meditation is the most powerful stress-relieving tool there is. Ohm.

➠ Exercise not only takes your mind off your problems, it reduces stress hormones. Hop and jump to it.

➠ Finding a good counselor is a good investment of your time and dollars. Not only will they help you get through this time, but can also equip you with tools to use when stress next crosses your path.

THYROID

WHAT IS IT?

The thyroid gland is one tricky customer. Once disturbed, it's the devil to restore to its preferred state of hormonal harmony. The thyroid gland is your body's internal thermostat, responsible for regulating temperature as well as governing metabolism. It does this by determining how quickly or slowly cells use and produce energy, the implication of this means that thyroid hormones affect all bodily functions. Hypothyroidism or low thyroid function is one of the most common hormonal deficiencies, especially for women.

SYMPTOMS

The classic sign of hypothyroidism is a goiter, or a swelling of the thyroid gland, which appears like a bulge or lump in the neck. However, many symptoms of low thyroid activity are less obvious and include one or more of the following:

- ☑ Puffy face and lips
- ☑ Dry skin
- ☑ Dry and thickened skin on shins
- ☑ Thinning hair
- ☑ Thinning of outer third of eyebrows
- ☑ Cold hands and feet
- ☑ Increased intolerance to cold temperatures
- ☑ Constipation
- ☑ Hoarseness of voice
- ☑ Depressed mood
- ☑ Poor concentration
- ☑ Fatigue
- ☑ Weight gain
- ☑ Difficulty in losing weight
- ☑ Decreased libido

IODINE AND HEALTH

Hypothyroidism is common in areas where there is little or no iodine in the soil. No iodine in the soil means no iodine in the food crops grown from this soil. Iodine deficiency is a common nutritional deficiency and acknowledged as a major public health concern. Not only can it cause hypothyroid disease, low iodine levels during pregnancy negatively impacts on the intellectual development of the unborn child. Public health policies in the past have been to "iodize" salt, and more recently iodine has been added to bread (except organic bread). A recent spike in hypothyroid cases may be attributed to two arbitrary causes. Alongside the emergence of the foodie culture, many consumers are opting for fancy-pants rock or sea salt in preference to dowdy old iodized salt. Additionally, milk has historically been an "accidental" source of iodine in the diet. Iodine is not normally found in large amounts in any dairy products. However, in a case of a happy incidental contamination, until recently dairy equipment was sanitized with iodine containing cleaning products, and so tiny amounts of iodine found its way into dairy foods. Dairy equipment is no longer cleaned in this way, meaning dairy foods have returned to their low iodine status.

WHAT CAUSES IT?

❏ Hashimoto's thyroiditis (a common form of hypothyroidism) is an autoimmune condition. Like many autoimmune conditions such as multiple sclerosis and rheumatoid arthritis, Hashimotos thyroiditis is thought to be hereditary, but its genetic manifestation will only likely appear after it has been triggered by an event such as a period of high stress or infection.

❏ After childbirth is a common time for this hypothyroidism to appear, called postpartum thyroiditis, quite possibly precipitated by the unborn babies extra requirements for iodine, and/or the extra stress on mother's body.

❏ Inadequate dietary intake of iodine is a major cause of hypothyroidism as the thyroid hormones require the mineral iodine, and if it's not in the diet, it's not available for thyroid hormone creation.

❏ Certain medications including lithium can interact with iodine levels.

❏ Past exposure to chemicals and pesticides.

❏ Radiation exposure.

❏ Stress. All the endocrine (ductless) glands are interconnected. Increased cortisol levels (the adrenal stress hormone) are implicated in lowering thyroid hormone function.

❏ Chronic infection or inflammation may precipitate hypothyroidism

WHAT TO DO?

As the thyroid is so sensitive, and has the potential to swing from an underactive to overactive state, it is wise to seek advice from your health practitioner before embarking on any course of treatment.

Testing Thyroid Levels

The standard blood test for ascertaining thyroid function is to look for levels of TSH (thyroid stimulating hormone released by the pituitary gland), T4, and T3 (both thyroid hormones). T4 is converted to T3 by the loss of an iodine molecule, and T3 is the more active form of the hormone. This occurs in the liver, muscles, and kidneys, and requires the presence of selenium and zinc. If there are low levels of thyroid hormone, the pituitary gland will increase TSH in order to stimulate the thyroid gland into producing more thyroid hormones.

If TSH is high and thyroid hormones are low, the diagnosis of hypothyroidism is made. In this case, thyroid hormones (thyroxine) will often be prescribed in order to re-establish hormonal order. However, in some cases TSH will be in the normal range, as will T3 and T4. Yet there are still signs and symptoms of low thyroid hormones (mentioned above.) It is believed that during some illnesses and times of stress, another form of T3 is produced, known as reverse T3 or rT3, alongside plain old T3. Reverse T3 is less active than T3. Normal blood tests for thyroid hormones don't look for the ratio of rT3 to T3, and it will seem that levels are normal, even though there may be symptoms of low thyroid activity. Certain laboratories do perform this test of rT3.

Test Your Resting Body Temperature

One low-tech method for ascertaining whether your might have low thyroid hormone levels is to chart your basal or resting body temperature. As mentioned previously, the thyroid gland is the body's thermostat, regulating temperature. Known as the Barnes Basal Temperature Test, you simply record your temperature for five days in a row, and take an average of the readings. If you record an average temperature 98 degrees Fahrenheit it may be an indication your thyroid hormone levels are low, and to seek advice from your health practitioner.

❏ Leave a thermometer next to your bed.

❏ First thing in the morning, as soon as you wake and before you get out of bed, place a thermometer under one armpit.

❏ Leave it there for a full ten minutes.

❏ Record your results for five days in a row. Then take an average. (Divide the sum of five readings by five).

❏ For women, start on day two of your menstrual cycle (second day of period).

❏ An average reading of below 98°F may indicate low thyroid hormone levels

Diet

❏ Increase food that is high in iodine, including shellfish, marine fish, seaweed, egg yolk, and iodized salt (unless you have high blood pressure, when increasing salt is not advised).

❏ There appears to be a connection between thyroiditis and gluten intolerance. It is worthwhile going gluten free for a month to see if this helps with your symptoms.

❏ Goitrogens (named after the symptom of goiter) are substances that prevent iodine from being utilized by the thyroid gland. Goitrogens are found in the Brassica family including broccoli, Brussels sprouts, kale, cauliflower, turnips, radishes, horseradish mustard greens, and rutabaga. Also found in soybeans, cassava root, peanuts, pine nuts, and millet. Goitrogens are only active in food eaten in the uncooked or raw state; cooking inactivates goitrogens.

❏ Increase foods containing zinc, selenium, and vitamin A to improve conversion from T4 to active T3. (See Appendix D for a list of these foods.)

Remedies

❏ Herbs that increase thyroid activity include bladderwrack, withania, and coleus.

❏ Take a supplement that includes iodine, selenium, vitamin A, and zinc.

❏ Stress is often the trigger to unbalance thyroid

BEHIND THE SCENES

The thyroid gland is an endocrine or ductless gland, meaning it secretes its gear inside the body (e.g., adrenal glands) compared to exocrine glands, which excretes outside the body (e.g., sweat glands). The endocrine glands, which include pituitary, pancreas, ovaries, testes, thyroid, and adrenal glands, are intimately connected. When something goes awry with one gland, this will impact on all the others. The treatment implication is twofold. First, tread carefully and slowly. Making small changes is the best way to treat this little gland. And secondly, by supporting other endocrine glands, this will have a positive impact on the others. In the case of the thyroid gland there is a special relationship with the adrenal glands, the glands that deal with stress. It is not uncommon, after a period of stress, and increased production of the stress hormones, adrenaline and cortisol, that the thyroid gland can "act up." By addressing the initial cause and pacifying the adrenal glands, this is likely to calm the thyroid gland and reverse symptoms.

function. The antistress adaptogen herbs are useful in long-term balancing of the endocrine glands, including the thyroid. These include rehmannia, withania, rhodiola, and licorice.

❑ Vitamins A and B complex will help you cope with stressful times.

Other

❑ To check whether your thyroid function may be low, chart your basal temperature. (See Test Your Resting Body Temperature above.)

❑ Stress needs to be kept under control. Take regular exercise and incorporate stress-relieving activities such as meditation, knitting, tai chi, or playing or listening to music.

AT A GLANCE

Diet

⟶ Thyroid hormones need iodine; eat iodine-rich foods including shellfish, marine fish, seaweed, egg yolk, and iodized salt.

⟶ Trial a gluten-free month. Evidence suggests a connection between gluten intolerance and thyroiditis.

⟶ Boil your veggies, at least the ones containing goitrogens. Goitrogens prevent iodine from being used by the thyroid gland to create thyroid hormones. Goitrogens are found in the following foods: broccoli, Brussels sprouts, kale, cauliflower, turnips, radishes, horseradish, mustard greens, and rutabaga. Also found in soybeans, cassava root, peanuts, pine nuts, and millet. As cooking inactivates goitrogens, avoid eating any of these foods in their raw or under-cooked state in the case of low thyroid.

Remedies

⟶ Several herbal remedies assist the thyroid gland to produce thyroid hormones; these include bladderwrack, withania, and coleus.

⟶ Take a supplement that contains iodine, selenium, vitamin A, and zinc.

Other

⟶ Chart your basal temperature to assess whether you might have low thyroid levels.

⟶ Play music, meditate, exercise—whatever it takes for you to lower your stress levels. Stress is the great thyroid unbalancer.

VARICOSE VEINS

WHAT IS IT?

Veins send blood to the heart and lungs to be re-oxygenated. Not as strong walled or elastic as arteries (which are designed to cope with the vigorous action of blood pumped from the heart), veins have valves, which in good times prevent the backward flow of blood. When times aren't so good, these valves lose their oomph, known as valvular incompetence (as in "you incompetent ninny"), causing blood to pool and veins to swell and become varicosed. Varicose veins are veins in the lower leg that have become enlarged, twisted, and swollen.

SYMPTOMS

- ☑ Most varicose veins occur in the superficial veins of lower legs.
- ☑ Heaviness and aching pain in the legs
- ☑ Swelling of the ankles
- ☑ Cramping of the legs
- ☑ A shiny brownish-blue discoloration around the ankles
- ☑ Ulceration may occur.

WHAT CAUSES IT?

- ❏ There is a very strong genetic predisposition; additionally, three times as many women are affected than men.
- ❏ Standing up all day, especially on hard floors.
- ❏ Sitting down for long periods and crossing the legs also impedes proper blood flow.
- ❏ Pregnancy often causes varicose veins due to the extra weight of the baby pressing down and congesting the venous return of blood from the lower body.

- ❏ Constipation and straining increase the pressure in the abdomen, constricting the flow of blood up from the legs.
- ❏ Prior trauma, surgery, immobilization, or deep-vein thrombosis.
- ❏ Being overweight adds more stress on the lower veins.
- ❏ Varicose veins point to poor circulation generally.

WHAT TO DO

Treating varicose veins takes considerable patience. Whether they can be saved depends on how badly the veins have been stretched. Treatment helps prevent future varicose veins.

Diet

- ❏ Foods containing bioflavonoids (including the pith of citrus fruits, cherries, blackberries, rye, blueberries, rosehip tea, and buckwheat) can help strengthen the veins.
- ❏ Foods that improve circulation include garlic, onion, ginger, and chili.
- ❏ Avoid sugar and white flour products.
- ❏ A high-fiber diet can help prevent constipation.

Remedies

- ❏ Take bioflavonoids (rutin and hesperidin in particular) to strengthen the veins. Vitamin C is also very good for this, and they are often sold in combination.
- ❏ The tissue salts calcium fluoride (calc. fluor.) and silicea are used primarily to give strength and elasticity to the vein walls.
- ❏ Bromelain, the enzyme from the pineapple,

can help reduce varicose veins that tend to be lumpy.

❏ Oligomeric proanthocyanidin complexes (OPCs) found in grapeseed and maritime pine bark are useful for strengthening collagen and vein walls.

❏ Herbs that are excellent in the treatment of varicose veins are horse chestnut, butcher's broom, ginkgo biloba, bilberry, and witch hazel.

❏ After your shower, massage in some cream containing one or more of horse chestnut, butcher's broom, citrus seed extract, and/or some of the essential oils mentioned below.

❏ If your legs are hot from standing, apply a cool compress of witch hazel lotion straight onto the veins. Keep a bottle in the fridge.

Other

❏ Exercise is vital as the muscles help pump the blood up the legs, improving circulation. Exercise daily. Choose from swimming, walking, dancing, and yoga. The inverted postures of yoga, where the legs are above the heart, are particularly good for varicose veins.

❏ Massage can help relieve and prevent varicose veins. If you can't afford to, or don't have the time to treat yourself to a weekly massage, all you need to do is master the simple technique of *effleurage*. The first stroke taught to massage students, effleurage is a gliding upward movement using a gentle but firm touch using the whole palm of your hand. The movement is from the feet towards the heart, encouraging the flow of blood up the veins, easing congestion and swelling. You can use baby powder, cold-pressed vegetable oil, or better still a cream containing herbs and nutrients mentioned above.

❏ A very simple and effective form of relief for the symptoms of varicose veins is to lie with both legs up against a wall for about fifteen minutes at the end of every day. If you work on your feet all day this is invaluable.

❏ Wear compression stockings, particularly on days where you need to stand or walk a lot or if you plan to journey by plane for many hours.

❏ Acupuncture and reflexology are effective modalities for treating varicose veins.

AROMATHERAPY

Blend the following oils into 20 grams of unscented vitamin E cream and apply to legs daily. Can also be used for bathing by mixing with Epsom salts.

❏ 3 drops of cypress oil—a renowned venous decongestant (an excellent choice in treating varicose veins)

❏ 2 drops of red myrtle oil—venous decongestant

❏ 4 drops of lemon oil—tonifying on the blood vessels

❏ 1 drop of geranium oil—stimulates circulation

DIET

→ Bioflavonoids strengthen collagen, the protein that forms blood vessels including veins. Foods containing the bioflavonoids include the pith of citrus fruits, cherries, blackberries, rye, blueberries, rosehip tea, and buckwheat.

→ Foods to improve general circulation include garlic, onion, ginger, and chili.

REMEDIES

→ Rutin and hesperidin are two bioflavonoids that will help strengthen veins. Take in combination with vitamin C, which plays a similar role.

→ Grapeseed and maritime pine bark contain oligomeric proanthocyanidin (OPC) complexes, which are helpful for strengthening collagen and vein walls.

→ Take herbs that assist in improving circulation and strengthening vein walls such as horse chestnut, butcher's broom, ginkgo biloba, bilberry, and witch hazel.

OTHER

→ It is important that you take regular exercise to improve blood flow. Swimming and yoga are particularly good. The inverted postures of yoga, where the legs are above the heart, are perfect for preventing varicose veins.

→ Massage, acupuncture, and reflexology are all good modalities in the prevention and treatment of varicose veins.

WARTS

WHAT IS IT?

Warts are caused by the human papillomavirus (HPV), of which there are more than 100 subtypes. Warts are generally painless and can appear anywhere on the body. If unsure, always check with your doctor or dermatologist to verify it is a wart.

Common Warts

Most often found on the hands. They can spread from one part of the body to another, but seldom from person to person.

Subungual or Perungual Warts

Found around and under fingernails and toenails.

Genital Warts

These are easily spread via unprotected sex. They can appear around and in the vagina, on the tip of the penis, around or in the anus, and also on the thighs. It is wise to have genital warts checked and attended to by your doctor or specialist. Women with genital warts are more susceptible to cancer of the cervix. Genital warts should not be treated at home.

Plantar Warts

These usually grow on the sole of the foot, and are often tender to the touch. If your wart does not respond to natural treatments, ask your doctor or podiatrist for more aggressive antiwart treatment.

SYMPTOMS

☑ Flat or slightly raised area on the surface of the skin

☑ Can be cauliflower shaped

☑ Colorless, white, or pink

WHAT CAUSES IT?

❏ You kissed a frog?

❏ Any viral condition, including warts, is a sign that your immune system is not firing from all cylinders.

WHAT TO DO

Diet

❏ Avoid sugar as it suppresses the immune system.

❏ Eat unprocessed fresh food centered on vegetables, fruit, whole grains, nuts, and seeds.

❏ Coconut oil contains lauric acid, which has antiviral properties. Coconut oil is a stable cooking oil; try it in stir-fries.

❏ Garlic is terrific for the immune system and has antiviral qualities. Raw is best.

Remedies

❏ Herbs to boost the immune system include echinacea, andrographis, thuja, cat's claw, and St. John's wort.

❏ Vitamin C and zinc are excellent in boosting your immune system.

❏ The topical application of a tincture or ointment containing licorice, cat's claw, St. John's wort, and/or lemon balm.

❏ The homoeopathic remedy thuja can be very effective.

❏ Apply salicylic acid (from the chemist) directly onto the wart.

Other

❏ Most warts disappear in their own good time; have patience.

❏ Apply a section of banana peel, squishy side, on wart, and cover with tape. Replace with a new peel daily until the wart has disappeared.

❏ Several trials have shown that warts disappear with daily application of a drop of tea tree oil.

❏ Cover wart with plain old sticky tape. Keep on for as long as possible. Not sure why this works. Perhaps warts have noses and suffocate.

❏ Don't pick or scratch. Warts can be spread.

❏ For painful plantar warts, place a corn pad or similar padding around the wart to take the pressure off when walking, and awaiting the disappearance of said wart.

AROMATHERAPY

Used in combination, 2 drops of tea tree oil and 2 drops of lemon-scented eucalyptus oil is an all-penetrating, antiviral, and antiseptic blend. Apply using a Q-tip or cotton swab directly to the wart. Cover with tape and leave for a few days then reapply the same treatment. Be patient; it is a slow process!

AT A GLANCE

DIET

→ Sugar suppresses your immune system. Avoid it.

→ Your diet needs to contain loads of fresh fruit and vegetables, whole grains, legumes, nuts, and seeds.

→ Lauric acid has antiviral properties. It can be found in coconut oil. Use in cooking or add to your muesli.

REMEDIES

→ Warts are caused by a virus. Boosting your immune system is a way of beating this virus. Antiviral herbs include echinacea, andrographis, cat's claw, and St. John's wort.

→ Vitamin C and zinc are excellent for boosting your immune system.

OTHER

→ Warts are contagious, so stop picking at them, and be cautious about what and whom you touch with your wart.

→ A daily drop of tea tree oil on the wart can be effective.

→ Place a piece of banana peel (the inside of the skin) onto your wart. Cover and replace with new peel daily.

APPENDIX A
ESSENTIAL OIL
THERAPEUTIC PROPERTIES

Abortifacient. Capable of inducing abortion.

Alterative. Cleanses the blood and corrects impure blood conditions.

Analgesic. Remedy or agent that deadens pain.

Anthelmintic. Destroying or expelling intestinal worms.

Anti-Allergic. An agent that reduces the symptoms of allergies.

Anti-Arthritic. An agent that combats arthritis.

Anticatarral. An agent that helps remove excess mucus from the body.

Antidepressant. An agent that is uplifting and counteracts melancholy.

Anti-Emetic. An agent that reduces the incidence and severity of vomiting.

Antihistamine. An agent that counteracts the physiological effects of histamine production in allergic reactions.

Anti-inflammatory. Alleviates inflammation.

Antimicrobial. An agent that resists or destroys pathogenic microorganisms.

Antiphlogistic. Checks or counteracts inflammation.

Antipruritic. Relieves sensation of itching or prevents its occurrence.

Antiseptic. Destroys and prevents the development of microbes.

Antispasmodic. Prevents and eases spasms or convulsions particularly in muscle tissue.

Antisudorific. An agent that reduces sweating.

Antitussive. An agent that relieves coughs.

Aperitif. Stimulates the appetite.

Astringent. An agent that contracts, tightens, and binds tissues.

Bactericide. An agent that combats bacteria.

Balsamic. Applies to resins—a soothing and healing agent.

Carminative. Soothes and settles the gut wall, thereby easing gripping pain and helping the removal of gas from the digestive tract.

Cephalic. Stimulating and clearing the mind.

Cholagogue. Increases bile production—stimulates the flow of bile from the liver.

Cicatrisant. Helping the formation of scar tissue.

Convulsant. An agent that causes convulsions.

Cytophylactic. Encouraging growth of skin cells.

Decongestant. Releasing nasal mucus.

Demulcent. An agent that soothes, softens, and allays irritation of mucous membranes.

Deodorant. An agent that helps destroy odors.

Depurative. Purifying the blood—also known as alterative.

Diaphoretic. An agent that produces or promotes sweating—aids in helping the skin eliminate waste from the body. (See also sudorific).

Digestive. An agent that aids digestion.

Disinfectant. An agent that aids in destroying germs.

Diuretic. An agent that increases the secretion and elimination of urine from the body.

Emetic. An agent that induces vomiting.

Emmenagogue. An agent that promotes and regulates menstrual flow.

Emollient. An agent used externally to soothe and soften the skin.

Estrogenic. An agent that stimulates the action of estrogen.

Expectorant. An agent that expels mucus from the respiratory system.

Febrifuge. An agent that cools and reduces high body temperatures.

Fungicide. An agent that destroys fungal infections.

Galactagogue. An agent that increases the flow of milk.

Germicidal. An agent that destroys germs or microorganisms.

Hemostatic. An agent that arrests (stops) bleeding.

Hepatic. An agent that stimulates and aids liver function.

Hypertensive. An agent that increases blood pressure.

Hypnotic. An agent that produces sleep.

Hypotensive. An agent that lowers blood pressure.

Immune-Stimulant. An agent that is stimulating to the immune system.

Insecticide. An agent that kills insects.

Laxative. An agent that aids bowel evacuation.

Mucolytic. Dissolving or breaking down mucus (see also expectorant).

Nervine. Reduces nervous disorders—beneficial effect on the nervous system.

Parturient. An agent that aids in the delivery in childbirth.

Prophylactic. An agent that prevents disease.

Relaxant. An agent that causes relaxation of the mind and/or body.

Restorative. An agent that helps strengthen and revive the body systems.

Rubefacient. An agent when applied to the skin in some form, will cause a gentle and localized increase in surface blood flow.

Sedative. An agent that reduces functional activity. Calms the nervous system; reduces stress and nervousness throughout the body.

Spasmolytic. See antispasmodic.

Stimulant. An agent that stimulates the physiological functions of the body.

Stomachic. An agent that relieves gastric disorders.

Styptic. An agent that aids in arresting external bleeding (See also astringent).

Sudorific. An agent that increases perspiration.

Tonic/Tonifying. An agent that improves bodily performance.

Uterine. An agent that is tonifying to the uterus.

Vasoconstrictor. An agent that aids in the contraction of blood vessel walls.

Vasodilator. An agent that aids in the dilation of blood vessel walls.

Vermifuge. An agent that aids in the expulsion of worms (see also anthelmintic).

Vulnerary. An agent that prevents tissue degeneration and arrests bleeding in wounds.

APPENDIX B
BACH FLOWERS

*Take no notice of the disease; think only of the outlook
on life of the one in distress.* —DR. EDWARD BACH

After many years of treating patients in London's famous Harley Street in the 1930s, gastroenterologist Doctor Edward Bach began to see a connection between people's emotions and their illnesses. His observations have been borne out by modern medical research, which has shown that stress and our emotions are involved in a range of illnesses, from those affecting our immune systems to diabetes and heart disease. Doctor Bach retired from medical practice to develop a range of remedies to help all sorts of emotional states. He drew on nature for his inspiration, sourcing the ingredients for most of his remedies from trees and flowers. He developed thirty-eight remedies in all, and they are known as "Bach flowers."

Rescue Remedy is the best known and most widely used of the Bach flowers. A mixture of five Bach flowers, it helps in most situations of fear or shock. It's a handy remedy to have in the glove box or first-aid kit. However, the Bach flowers offer much more than rescue remedy. Within the thirty-eight remedies you will find four or five (or more on a bad day) to suit your emotional repertoire. I try to combine a here-and-now remedy targeted to whatever problems a person is facing, with a "constitutional" remedy that suits them whatever stage of life they are in.

These constitutional Bach flowers are tailored to the main personality characteristics of the person. For example, a water violet person will never be the life of the party. A rock water person will always need to be aware of their tendency to be hard on themselves. A vervain person will always need to be careful of taking on too many tasks. An oak person will always need to remind themselves to stop pushing to the point of exhaustion. We are born with certain personality traits, and in getting to know and accept ourselves, we are better able to adjust to life's circumstances instead of reacting; we can respond according to our nature.

The list of Bach flowers in this appendix describes the personality types and emotional states that each remedy is helpful for. It is important to remember that the characteristics can often be a two-edged sword. For instance, a beech person can be intolerant and critical, yet on the positive side this attribute means that when they do a job they do it perfectly, all t's crossed and i's dotted. These are the people that make great real estate agents or lawyers. Although some of the characteristics targeted by the Bach flower remedies may soundnegative, they should only be considered negative if that attribute is causing you unhappiness or difficulty in your life.

The Bach flower remedies come in little bottles of "stock" or concentrate. You add two drops of the stock to another bottle containing 15 ml of a mixture of spring water and 10 ml brandy.

(The brandy is not medicinal; it helps preserve the mixture so it doesn't go bad. For those with an aversion to or would prefer to avoid alcohol, gently heat the brandy to just before boiling point to allow the alcohol to evaporate.) The usual way to take Bach flowers is to pop 7 drops of this mixture under your tongue three or four times a day. You can also put 10 drops of Bach flowers in the bath or rub two or three drops on your wrist. You can't overdo them, so you are the judge of how often and how long you need to take them, but give it at least a week.

Whereas you might take a herb or a drug to treat a particular symptom, the actions of Bach flowers are more indirect and subtle. You can never predict how a person will change once they start taking Bach flowers, and the beauty is that the change will bring out the best in the person to help them deal with any given situation. Bach flowers help you to be more in control. If you find that you love using them, it's worthwhile making an investment and buying all thirty-eight stock bottles.

Agrimony (Brave face)

The agrimony person is often the life of the party. Most people would be surprised that behind the happy-go-lucky exterior lies a tortured soul with a turbulent state of mind. The agrimony person conceals their worrying from others, and often seeks excitement or company in order to escape and take their mind off things that are troubling them. Sometimes they resort to alcohol and drugs to drown their worries.

You know you're an agrimony person if your best and dearest friends know you are putting on a happy front, while the outside world has no idea. You can keep up appearances but the emotional cost is high: the bigger the difference between the real you and the pretend you, the bigger the pain.

Agrimony will not rip the mask away, but will allow you to integrate the two yous. You will be surprised that this will give you strength rather than making you more vulnerable. Remember, it is very lonely behind the mask.

Beech (Intolerance)

The beech person tends to be critical and a hard judge of others. They lack tolerance, and can become annoyed at others over insignificant things such as their mannerisms or habits. Beech people like order, and if everything isn't "just so" they get annoyed and cranky. A beech person can also be highly critical of themselves. The good side of the beech person is that they get things done in an orderly and correct way. Taking beech will help them relax a little.

Centaury (Can't say no)

Centaury people tend to be walked over—used as doormats by unscrupulous people. They have trouble saying no and standing up for themselves, may appear to be weak-willed and submissive, and tend not to follow their own path if it looks like it will trouble someone else. The remedy will help them stand up for themselves.

Cerato (Lack of trust in own judgment)

Cerato people always ask the advise of others. It can be nice to be the one asked—until you realize they ask everyone. All too often the Cerato person is misguided, which can lead to all sorts of problems. They might be a little draining on others. Taking Cerato will help them to learn to trust and follow their gut instinct.

Cherry Plum (Desperation)

The cherry plum state is an awful place to be: verging on a breakdown, fearing that you might do something dreadful to yourself or others. Cherry Plum is for fear of losing control and reason, fear of insanity, and fear of succumbing to sudden, violent impulses, possibly murderous or suicidal. Taking Cherry Plum will ease some of their terror and give them some peace where they can decide what course of action is best.

Chestnut Bud *(Groundhog Day)*

Chestnut Bud is for people who keep making the same mistake over and over. Regardless of changing circumstances they keep going down they same path; there is a pattern in their life that needs breaking. Chestnut Bud will help them to learn from their experiences instead of constantly repeating the same error. It can be of use in treating physical conditions that keep recurring.

Chicory *(Why me?)*

A chicory person feels hard done by, as though everything is stacked up against them and things aren't fair. Chicory people very easily feel hurt or offended and rejected, and may become overly possessive of a friend or loved one. They might be a bit sulky when not given attention, and might tend to think of themselves before others. Taking Chicory will help them to see that the cup is half full instead of half empty.

Clematis *(Dreaminess, inattentiveness)*

Clematis people are dreamers. They withdraw into their own world, are absentminded, and can appear indifferent and listless. Clematis folk are a little fey, and not inclined to get involved in practical day-to-day matters. Taking Clematis will help to keep them grounded and more focused.

Crab Apple *(Shame)*

Crab Apple people don't like themselves very much. In fact, self-hate might be closer to the heart of the matter. Crab Apple can be an effective remedy when a person feels ashamed about their physical appearance or self in general, or when they feel unclean, mentally and physically. It's often good for people with eating disorders. It can also be of use when a physical condition causes a patient to feel dirty, unclean, or embarrassed.

Taking Crab Apple is one step on the path to self-love.

Elm *(Overwhelmed)*

Elm is for people who are usually capable but temporarily feel overwhelmed by a situation, or inadequate to tasks they usually breeze through. Elm people are often very good at what they do, but sometimes when they view the enormity of a task or their responsibilities, suddenly feel unable to cope. Taking Elm will ease this feeling of burden.

Gentian *(Discouraged, melancholy)*

Gentian is for feelings of discouragement. It is helpful when a person's outlook is negative, they are suffering from a deep depression, or they feel down about setbacks and difficulties. Taking Gentian will allow a little light to shine on these feelings of discouragement.

Gorse *(Loss of all hope)*

Gorse is for feelings of despair that things will never improve and nothing can be done. It is useful when a person has lost heart and feels they are condemned to a lifetime of suffering. Taking Gorse will allow hope into the situation.

Heather *(Self-absorption)*

To Heather people it's as though the world revolves around them. They are talkative, but usually talk about themselves, and tend to be poor listeners. That's enough about me, what do you think of me? A Heather person may also be lonely. Taking Heather will broaden their horizons—taking an interest in others often improves their outlook.

Holly *(Hate)*

Holly is for feelings of anger, intense hatred, jealousy, suspicion, and rage. The Holly person can be physically or verbally aggressive and might have temper tantrums. There may or may not be a "good" reason for hateful feelings occurring, but such strong emotions can tear you apart. Hatred is absence of love, and it is usually the one who hates the most who feels love the least. Taking Holly will open the heart to some rays of love and compassion. Great remedy for small children prone to tantrums.

Honeysuckle *(Regret)*

Honeysuckle is for those who look back, thinking "I'll never be as happy as I was when . . ." The Honeysuckle person lives in the past and this might be affecting their life now. Always looking back in sadness means they are less able to build a happy future, or be in the present. Honeysuckle is of use when a person suffers from homesickness, or is missing a past relationship or an earlier time in their life. It might also be of use when a person is unable to move on after a period of grieving.

Hornbeam *(Weariness)*

Sometimes called the "Monday morning" remedy, Hornbeam treats feelings of weariness. A person in need of Hornbeam feels doubtful they have the strength to cope with things, but manages. They are just plain tired. Hornbeam is also a useful remedy when a person is convalescing.

Impatiens *(Frustration, irritability)*

Impatiens people like everything done quickly. They tend to get irritated easily, finish other people's sentences, and tap their feet. Impatiens people are impatient with themselves, others, and situations. Taking Impatiens will slow things down allowing time to smell the roses.

Larch *(Lack of confidence)*

The Larch person believes they won't succeed in life, and anticipates failure. They are not envious of other people's success, they're just convinced they can't do well themselves. Larch is the classic self-esteem remedy.

Mimulus *(Fear)*

Mimulus is the remedy for fear when you know exactly what you are frightened of, for example, spiders or public speaking. Mimulus people tend to blush easily. Don't try things for fear of failing. Mimulus is good for "fraidy cats."

Mustard *(Depression)*

Mustard is helpful for depression that descends like a black cloud and has no known cause. It's like a black hole that you can't see a way out of. Taking Mustard will help lift the depression so you see your way forward.

Oak *(Determined)*

Oak is for people who are terribly strong, like the oak tree. Oak people are plodders whose efforts are relentless. They can sometimes be obstinate. They keep going and going, and never give up—even when they should. Oak helps you know when to throw in the towel, before you drop from exhaustion. Oak can also be of use for long-standing medical conditions.

Olive *(Total exhaustion)*

Olive people have fought a long hard battle and are totally wiped out. They have no reserve strength. Everything is an effort, and nothing brings them pleasure any more. They have gone past the point of no return, and are exhausted to the point of tears. Olive helps them turn the corner.

Pine *(Guilt, self-reproach)*

Pine people tend to take responsibility for everything. They are ready, willing, and able to take the blame when things go wrong. If they trip over a chair, they will apologize. Always on a mission to improve themselves, they tend to be conscientious but are never happy with their achievements. *Mea culpa!* Taking pine helps put things into perspective. Guilt really gets in the way of progress.

Red Chestnut *(Worry about others)*

Red Chestnut people worry excessively about the people they care for, and are fearful that things will happen to hurt their loved ones. This can cause heartache for them and their beloved. There is concern, and then there is worry.

Rock Rose *(Panic)*

When there is a feeling of terror, or panic, or a feeling like being in a nightmare, taking Rock Rose replaces the panic in the air with a sense of calm.

Rock Water *(Hard taskmaster)*

Rock water people tend to be extremists or purists who are rigid in outlook and hold strong opinions. They push themselves hard, and set extremely high standards for themselves. Hair shirts were made for Rock Water people. Taking Rock Water will replace their hair shirts with silk!

Scleranthus *(Butterfly mind)*

Which dress shall I wear—the red or the blue? Scleranthus just cannot decide—not just about clothes but about anything. They are very changeable in mood and opinions. Scleranthus can be of use when a person's physical symptoms change frequently.

Sweet Chestnut *(Limit of endurance)*

Sweet Chestnut helps a person who has reached the limit of what they can endure. They are in a state of mental torture and despair where the future is complete darkness. No hope, no peace. Sweet Chestnut is referred to as the "dark night of the soul" remedy. Taking Sweet Chestnut will let some morning light shine in.

Vervain *(Busy bee)*

The Vervain person has an extremely high level of mental energy and a strong will. They tackle too many jobs at the same time, and are always thinking ahead. Sensitive to injustices, they are fond of worthy causes, and can be enthusiastic to a fault. They are often highly strung and unable to relax. Taking Vervain will help them chill.

Vine *(Dominance)*

What Vine people want they usually get. They tend to be pushy and ride roughshod over other people's opinions. While this makes them high achievers, it can be at some cost to the feelings of others. Strong-willed and dominant, they demand obedience. Taking Vine will assist them to see both sides of an argument and be more forgiving of other people's faults.

Walnut *(Protection)*

Walnut provides protection from a tendency to be overly influenced by situations, people, and feelings. It is particularly good if you are an ultrasensitive person who is overly affected by others. It is also good protection against the effects of change and transition, allowing you to move from one stage of life to another—for example, changing career or relationships, or at times of life such as menopause and puberty.

Water Violet *(Aloofness)*

Water violet people can appear distant, proud, or even aloof to others, but it's just because they don't reveal their feelings. Others may find their detached attitude condescending, but this is not the case. Water Violet types are usually very good at what they do, but they don't blow their own trumpet.

White Chestnut *(Constant unwanted thoughts)*

White Chestnut is good for people plagued by obsessive thoughts that go around and around in their minds like a mouse in a wheel. White Chestnut can help free them from this constant mind chatter, which is exhausting and can affect their work and sleep.

Wild Oat (Direction finder)

Wild Oat illuminates the path you should take, and is useful when you are uncertain about what to do in a particular situation or in life generally. It counteracts any feeling of unhappiness about what direction to take, and helps you to focus on your life's purpose.

Wild Rose (Apathy)

The Wild Rose is apathetic. Everything seems too hard for them. Lacking drive, ambition, and vitality, they are resigned to whatever life hands them. Wild Rose will improve their day-to-day focus on what is important.

Willow (Resentment)

Willow is a useful remedy for a person who's feeling sorry for themselves. This person is jealous and bitter about other's good fortune, and nothing pleases them—wet blanket. Willow will help them get over these awful feelings.

RESCUE REMEDY

Rescue remedy, a combination of five Bach flowers, helps you to deal with emergencies. It is also good to take before an exam or job interview or when you are very stressed. Place 5 drops under the tongue when necessary.

Rescue remedy, although a mixture of five Bach flowers, is sold as a single remedy. It contains:

❑ Star of Bethlehem—for shock

❑ Rock Rose—for panic

❑ Impatiens—for tension

❑ Cherry Plum—for desperation

❑ Clematis—for feeling "out of body"

Rescue remedy is a good all-purpose emergency remedy. If you have used it in the past and did not find it useful, it might be because the mixture of Bach flowers did not fit your experience of the situation. In that case it would be preferable to create your own tailor-made blend of Bach flowers suitable to your particular needs.

MAKING REMEDIES

Plants are mankind's oldest medicine. And they still work a treat. Originally, man would have simply picked the flowers, leaves, or seeds from a plant, and eaten them. Still not a bad method. Or scrunched up a few leaves and applied them directly on a wound to staunch the bleeding. The most natural way to use plants is straight from the garden. However, plants have a short season, and your need for their healing power may not coincide with the growing cycle, so a means of preserving is needed. Drying herbs, making a tincture, ointment, or infused oil, are all means of preserving plants for medicinal use. The life of the herb is extended by as much as three years by using these methods.

Methods to preserve and administer plant medicine have not changed much over the centuries. What follows is an exposition of how to make your own medicine from plants you have grown. If you have had a failed crop or don't have the time to make your own medicine, but are keen to use medicine grown from the earth, research organic herb sellers in your area or get referrals for a local herbalist. Additionally, there are some very fine proprietary products available in supermarkets, health food shops, and online.

GATHERING

Different parts of a plant are used for medicine—the leaf, the root, bark, or flowers. Just what part is the best to use for each particular remedy has usually been established through hundreds of years of practice by village herbalists, and has more recently been confirmed by scientific studies.

The rule of thumb is that plants are gathered at the peak of their growth, which usually occurs around spring and summer. The best time is early morning, after any dew has evaporated. Herbal lore recommends harvesting when the moon is on the wane. This is not about tiptoeing around the yard at midnight in a flowing robe; it's a time when there is less sap in the leaves and stems, making for speedier drying. Discard any leaves or flowers that are damaged, choosing the freshest, greenest, and most healthy-looking plants for medicine. Follow these guidelines:

❏ **Leaves.** Young unblemished leaves picked before the flowers open are the richest in medicinal properties.

❏ **Flowers.** Pick as soon as they open if you can get there in time.

❏ **Seeds.** Best if sun-ripened and gathered before they are dispersed by wind, eaten by birds, or drop on the ground.

❏ **Bark.** Harvested early spring or late autumn. Take care to take only small pieces so as not to damage the plant.

❏ **Roots.** Harvest autumn or when the aerial

parts are dying off. Dig deep into the soil to lift the entire root without bruising. Brush and wash thoroughly, snipping fine rootlets off with scissors.

The best time to cut plants for drying is just before they flower. Be sure to cut early in the morning, and if you want the plant to continue growing, some leaves should be left on the stems. After you have cut your herbs, you can make your medicine immediately or you may wish to dry them for future use.

DRYING

Plants can be dried in bunches, hanging upside down from a roof or shelf in a dry room. To protect hanging plants from the light and dust, cover them with perforated brown paper bags. They are ready when the leaves come off the stems easily.

Leaves, petals, and roots are best dried on a wire tray. A clean flywire (window) screen makes an excellent tray. Place the wire tray where air can circulate above and below it, and spread the plant matter out in a single layer. If necessary, trays can be stacked on top of one another. Turn the plant material daily for about four days.

After herbs are dried, put them in airtight containers; glass is the best, but metal or plastic can be used. You can store leaves whole or crushed. Crush the leaves in a coarse strainer, or with a mortar and pestle. Label and store the glass jars out of direct sunlight to preserve the color and retain the flavor of the herbs.

Freezing plants is a good alternative to drying. Use only the healthiest leaves, as wilted leaves won't have the full flavor after freezing. Cut and clean the plant and put in plastic sandwich or freezer bags. Remember to identify the plant and date it. Once thawed the plant matter can be used as per fresh plant for making medicine.

TEA

Also known as a tisane or infusion, tea is the simplest way to make a remedy. If you are new to the herbal tea game, you might be surprised at how good they taste, and you may choose to replace a coffee, soft drink, or alcohol with a cup of herbal tea. Or not.

Preparation

❑ One teaspoon dried or two teaspoons of the fresh plant (chopped or ground) to one cup of boiling water.

Process

❑ In a teapot or coffee plunger add plant and boiling water. Allow to steep for five minutes or more. Honey can be added, but not milk, as it may curdle.

No more needs to be done if using leaves or flowers as they will release their therapeutic goodies easily enough. However, if your medicine is a seed, stem, root, or bark, this will need to be lightly ground to increase the surface area. Use a mortar and pestle or a couple of whizzes in a coffee grinder kept specifically for your herbs and spices.

A decoction is a tea that has been simmered for ten minutes or so. This is recommended if the plant matter is extremely hard or woody, or if you want a stronger form of tea. Any tea can be made into a gargle, mouthwash, eyewash, footbath, hand bath, bath, and compress.

Make tea fresh each time or plan to use within twenty-four hours so it doesn't go off. In a twenty-four-hour period it can be reheated or drunk cold without a reduction in therapeutic quality.

TINCTURES

Alcohol-based plant remedies have been used for centuries. Nicholas Culpepper, a seventeenth-century botanist and herbalist, frequently recommended herbs to be steeped in wine. Alcohol is a very efficient preserving agent, preventing bacterial and fungal spoiling. In this way the remedy can be kept for months to years. Additionally, alcohol is a good solvent. A solvent is a substance within which another substance can dissolve, in this case the therapeutic compounds in the plant.

Don't like drinking alcohol? The amount of alcohol in a dose of tincture (a dose is usually 5 ml) works out to be less than a sixth of a standard glass of wine or beer. This amount can be tolerated by most people. However, if the liver is severely compromised (e.g., with cirrhosis), the person is an ex-alcoholic, or there are religious reasons, teas and tablets may be taken instead. Or else the tincture can be heated to evaporate the alcohol. Tinctures can be made from fresh or dried plant material. An extract is a more concentrated form of tincture, and requires special equipment not easily applicable to a home environment.

TEA VERSUS TISANES

Traditional tea is made only from the leaves of a bush called *Camellia sinensis*. "Teas" can also be made from the flowers, leaves, seeds, and roots of various herbs. For instance, dandelion tea is made from dried dandelion root, chamomile tea from chamomile flowers, and peppermint tea from peppermint leaves. However, as they are not made from leaves of the *Camellia sinensis* bush, they should not really be called tea at all. Instead, they should be called herbal "infusions," or to use the French, "tisanes" (pronounced *tizz-ahn*).

Preparation

❏ 1 part plant (fresh or dried) to 3 parts liquid

❏ Liquid—30 percent high-proof vodka and 70 percent water—that is, for 100 grams of plant matter you will need 300 ml of liquid or for 500 grams plant matter you will need 1.5 liters of liquid.

Process

❏ Place all the liquid into a good powerful blender. If you have a large amount, this is best done in smaller batches. Add plant matter gradually, breaking it up into small pieces so that the blender doesn't have to work too hard. If stalks and stems are too tough, discard them or you'll risk breaking your blender. Pour into a jar with lid. Mark on a label the date and plant, as all tinctures look the same. Leave in a dark cool place for three months. Every few days throughout this time, check the tincture to make sure plant matter hasn't risen above the liquid; if it does, stir it in and add more liquid if necessary.

At the end of three months all the precious compounds have been dissolved from the plant matter and into the liquid. Into a large jug, strain the liquid through two layers of butter muslin (available from a haberdashery or fabric shop), and squeeze thoroughly. Pour into an amber or dark glass bottle with lid; label once again. The tincture should last two years. Keep in dark, cool place.

TABLETS AND CAPSULES

Modern herbal medicine has embraced the use of tablets and capsules as they don't taste bad—a common complaint about tinctures and some teas. They are convenient—just place them in your bag or pocket, and you take them wherever you are. The machinery needed to make a tablet is usually beyond the humble home medicine maker; however, capsules are simple to make, if a little fiddly.

Preparation

❏ The plant material needs to be in a dry form and very finely ground into a powder. A coffee grinder is ideal for this. Purchase 00 size capsules from pharmacy or on the Internet.

Process

❏ Clean your hands thoroughly and/or wear surgical gloves. Place the powdered plant in a shallow dish. Separate the halves of the capsule and move them together through the powder, filling them in the process, then push the halves together. Place in labeled jars.

TOPICAL MEDICINE

Creams, infused oils, poultices, and compresses are topical or external medicines. The skin is our largest organ, with plenty of surface area to absorb medicine. These topical applications can be used to treat a skin problem or wound, as well as treating the body beneath the skin. Some plants can cause a reaction on the skin. It is best to dab some on your wrist or inner elbow for a few minutes to test, before applying the whole mixture.

Compress

A compress is an excellent way to bring the healing plant to the site of the problem. They can be made from herbal teas, decoctions, or diluted tinctures. Dilute at 1 part tincture to 10 parts water. Compresses are good for skin problems such as eczema or boils, or to relieve pain internally—for example, period cramps, arthritis.

Preparation

❏ You will need a towel and a number of soft cotton material strips cut from a sheet or pillow-case, or you can use muslin. The liquid can be a strong tea, a decoction, or diluted tincture.

Process

❏ Dip one thick or two thin strips of material into the liquid. Squeeze off excess liquid. Apply to the area, covering as much of the affected part as possible. Wrap with plastic wrap. Cover with a towel to avoid dripping. Keep the compress on the affected for twenty to thirty minutes. Reapply as needed.

NOTE: A word about plastic wrap. Plastics are an integral part of life in the twenty-first century. And very handy, particularly in this application of keeping the heat and liquid in. However, there is some evidence that the breakdown products of plastic may not be fabulous for our health, and it is best to avoid drinking or eating directly from plastic containers, particularly when heated. Always ensure that there is a layer of material between your skin and the plastic wrap.

Poultices

A poultice is similar to a compress, but instead of using a liquid, the plant material itself is used. It is often used warm and can be used to draw out toxins, impurities, and pus.

Preparation

❏ You will need a towel and a number of soft cotton material strips cut from a sheet or pillow-case, or you can also use muslin.

Process

❏ Chop or grind your chosen herb finely, and simmer in a small amount of water until it thickens to a paste or jelly.

❏ Add some olive oil just before spreading onto strip of material.

❏ Apply the affected area, cover with plastic wrap, and then cover this with a towel for twenty minutes or so until cooled.

Creams

The easiest way to make a cream at home is to add either herbal tinctures, infused oils, and/or essential oils into an already prepared base cream.

Preparation

❏ Buy from pharmacy or online a white, vegetable-based moisturizing cream, low allergen, with no color or fragrance. These can be based on beeswax, coconut butter, shea butter, glycerin, or cold-pressed oils.

❏ Your choice of tincture, infused oil, and/or essential oil.

Process

❏ Simmer 100 ml of tincture until it is reduced down to a concentrated 20 ml; stir this into 100 grams of cream. Add more or less tincture or oil to create the right consistency of cream— that is, not too runny.

❏ Add 20 ml infused oil to 100 grams cream.

❏ Add 10 drops essential oil to 100 grams cream.

Keep your mitts out of your concoction. Try not to dip your fingers in the cream to avoid contamination; instead use a small, clean plastic or ceramic spatula.

Balms

Preparation

❏ 15 to 20 grams beeswax or cocoa butter (available from the health food store)

❏ 20 to 100 drops (approximately 1 to 5 ml) of pure essential oil blend

❏ 80 to 85 ml vegetable oil

Sweet almond oil, apricot oil, or jojoba oil are the best oils of choice as they remain relatively stable when heated. Olive oil and coconut oil may also be used; however, their consistency is thicker and they are not as easily absorbed by the skin.

Alternatively, you can use 100 grams shea butter in lieu of the above ingredients. Vegetable oil, beeswax, and cocoa butter are relatively inexpensive, but shea butter is very soothing and softening to the skin.

Process

❏ Melt the beeswax or cocoa butter with the vegetable oil (or shea butter).

❏ Once the mixture starts to cool, add your essential oils and stir thoroughly—if essential oils are added while the mixture is too hot they will vaporize.

Pour into sterile container, rest lid on top to cover. Do not seal the container until the balm is cool as the remnant heat may condensate on the lid, which could cause mold to grow and contaminate the balm. Don't forget to label your balm with the contents and date.

ESSENTIAL OILS

The use of essential oils to relax and heal goes back in time to ancient Greece, Egypt, and Rome. Think of all those glistening, well-oiled gladiators! While the term is essential *oil,* these oils are not oily like olive oil. Essential oils are highly concentrated oils extracted from aromatic plants. They are often added to base oils such as almond, jojoba, or olive oil, as in the case of the Romans. Essential oils such as lavender, neroli, and rose that are used in massage and cosmetic treatments are often selected for their beautiful smell. But the science of aromatherapy shows that various essential oils have medicinal properties. For instance, tea tree oil contains terpenes, which is antifungal and antiseptic for skin conditions like tinea. Lavender contains linalool, a mild sedative and an antispasmodic.

Producing essential oils is not difficult, but requires making or buying a purpose-made still,, and this is beyond the resources and interest of many home medicine makers. However, the basic principles are as follows. In a closed metal container, plant material is placed on a grate, similar to a vegetable steamer, over boiling water. As the water boils, vapor containing the essential oil is collected and cooled in a condenser. Most important is the next step, where a separator separates the essential oil from the water vapor. The essential oil is then bottled and lasts around two years. Depending on the original plant, the left over hydrosol (water vapor cooled, minus the essential oil), is used in cosmetics and food such as rosewater and lavender water.

How to Use Essential Oils

Add some to your bath, footbath, or hand bath. Use in a steam vaporizer or essential oil burner. They can also be added to creams. (See Creams, earlier.)

NOTE: Just a word of caution. Essential oils are very strong and should be used sparingly, and you never take them internally. As little as one teaspoon of essential oil, if swallowed, could cause permanent liver damage.

Oil Infusion

Oil infusions are different from essential oils. Firstly, all the plant is used, not only the aromatic molecules being vaporized and condensed. The whole plant is macerated or steeped in a carrier oil, so a variety of the herbs medicinal properties are imparted to the oil. Infused oils are less aromatic, but more complete in their plant profile. A few drops of essential oil can be added to infused oil to magnify a certain effect if necessary.

Preparation

❏ Immerse fresh or dry herb in almond oil and cover to about two to three inches above the plant matter.

Process

❏ Pour contents into an airtight glass jar. It's best to make up a quantity that reaches almost to the top of the jar so that there is as little air as possible above the oil.

❏ Leave in a warm, dark place.

❏ To maintain the quality of your oil, you need to check regularly to ensure that plant matter is completely immersed. If it isn't, push plant matter down and if necessary, add extra oil to cover.

❏ If mold develops this may mean that there is too much air between the oil and the top of the jar, and/or that it is in too warm a place. Carefully and thoroughly skim the mold off and top up your jar or bottle with more oil. Move to a cooler place if necessary.

❏ Leave to steep for six weeks.

❏ Strain into a jug through muslin. Pour into a bottle with a screw-top lid and store in the fridge.

❏ Infused oil can be added to creams and poultices.

APPENDIX D
FOOD SOURCES

Foods High in Vitamin B$_6$

- avocado
- banana
- bell peppers (capsicums)
- bran (rice and wheat)
- Brussels sprouts
- cauliflower
- chicken
- dried herbs and spices: chili, paprika, garlic, tarragon, sage, spearmint, basil, chives, savory, turmeric, bay leaves, rosemary, dill, onion powder, oregano, marjoram
- fish: tuna, salmon, cod
- halibut
- hazelnuts
- kidney beans
- leek
- lentils
- liver
- molasses and sorghum syrup
- peas
- pistachios
- potatoes
- raw garlic
- shiitake mushrooms
- spinach
- squash (pumpkin)
- sunflower and sesame seeds
- sweet potato
- turkey
- turnip greens
- venison
- whole grains

Food Sources High in Vitamin C

- blackcurrants
- broccoli
- Brussels sprouts
- cabbage
- cauliflower
- capsicum (green and red)
- chilies (red, green)
- guava
- kiwi fruit
- lychees
- mango
- oranges
- papaya
- parsley
- rock melon
- rosehips
- strawberries
- tomato
- watermelon

Foods High in Beta-Carotene

- apricots
- beet greens
- butternut squash/pumpkins
- cabbage
- carrots
- collards
- dried herbs: basil, parsley, marjoram, oregano, sage, coriander, thyme
- kale
- lettuce (red leaf)
- mango
- mustard greens
- red capsicum
- rock melon
- spinach
- sweet potato
- turnip greens

Foods High in Bioflavonoids/Flavonols

General bioflavonoids:
apricots, berries, blackcurrants, buckwheat, capsicum, tomatoes, cherries, citrus fruits, fresh fruits and vegetables, grapes, papaya, green tea, prunes

Subcategories:
- anthocyanidins—cherries, red grapes, red wine
- apigenin—celery, artichokes
- apigenin—parsley
- catechin—blackberries, black grapes, apples, pears, plums, peaches, apricots, soya beans, dark chocolate, black tea, red tea, green tea
- cyanidin—cherries, red grapes, bananas
- daidzein—soya beans
- delphinidin—bananas, black beans, kidney beans
- epicatechins—blackberries, black grapes, apples, pears, plums, peaches, apricots, fava beans, pinto beans, snap beans
- epigallocatechin—fava beans, pinto beans, snap beans, black tea, red tea, green tea
- eriodictyol—citrus fruits (grapefruit, lemons, limes, oranges)
- flavones—celery, artichokes
- genistein—soya beans
- hesperidin—citrus fruits (grapefruit, lemons, limes, oranges), cumin, peppermint
- isoflavones—soya beans
- isorhamnetin—dill, parsley
- kaempferol—black beans, kidney beans, snap beans, okra, broccoli, capers
- luteolin—celery, artichokes, peppers, tomatoes, eggplants, thyme
- malvidin—black beans, kidney beans
- myricetin—blueberries, blackberries, snap beans, okra, broccoli, red wine
- naringenin—citrus fruits (grapefruit, lemons, limes, oranges)
- petunidin—black beans, kidney beans
- quercetin—blueberries, blackberries, peppers, tomatoes, eggplants, red onions, green onions, snap beans, okra, broccoli, dill, capers, red wine, apples
- thearubigin—black tea, red tea, green tea

Foods High in Boron

- almonds
- avocados
- bananas
- beans
- beets
- broccoli
- carrots
- cherries
- chick peas
- clams
- dark chocolate
- hazelnuts
- honey
- licorice
- mussels
- onions
- oranges
- parsnips
- peanuts
- pears
- pecans
- popcorn
- potatoes
- prunes
- raisins
- red apples
- red grapes
- red wine
- scallops
- swedes
- walnuts

Foods High in Calcium

- almonds and almond butter
- brazil nuts
- cheeses (in order of highest to lowest): parmesan, Romano, gruyere, mozzarella, Swiss, cheddar, hard goat's cheese, and provolone
- dark leafy greens (in order of highest to lowest): raw turnip greens, dandelion greens, kale, mustard greens, collard greens, spinach
- flax seeds
- globe artichokes
- goat's milk
- grass-fed cow's milk
- herring
- parsley
- sardines
- sesame seeds (highest when roasted or dried) and sesame paste (tahini)
- sprouts
- tinned salmon
- tofu
- whitebait
- whole-grain wheat
- yogurt

Foods High in Chromium

- apples
- bananas
- brewer's yeast
- broccoli
- cheese
- corn on the cob
- eggs, organic
- mushrooms
- onions
- organ meats
- oysters
- potatoes
- spinach
- sweet potato
- tomatoes
- whole grains

Foods High in DHA/EPA

- avocado (omega-6)
- fish (in order of highest to lowest): salmon, sardines, mackerel, herring, and tuna
- flaxseeds
- grass-fed beef
- halibut
- omega-3 fish: mackerel, tuna, salmon, herring, sea mullet, redfish, flounder, trevally, tailor, tarwhine, Sydney rock oysters, blue mussel, rainbow trout, whiting
- omega-3 oils include: flaxseed, hemp seed, canola, soybean
- omega-6 fish: swordfish, salmon, silver perch, mackerel, gemfish, herring, brown trout (hetchman)
- omega-6 oils include: safflower, sunflower, corn, soybean, sesame, canola
- pumpkin seeds (omega-6)
- scallops
- shrimp
- soya beans
- tofu
- walnuts

Foods High in Folic Acid/Folate (Vitamin B$_9$)

- asparagus
- beans (pinto, garbanzo, mung)
- broccoli
- dark leafy green vegetables (spinach, turnip greens, collards)
- dried herbs (in order of highest to lowest): spearmint, rosemary, basil, chervil, coriander, marjoram, thyme, bay leaf, parsley
- edamame (dry roasted soybeans)
- enriched/fortified cereals
- legumes
- lentils
- lettuce
- liver
- nuts (peanuts)
- orange juice
- sunflower seeds
- wheat germ
- yeast extract spreads

Foods High in Iron

- baked beans
- dark chocolate and cocoa powder
- dhal
- dried apricots
- enriched/fortified cereals
- green leafy vegetables (spinach, Swiss chard)
- Jerusalem artichokes
- lentils
- liver and organ meats
- molasses
- mollusks (clams, mussels, oysters, shrimp)
- nuts (highest to lowest): almonds, walnuts, pecans, cashew, pine, hazelnut, peanut, pistachios, and macadamia.
- prune juice
- red meats
- sardines
- sesame seeds
- squash and pumpkin seeds
- tofu
- tomato paste

Foods High in Iodine

- artichokes
- citrus fruits
- dried seaweeds (kelp is richest)
- egg yolk
- garlic
- grass-fed cow's milk and mozzarella cheese
- navy beans
- ocean fish: haddock, mackerel, cod
- pineapples
- potato with skin
- shellfish
- spinach
- strawberries
- tuna
- turkey breast
- watercress
- yogurt

Foods High in Magnesium

- almonds
- avocado
- blackberries
- buckwheat
- cabbage
- cashews
- cocoa
- corn
- edamame (dry roasted soy beans)
- eggplant
- garlic
- grapes
- green leafy vegetables
- legumes
- lima beans
- millet
- mineral water
- molasses
- muesli
- mushrooms
- pineapple
- potato with skin
- seeds (particularly squash, pumpkin, watermelon seeds, flax, sesame, and sunflower)
- soy flour
- tomato
- whole grains

Foods High in Manganese

- apricots
- barley
- blackberries
- Brazil nuts
- brown rice
- buckwheat
- bulgur
- grapefruit
- hazelnuts
- kelp
- lima beans
- oat bran
- peas
- pineapple
- raisins
- raspberries
- raw egg yolk
- wheat germ
- whole-grain flour

Foods High in Oligomeric Proanthocyanidin

- apples
- bilberry
- black tea
- blackcurrant
- cinnamon
- cocoa beans
- coconuts
- cranberries
- grapeseed
- green tea
- red grapes
- acai

Foods High in Quercetin

- apples
- blackberries
- blueberries
- broccoli
- capers
- chamomile
- dill
- eggplants
- green onions
- lovage
- okra
- peppers
- red onions
- red wine
- snap beans
- tomatoes

Foods High in Resveratrol

- acai and goji berries
- dark berries
- dark chocolate and cocoa/ cacao
- peanuts with skins on
- pistachios
- red and purple grapes

Foods High in Selenium

- apple cider vinegar
- barley
- Brazil nuts
- broccoli
- brown rice
- cashews
- caviar
- eggs
- garlic
- hazelnuts
- lobster, shrimp, and crab
- molasses
- mushrooms
- organic onion
- pecans
- poultry
- radish
- scallops
- shellfish and fish such as tuna, anchovies, swordfish, pickled herring, tilefish
- sunflower seeds
- turnips
- whole grains

Foods High in Silica

- avocado
- bananas
- barley
- beer
- carrots
- cucumber
- dandelion
- dark leafy greens
- green beans
- lettuce
- mineral water
- oats
- onions
- potatoes
- raisins
- root vegetables
- strawberries
- whole-grain cereals

Foods High in Soluble Fiber

- psyllium seeds
- legumes, especially lima and kidney beans followed by pinto, navy, black, and northern beans
- whole grains, especially oats and barley
- prunes
- pears
- citrus fruits
- nectarines
- peaches
- apples
- bananas
- blackberries
- lentils
- chickpeas
- flaxseeds
- artichokes
- Brussels sprouts
- jicama
- chili peppers
- carrots
- corn
- green cabbage
- cauliflower
- asparagus
- bok choy
- broccoli
- beets
- eggplant
- celery
- romaine lettuce
- iceberg lettuce

Foods High in Vitamin A

- carrots
- cheese
- cod liver oil
- collard greens
- cornmeal
- cream
- egg yolks
- kale
- liver and organ meats
- mustard greens
- poultry
- romaine lettuce
- spinach
- sweet potato
- Swiss chard
- turnip greens
- winter squash

Foods High in Vitamin B$_{12}$

- liver
- kidney
- lamb
- venison
- beef (grass-fed)
- molasses
- poultry
- crustaceans (scallops, shrimp)
- fish (sardines, salmon, cod, halibut)
- fortified cereals
- eggs
- dairy (yogurt)
- soy milk

Foods High in Vitamin B$_3$ (Niacin)

- yeast extract spread
- rice and wheat bran
- liver
- red meat (beef, organ meats, veal)
- fish (anchovies, tuna, salmon, sardines, sword-fish, white fish)
- chicken
- turkey
- halibut
- wheat germ
- peanuts
- legumes
- brewer's yeast
- mushrooms
- brown rice
- bulgur wheat
- sesame and sunflower seeds
- whole-meal pasta
- buckwheat
- dried peaches
- sun-dried tomatoes
- paprika

Foods High in Vitamin D

- butter
- caviar (red and black)
- cod liver oil
- eggs
- fortified milks (dairy and soy)
- herring
- kipper
- mackerel
- mushrooms
- oysters
- tinned salmon and sardines
- tuna

Foods High in Vitamin E

- almonds
- asparagus
- avocado
- brown rice
- cashews
- dried apricots
- dried herbs: paprika, red chili powder, oregano, and basil
- greens (Swiss chard, turnip greens, mustard greens, collard greens)
- papaya
- peanuts
- pickled green olives
- pine nuts
- soybean oil
- spinach (cooked)
- sunflower seeds
- taro root (cooked)
- walnuts
- wheat germ and wheat germ oil

Foods High in Vitamin K (Phylloquinone)

- asparagus
- broccoli
- Brussels sprouts
- cabbage
- darky leafy greens (kale, dandelion greens, collards, cress, spinach, turnip greens, mustard greens, beet greens, Swiss chard, broccoli, kohlrabi, radicchio, lettuce)
- dried herbs: basil, sage, thyme, parsley, coriander, marjoram, oregano
- green beans
- liver
- pickled cucumber
- prunes
- soybeans
- spring onions
- tomato

Foods High in Zinc

- almonds
- dark chocolate cocoa
- dhal
- fish (sardines,
- ginger root
- tomato sauce and paste
- oysters
- peanuts
- pecans
- pepitas (pumpkin seeds)
- popcorn
- red meat (liver, beef, lamb)
- sesame seeds
- shellfish (crab, scallops, shrimp)
- split peas
- sunflower seeds
- turkey
- walnuts
- wheat germ
- whole grains

ACID-FORMING FOODS

Our body likes to be in a state of steady balance (homoeostasis). We prefer our blood pressure to be within a certain safe range, same goes for blood sugar levels, hormone levels, temperature, and pH levels.

The pH is a measure of acid and base (alkalai) levels. Different parts of the body need to have differing pH. For instance, blood needs to hover around a pH of 7.4 (slightly alkaline) whereas stomach acid should be a corrosive 2 to 3, in order to start the digestion of protein, and to kill bacteria and parasites that might hitch a ride alongside food and water.

Although there is little research so far in this interesting area, for decades, natural health practitioners have recommended a diet that "alkalizes" the bloodstream. Basically the premise is that many diseases, including cancer, osteoporosis, arthritis, gout, and many others are influenced considerably by the dietary acid-alkaline balance. For example, osteoporosis may be the result of a chronic intake of acid-forming foods consistently outweighing the intake of alkaline foods leading to the bone being constantly forced to give up their alkaline minerals (calcium and magnesium) in order to buffer the excess acid.

Establishing pH Balance

In regards to proper pH balance, the dietary goal is quite simple—make sure that you have a higher intake of alkaline-producing foods than acid-producing foods. Basically, an alkaline diet is one rich in vegetables, fruit, and legumes while avoiding overconsumption of grains, meat, dairy, and some nuts. There is a difference between acidic foods and acid-forming foods. For example, while foods like lemons and citrus fruits may *taste* acidic, they actually have an alkalizing effect on the body. What determines the pH nature of the food in the body is the metabolic end products when it is digested (sometimes called "metabolic ash"). For example, the citric acid in citrus fruit is metabolized in the body to its alkaline form (citrate), and may even be converted to bicarbonate—also alkaline. I hope this is not too confusing; it's important to remember that, like everything in life, it's about balance. We need to eat some acid-forming foods too.

This table shows the acid-forming potential of various foods. The more acid forming, the higher the A value. The acid-forming potential or potential acidic load related to various proteins and minerals found within the food. The more alkaline or base forming a food is, the higher the B value. Remember, life is a balance, we need to include both A and B (acid forming and alkalining—or base—forming) foods for good health. It is only when you have a condition such as arthritis you might consider reducing some high acid-forming foods if they happen to be a big part of your diet.

ACID-FORMING POTENTIAL OF VARIOUS FOODS

FOOD	EFFECT	POTENTIAL ACIDIC LOAD	FOOD	EFFECT	POTENTIAL ACIDIC LOAD
BEVERAGES			**GRAINS AND FLOUR**		
Apple juice, unsweetened	B	−2.2	Barley (whole meal)	A	5.0
Carrot juice	B	−4.8	Corn (whole grain)	A	3.8
Coca-Cola	A	0.4	Oat flakes	A	10.7
Coffee	B	−1.4	Rice, brown	A	12.5
Orange juice, unsweetened	B	−2.9	Rice, white	A	4.6
Red wine	B	−2.4	Wheat flour, white	A	6.9
Tomato juice	B	−2.8	Wheat flour, whole meal	A	8.2
FATS, OIL, AND NUTS			**PASTA AND BREAD**		
Almonds	A	4.3	Spaghetti, white	A	6.5
Hazelnuts	B	−2.8	Bread, wheat flour, whole meal	A	1.8
Peanuts, plain	A	8.3			
Pistachio	A	8.5	Bread, white wheat	A	3.7
Walnuts	A	6.8	**LEGUMES**		
FISH AND SEAFOOD			Beans, green / French beans	B	−3.1
Halibut	A	7.8	Lentils, green and brown, whole, dried	A	3.5
Salmon	A	9.4			
Shrimp	A	7.6	Peas	A	1.2
Tiger Prawn	A	18.2	Soy beans	B	−3.4
FRUITS			Soy milk	B	−0.8
Apples	B	−2.2	Tofu	B	−0.8
Apricots	B	−4.8	**MEAT AND SAUSAGES**		
Bananas	B	−5.5	Beef, lean only	A	7.8
Figs, dried	B	−18.1	Chicken, meat only	A	8.7
Grapefruit	B	−3.5	Turkey, meat only	A	9.9
Grapes	B	−3.9	Veal, fillet	A	9.0
Kiwi fruit	B	−4.1	**MILK, DAIRY PRODUCTS AND EGGS**		
Orange	B	−2.7	Cheddar-type, reduced fat	A	26.4
Peach	B	−2.4	Cottage cheese, plain	A	8.7
Pear	B	−2.9	Egg	A	8.2
Raisins	B	−21.0	Egg, white	A	1.1
Strawberries	B	−2.2	Egg, yolk	A	23.4

ACID-FORMING POTENTIAL OF VARIOUS FOODS (continued)

FOOD	EFFECT	POTENTIAL ACIDIC LOAD	FOOD	EFFECT	POTENTIAL ACIDIC LOAD
MILK, DAIRY PRODUCTS AND EGGS (continued)			**VEGETABLES (continued)**		
Emmentaler Cheese full fat	A	21.1	Celery	B	–5.2
Fresh cheese (Quark)	A	11.1	Eggplant	B	–3.4
Milk, whole, evaporated	A	1.1	Fennel	B	–7.9
Milk, whole, pasteurized, and sterilized	A	0.7	Kale	B	–7.8
Parmesan	A	34.2	Lettuce, iceberg	B	–1.6
Processed cheese, plain	A	28.7	Mushrooms, common	B	–1.4
Rich, creamy full-fat cheese	A	13.2	Onions	B	–1.5
Skim milk	A	0.7	Peppers, green bell	B	–1.4
Whey	B	–1.6	Potatoes	B	–4.0
Yogurt, whole milk, fruit	A	1.2	Radish, red	B	–3.7
Yogurt, whole milk, plain	A	1.5	Rucola	B	–7.5
SWEETS			Sauerkraut	B	–3.0
Chocolate, dark	A	0.4	Spinach	B	–14.0
Chocolate, milk	A	2.4	Tomato	B	–3.1
Honey	B	–0.3	Zucchini	B	–4.6
VEGETABLES			**HERBS AND VINEGAR**		
Asparagus	B	–0.4	Apple vinegar	B	–2.3
Broccoli, green	B	–1.2	Basil	B	–7.3
Brussels sprouts	B	–4.5	Chives	B	–5.3
Carrots	B	–4.9	Parsley	B	–12.0
Cauliflower	B	–4.0	Wine vinegar, balsamic	B	–1.6

Reference: Vormann, J., Worlitschek, M., Goedecke, T., and Silver, B. "Supplementation with Alkaline Minerals Reduces Symptoms in Patients with Chronic Low Back Pain." *J Trace Elem Med Biol.* 2001;15(2–3):179–83.

APPENDIX F
BUTEYKO
BREATHING

WHAT IS IT?

While researching heart disease in the 1950s, Konstantin Buteyko, a Russian doctor, developed a breathing technique that not only helped reduce high blood pressure, but also a variety of conditions including asthma and anxiety. The premise of the technique is that many conditions are the result of "overbreathing" or chronic hyperventilation. Completely at odds to the popular view that taking big deep breaths of air is "good" breathing, the Buteyko way is to minimize intake, reducing and calming the breath toward normal. Not so different from ancient yogic pranayama or Hatha yoga breathing, whereby a man could breathe one breath per minute for the duration of one hour.

Buteyko believed that we need to increase carbon dioxide levels in the body. Carbon dioxide is often thought of as a "waste" gas, but carbon dioxide is vital to life. While it is true that we breathe to get rid of excess carbon dioxide, it is also important that we retain a quotient of this gas. Depending on our genetic predisposition, the habit of breathing too much causes a reduced concentration of carbon dioxide in the blood, resulting in narrowing of the airways and blood vessels. Conversely, a slight rise in carbon dioxide toward normal has several beneficial effects in the body, including relaxing smooth muscle, increasing oxygenation, switching on the relaxing nervous system, and increasing the body's production of nitric oxide.

Smooth Move

Smooth muscle surrounds and lines all hollow structures in the body, including the airways, blood vessels, bowel, bladder, and uterus. A slight increase in carbon dioxide serves to relax smooth muscle. In the case of smooth muscle lining the blood vessels, this will dilate or widen the arteries, improving circulation and helping lower blood pressure, and the effect on the blood vessels in the head will reduce the incidence of headaches. For the respiratory system, relaxation of the bronchi and smaller airways (bronchioles), will improve air flow and markedly reduce airway spasms associated with asthma. In the case of the bowel wall, relaxed smooth muscle means relief from symptoms of irritable bowel syndrome, constipation, and reflux.

Oxygen Increase

It seems counterintuitive that higher carbon dioxide levels will increase oxygenation in the body. Yet it's true. In fact, the Danish professor of physiology Christian Bohr figured out how this works in 1904, and the Bohr effect has been named in his honor.

As air is inhaled into the lungs, oxygen crosses over the alveolar membrane. Oxygen travels around by "sticking" to hemoglobin molecules, themselves attached to red blood cells. An increase in carbon dioxide "tells" hemoglobin to let go of the oxygen molecules, encouraging the precious oxygen cargo to be delivered to the organs and tissues where it is most needed. The Bohr effect proves that a slight increase in carbon dioxide levels increase oxygenation throughout the body—oxygen needed for muscles to work, energy to be produced, and the brain to function at optimum efficiency

Rest and Relax

The autonomic nervous system is comprised of two parts, the sympathetic nervous system (SNS), fueled by adrenaline and known as the "fight-or-flight" response, and the parasympathetic nervous system (PNS), which has the opposite effect, and has been coined the "rest and digest" response. Most people today have an overabundance of "fight-or-flight" hormone due to the many stresses of modern life. Increasing carbon dioxide levels helps to dampen down the SNS response and switches on the PNS. Which makes Buteyko breathing perfect for anyone who feels stressed and anxious. In the "old days," a person experiencing a panic attack was advised to breathe into a paper bag. What did this do? Increase carbon dioxide levels, switch on the PNS, and switch off the SNS.

Dr. NO

Nitric oxide (NO) is a naturally produced gas that medical scientists want to capture into saleable capsules as it has so many health benefits. At a cellular level, NO works as an antioxidant and anti-inflammatory, helping in the prevention of heart disease, cancer, and diabetes. Nitric oxide improves the immune response as well as increases blood and oxygen flow throughout the body, including the brain. Large amounts of NO are produced at the time of sexual climax. Increased carbon dioxide increases natural NO production. Bring on Dr. NO.

Breathing Boot Camp

All breathing exercises taught in Buteyko breathing have one goal—to decrease breathing volume toward normal, thereby increasing carbon dioxide levels toward normal. As seen previously, reduced breathing volume does not decrease oxygen levels; in fact, it's the reverse. Individuals who breathe heavily, with noticeable breathing during rest, or who mouth breathe or sigh regularly, are usually more tired, stressed, and are not as healthy as their nasal- and quiet-breathing peers.

Each Buteyko school and teacher has their own set of preferred exercises. The exercises retrain the brain to accept a higher amount of carbon dioxide than it is used to, if overbreathing is the problem. The Buteyko course itself is like a breathing "boot camp" with homework and daily practice to improve breathing technique. Generally, once the brain has reset to accept the correct levels of carbon dioxide, and symptoms have improved, you will not need to practice any special breathing exercises.

The best results are obtained by enrolling in a course. However, following are three simple suggestions that will help restore better breathing habits and reduce symptoms of overbreathing.

DID YOU KNOW?

A study of people with asthma, reported in the *Medical Journal of Australia*, showed that after three months, people practicing the Buteyko technique had decreased their requirement for reliever medication by 90 percent and the use of inhaled corticosteroids by 49 percent. Buteyko breathing can have remarkable effects on a variety of conditions as well as helping to prevent a host of others.

OVERBREATHING

If you regularly experience any of the following symptoms, you are overbreathing:

- ❏ breathing through the mouth
- ❏ snoring
- ❏ coughing
- ❏ sniffing
- ❏ heavy breathing at night
- ❏ holding of breath (apnea) during day, or sleep apnea

- ❏ sighing regularly
- ❏ wheezing
- ❏ yawning
- ❏ taking large breaths prior to talking
- ❏ hearing breath during rest

1. Always breathe through your nose. You were given a nose for a very good reason. To breathe. Mouth breathing is the biggest cause of overbreathing, and is also quite unattractive. Other reasons for nose breathing include:

- ❏ **Filter.** Breathing through the nose filters bacteria, dust, and pollens, allowing them to be eliminated via mucous membranes.

- ❏ **Heat and hydrate.** Air entering the nostrils at 43°F will, by the time it has traveled through the turbinates, be heated to a cozy 86°F, and be up to body temperature 98.6°F by the time it enters the lungs. Air is also moistened along the way. Cold, dry air is a common trigger for sinusitis and asthma.

- ❏ **Volume.** The nostrils offer a smaller surface area than an open mouth, reducing the volume of air.

Throughout the day, be aware of your breath, and always try to breathe through your nose. You will find nose breathing easier to do if you place your tongue at the roof of the mouth, with three quarters of your tongue resting on the upper palate, and the tip nestled just behind the front teeth.

2. Small breath holds. Small breath holds is a simple exercise that helps increase carbon dioxide levels and is incredibly calming and safe for all. It is usually done in four-minute intervals, but can be conducted for a longer period of time, as often as you like. Sit comfortably, with your back straight and both feet resting on the ground. Close your eyes. With your mouth closed, take a small breath in and a small breath out. Gently hold your nose closed with thumb and forefinger for five seconds. Release your grip, and continue breathing gently through your nose for a further ten seconds. Repeat the process for four minutes. Signs that the parasympathetic nervous system has been switched on AND that the brain is relearning to accept slightly higher carbon dioxide levels include one or more of the following: increased saliva, glassy or moist eyes, slight flushing of the skin, feeling warmer (especially hands and feet), and a sensation of calm and relaxation.

Small breath holds can be done at night if you have trouble sleeping or whenever you have some time on your hands (e.g., on the phone to a Verizon rep). You don't need to close your eyes, so it can be done while watching TV or travelling to work in the bus or train.

And if you feel odd holding your nose in public, just hold your breath for a count of five instead.

3. Taping up. One of the more controversial Buteyko techniques is taping your mouth shut at night. When you sleep you have no control over the way you breathe, and snoring and mouth breathing are very common and will undo a lot of the good work you have achieved by nose breathing throughout the day. First of all, cut a strip of surgical tape about five inches long and one-inch wide. Paper tape, which is kind to the skin, can be purchased at any pharmacy. Fold a tab over at each end to ensure easy removal. Say your goodnights, then tuck both lips inwards and apply the tape. Not only will taping up reduce snoring and mouth breathing, your sleep will be deep and untroubled. If the idea of taping up is frightening, take some time during the evening to tape up while reading or watching TV.

Conditions that can be helped by Buteyko breathing:

❏ asthma

❏ snoring

❏ sleep apnea

❏ breathlessness

❏ lightness in chest

❏ stress

❏ poor concentration

❏ fatigue

❏ insomnia

❏ fibromyalgia

❏ constipation

❏ muscle cramps

❏ gum disease

❏ sinusitis

❏ anxiety

❏ pins and needles

❏ impotence

❏ headaches

CARRIER OILS

Sweet Almond Oil

Made from almond kernels. A source of vitamins A, D, and E as well as B_1, B_2, and B_6. A light textured oil that is easily absorbed. Good for sensitive, dry, inflamed skin. Good for nourishing the skin and preventing wrinkles. It can be used as a massage oil, and works well as a carrier oil for aromatherapy oils.

Apricot Kernel Oil

Made from apricot kernels. A light textured oil that is often used in cosmetic products to soften the skin. Good for dry and prematurely aged skin. Has moisturizing and nourishing properties, and is good for preventing wrinkles and treating inflammation. An excellent carrier oil for aromatherapy.

Grapeseed Oil

Made from washed and dried grape seeds. Light and nongreasy. Contains vitamin E and antioxidants that may reduce the appearance of stretch marks. Can be used as a carrier oil for aromatherapy.

Macadamia

Made from the macadamia nut. A pale yellow, nutty-smelling oil. Good for dry, mature, and ageing skin. Contains the same components found in human sebum. This oil is softening and rejuvenating. Easily absorbed by the skin and can be used as a carrier oil for aromatherapy.

Sesame

Made from sesame seeds. An oil used extensively in Ayurvedic massage and medicine. A light golden-colored oil containing vitamins A, E, and lecithin. An excellent oil for sun-damaged and dehydrated skin. Also therapeutic for eczema and psoriasis. A carrier oil for aromatherapy.

Sunflower

Made from sunflower seeds. Choose cold-pressed. A golden-colored, odorless oil that is a good carrier oil for aromatherapy. Suitable for all skin types.

Base Oils

These oils can be used by themselves or added to a carrier oil with possible the addition of aromatherapy oils.

Arnica

Made from the arnica flower. For external use only; very effective for bruising, muscular aches and pains, sunburn, and diaper rash. Do not use if skin is broken.

Avocado

From the dried flesh of avocado fruit. A deep green, herbaceous-smelling oil. Rich in essential fatty acids and vitamins A and D. Good for eczema and psoriasis. Helpful for dehydrated and prematurely lined skin.

Borage

Made from the seeds of the borage plant. High in gamma-linoleic acid. A pale golden-yellow oil. Good for dry and prematurely aged skin. Helpful for eczema and psoriasis.

Calendula

Made from the flowers of calendula or marigold plant. A golden yellow color. Not used as a massage oil, but can be used externally for broken veins, eczema, sunburn, insect bites, burns, abrasions, and wounds. It is anti-inflammatory and healing.

Carrot

From the carrot root vegetable. Bright orange color and high in vitamins A, B, C, and D. Good for dry and mature skin; helps reduce scarring and itching.

Evening Primrose

Made from the seeds of the evening primrose. Light yellow oil very helpful for dry, flaking, and fragile skin. A moisturizing and soothing oil. Good for itching, eczema, scarring, and psoriasis.

Jojoba

From the jojoba bean. Jojoba is not an oil, but a light-colored liquid wax, similar in structure to the skin's own sebum. Doesn't oxidize. Excellent for inflamed skin, mature or oily. Good for acne, eczema, stretch marks.

Rosehip

From the berries or rosehips after the rose has flowered. High in vitamin C. Excellent for damaged, mature, and sun-damaged skin. Helps to treat burns, scar tissue, and wrinkles.

Wheat Germ

Made from the germ of the wheat grain. Particularly high in Vitamin E. Has a strong odor and orange-yellow color. Excellent for mature and prematurely aged skin. Good for eczema, psoriasis, and treating scar tissue. Recommended for dry, devitalized skin.

INDEX

Acetaldehyde, 183

Acetylcholine, 223

Acidity, 22

Acidophilus, 75

Acne, 6–9

Acrylic acid, 75

Acupressure, 236

Acupuncture, 25, 29, 70, 142, 165, 174, 181, 186, 236, 238, 289

Adaptogens, 92, 167, 223, 247, 281, 287

Addictions, 14, 17

Adenine, 173

Adhatoda vasica, 32

Adrenal exhaustion, 278

Adrenal glands, 17, 18, 145, 146, 226, 227, 278

Adrenaline, 17, 66, 127, 276, 278, 279, 286

Affirmations, 20

Aging, 37, 79, 221

Air conditioning, 109

Airways, 31

Albizia, 155, 178

Alcohol, 11, 18, 37, 54, 61, 62, 84, 91, 94, 98, 102, 119, 124, 127, 129, 134, 138, 144, 147, 156, 161, 173, 178, 181, 183, 188, 196, 198, 207, 208, 221, 226, 230, 232, 237, 241, 246, 250, 251, 253, 263, 272, 274, 281, 303

Alexander Technique, 25, 34

Allergens, 180, 272
    airborne, 177–178

Allergic rhinitis. *See* Hay fever.

Allergies, 9
    addictive, 153–154
    desensitization, 34, 180, 272–273

food, 22, 23, 27, 28, 31, 91, 119, 127, 134, 137, 138, 152–156, 157, 158, 178, 211, 222, 238, 263, 272, 274

food avoidance/challenge program, 154–155, 157, 158, 159

See also Hay fever.

Allium cepa, 99

Allopurinol, 173

Aloe vera, 82, 95, 139, 156, 171, 190, 204, 230, 251, 264, 267

Alopecia. *See* Baldness.

Alopecia areata, 42, 43

Alopecia universalis, 42

Apha-lipoic acid, 125

Alzheimer's disease, 223, 280

Anal fistulas, 202

Anaphylaxis, 152, 153

Andrographis, 41, 49, 64, 70, 82, 91, 94, 98, 99, 131, 132, 134, 167, 176, 204, 230, 290

Anemia, 10–13, 43

Angelica, 41

Angiogenesis, 60, 65

Aniseed, 110, 213

Anorexia nervosa, 13–16, 197, 240

Anthocyanidins, 173

Antibiotics, 73–74, 127, 149, 160

Antidepressants, 58, 119, 145

Antifungals, 75

Anti-inflammatories, 23, 28, 65, 179, 232

Antioxidants, 38, 64, 77, 87, 188, 198–199, 232, 253

Antiperspirants, 47

Anus, 189

Anxiety, 17–21, 46, 56, 118, 129, 206, 222
Aphrodisiacs, 144–145
Apis, 29
Apoptosis, 60, 65
Appendix, 202
Appetite control, 57
Apples, 128, 175
Aquarobics, 25
Arginine, 94, 200
Arnica, 30, 54, 68, 188, 215
Aromatherapy, 121, 145, 224
    See also Carrier oils; Essential oils.
Arsenicum album, 129, 234
Arteries, 36, 37, 38, 87, 194
Arthritis
    osteo-, 22–26
    psoriatic, 263
    rheumatoid, 26–30
Artichoke leaf, 41
Artichokes
    globe, 37, 38, 68, 71, 88, 164, 167, 237
Aspartame, 182
Aspirin, 23
Assertiveness, 29
Asthma, 31–35, 320
Astragalus, 29, 32, 37, 38, 68, 70, 71, 82, 91,
    92, 223, 233, 281
Atheroma, 87
Atherosclerosis, 36–38, 88, 144, 192
Athlete's foot, 160, 162
Athletes, 243
Ausberger's rule, 4
Autoimmune diseases, 27, 29, 169, 231–233,
    261, 263, 264, 280, 285

Bach, Edward, 295
Bach flowers, 295–300
    Agrimony, 296
    Aspen, 208, 220, 281–282
    Beech, 296
    Centaury, 296
    Cerato, 296
    Cherry Plum, 296–297, 300
    Chestnut Bud, 247, 297
    Chicory, 114, 165, 297

Clematis, 224, 297, 300
Crab Apple, 15, 145, 247, 297
Elm, 297
Gentian, 297
Gorse, 120, 200, 297
Heather, 297
Holly, 259, 297–298
Honeysuckle, 298
Hornbeam, 298
Impatiens, 139, 298, 299
Larch, 145, 298
Mimulus, 15, 208, 220, 270, 282, 298
Mustard, 120, 259, 298
Oak, 298
Olive, 91, 147, 167, 298
Pine, 213, 298
Red Chestnut, 299
Rescue Remedy, 18, 20, 46, 68, 215, 237,
    281, 295, 300
Rock Rose, 20, 208, 299, 300
Rock Water, 15, 299
Scleranthus, 299
Star of Bethlehem, 30, 68, 282, 300
Sweet Chestnut, 282, 299
Vervain, 213, 299
Vine, 299
Walnut, 15, 228, 259, 299
Water Violet, 299
White Chestnut, 15, 208, 213, 282, 299
Wild Oat, 300
Wild Rose, 300
Willow, 114, 165, 259, 300
Back, 34, 149, 151, 183, 240
Bacon, Francis, 67
Bad breath, 39–42
Baldness, 42–45
Balms, 305
Banana peels, 291
Baptisia, 29, 167
Barberry, 161
Barley grass, 46
Barley water, 113
Barnes Basal Temperature test, 285–286
Barometric changes, 31
Barrett's esophagitis, 266

Base oils, 323–324
Baths and bathing, 47, 82, 84, 92, 114, 181, 208–209, 228, 282
    communal, 160, 161
    foot, 100, 228
    steam, 100, 270
Bats, 22, 25
Bayberry, 84
Bedrooms, 209
Bee pollen, 179
Beer, 119, 262
Benign prostatic hyperplasia (BPH), 261
Bergamot, 21
Beta-carotene, 64, 77, 87, 185, 204, 308
Beta-glucan polysaccharides, 65
Betaine hydrochloride, 151
Bicarbonate of soda, 58, 82, 114, 230
Bilberry, 44, 54, 64, 77, 84, 125, 176, 269, 289
Bile, 107, 164, 165, 237
Bile duct, 163
Bingeing, 56, 57
Bioflavonoids, 54, 161, 173, 189, 190, 199, 255, 288, 308
Biotin, 116
Birch, 174
Bitter melon, 125, 150
Black cohosh, 184, 185, 227, 228
Bladderwack, 286
Blepharitis, 102
Blood, loss of, 10, 141
Blood pressure, 192
    high, 33, 36, 37, 38, 86, 184, 192–195, 261
    low, 192
Blood sugar. See Glucose.
Blue flag, 79
Blueberries, 125, 173
BMI. See Body mass index (BMI).
Body fat, 60–61, 78, 226
    abdominal, 125
    fear of, 14
Body image, 243
    disordered. See Dysmorphia, body.
Body mass index (BMI), 243
Body odor (BO) 45–48
Body temperature, 99, 208–209, 284

basal, 285–286, 287
Bohr, Christian, 319
Bohr effect, 33, 319
Boils, 48–50
Bone, Kerry, 90, 92, 167
Bones, 22, 205, 240–242
Boron, 29, 309
Boswellia, 24, 29, 174
Bowel movements, 104, 107, 131, 189, 211, 255
Bowels. See Intestines.
BPH. See Benign prostatic hyperplasia (BPH).
Brahmi, 221, 222
Brain, 222, 224
Bran, 11, 87, 165
Breakfast, 222, 246, 251
Breast-feeding, 142, 254, 255
Breasts, 227, 258
Breath holds, 19, 33, 320, 321
Breathing and breathing techniques, 19, 20, 21, 34, 41, 52, 149, 320–322
    belly, 19, 87, 107, 205, 209, 282
    mouth, 175, 176
    See also Buteyko breathing.
Breckman, Israel, 92
Broccoli, 87
Bromelain, 51, 54, 110, 288
Bromhidrosis. See Body odor.
Bronchi, 51, 109
Bronchioles, 34
Bronchitis, 51–53, 109, 196
Bronchodilators, 32
Bruising, 53–55
Bryonia, 29
Buckwheat, 189
Bulimia, 56–59
Bupluerum, 29, 68, 233
Burdock, 8, 46, 49, 71, 79, 138, 264
Butcher's broom, 54, 190, 216, 269, 289
Buteyko, Konstantin, 33, 319
Buteyko breathing, 19, 33, 34, 38, 41, 52, 111, 176, 179–180, 182, 184, 186, 194, 213, 224, 273, 275, 282, 319–322
Butyric acid, 63

Cabbages, 251

Caffeine, 18, 32, 91, 105, 119, 141, 147, 182, 194, 197, 207, 226, 258, 261, 281

Calcium, 11, 18, 193, 194, 207, 208, 219, 240, 241, 242, 254, 255, 309

Calendula, 8, 29, 41, 46, 49, 75, 79, 82, 84, 102, 134, 138, 139, 156, 161, 164, 167, 190, 204, 230, 237, 252, 267, 270

Californian poppy, 185, 207, 215, 227

Calories, 63, 244, 248

Cancer, 60–67, 243
  breast, 65, 228
  prostate, 65, 261
  stages, 62
  treatments, dealing with, 67–72

Candida, 73–76, 91, 134, 138, 149, 151, 263, 272

Candida albicans, 45, 46, 73–76, 90, 91, 113, 134, 138, 149, 151, 160, 263, 272

Canker sores. *See* Ulcers, mouth.

Cannon, W. B., 277

Cantharis, 114

Capillaries, 268, 269

Caprylic acid, 161

Carbohydrates, 86, 123, 132, 230, 245, 248, 261

Carbon dioxide, 19, 33, 52, 111, 194, 273, 319

Carnitine, 247, 254

Carotenoids, 77

Carrier oils, 323–324

Cartilage, 22, 23

Cascara, 106

Casein, 7, 156, 157

Cat's claw, 29, 68, 70, 82, 94, 98, 131, 132, 167, 176, 204, 230, 233, 291

Cataracts, 76–78

Catechins, 199

Cayenne, 44

Celery and celery seeds, 24, 79, 88, 174

Celiac disease. *See* Gluten intolerance.

Cells, 60, 71, 123
  endometrial, 141, 142
  white blood (WBC), 70, 98, 166

Cellulite, 78–80

Cellulitis, 78

Cereals, 11

CFS. *See* Chronic fatigue syndrome (CFS).

Chakras, 221, 145

Chamomile, 20, 25, 58, 64, 95, 102, 106, 129, 132, 171, 194, 204, 207, 213, 215, 236, 252, 255, 281

Champagne, 216

Chaste tree, 7–8, 199

Cheese, 161

Chelation, 12, 242

Chelidonium, 88, 164, 237

Chemical sensitivities, 158–159

Chemobrain, 222

Chemotherapy, 43, 69–71, 196, 222, 235
  post- , 71

Chen pi, 236

Cherries, 173

Chewing, 105, 131, 132, 148, 149, 150, 175, 212, 267

Chia seeds, 7, 41, 87, 89, 107, 108, 124, 132, 165, 190, 198, 203, 222, 253, 258

Chickenpox, 81–82, 94

Chickweed, 82, 139, 252

Chilblains, 83–85

Childers, Norman F., 23, 28

Children, 4, 20, 34, 81, 135, 158, 166, 206, 207

Chilies, 79, 84, 98, 269

Chlorella, 46

Chlorine, 74, 75, 117

Chlorophyll, 46, 147

Chocolate, 258

Cholecystectomy, 164

Choleretics, 164

Cholesterol, 88, 86–89, 124, 280
  high density lipoprotein (HDL), 87, 124
  low density lipoprotein (LDL), 38, 87

Chondroitin, 24

Chromium, 119, 125, 182, 258, 309

Chronic fatigue syndrome (CFS), 90–93

Cilia, 109

Cinnamon, 98, 110, 125, 129, 161, 236, 272

Circadian rhythms, 206, 215

Circulation, 43, 44, 45, 70, 77, 79, 83–85, 116, 125, 141, 145, 221, 222, 288, 289

Citrate, 219

Clivers, 8, 46, 49, 79

Clothes, 47, 80, 82, 114, 116, 120, 139, 200, 216, 228, 256

Cloves, 161

Cocooning, 20

Codonopsis, 12, 125

Coenzyme Q10 (CoQ10), 41, 64, 88, 91, 147, 176, 270

Coffea, 184, 208

Coffee, 11, 32, 39, 40, 94, 105, 113, 124, 129, 156, 183, 215, 222, 230, 232, 241, 258, 263

Cognitive behavioral therapy (CBT), 20

Cold sores, 94–96, 230

Colds, 97–101, 194, 216, 238, 271, 274

Coleus, 125, 264, 286

Colitis, ulcerative, 27, 127, 201

Collagen, 79, 176, 241

Colocynth, 131

Colon, 130

Colonic irrigations, 47

Colonoscopies, 106

Compassion, 57

Compresses, 138, 304
  castor oil, 24, 29, 165, 238
  cold, 54, 95, 235, 236, 237, 238
  Earl Grey tea, 82, 95
  ginger, 24, 29, 132, 165, 238
  hot, 49, 238

Compression stockings, 289

Concentration, 70, 221–225

Congeners, 183

Conjunctivitis, 102–103

Constipation, 6, 12, 13, 38, 40, 41, 47, 70, 104–108, 131, 137, 149, 184–185, 189, 245, 255, 288

Contraceptive pills, 74, 113, 164

Cooking, 57, 119, 281

Cookware, 188

Copper, 11, 25, 29

CoQ10. *See* Coenzyme Q10 (CoQ10).

Corn silk, 113, 219

Corticosteroids, 205

Cortisol, 17, 66, 86, 118, 206, 221, 222, 223, 226, 244, 247, 248, 276, 278, 279–281, 282, 285

Cortisone, 32, 74, 196, 240, 244, 279

Corydalis, 142

Cosmetics, 103, 138

Couch grass, 174, 219

Cough, 52, 109–112

Counseling. *See* Therapy, psychological.

Cradle cap. *See* Dermatitis, seborrheic.

"CRAFT disease," 221

Crataeva, 219, 262

Cravings, sweet, 8, 258, 281

Creams, 305

Crohn's disease, 127, 201

Cryptosporidium, 127

Culpepper, Nicholas, 303

Curcumin, 24, 28, 65, 188, 199, 232

Cystic fibrosis, 196

Cystitis, 112–115, 218

Cytotoxic blood test, 159

Daidzein, 261

Dalai Lama, 224

Damiana, 119, 145, 147, 199, 215, 247

Dandelion, 8, 41
  leaf, 79, 174, 194, 219, 259
  root, 12, 46, 49, 70, 73, 90, 107, 150, 167

Dandruff, 115–117

DASH (Dietary Approaches to Stop Hypertension), 193, 194

Deep vein thrombosis (DVT), 215–216

Dementia, 221, 223

Dental care, 41, 58–59, 176

Dental devices, 39, 131

Deodorants, 47

Depression, 56, 58, 118–121, 144, 206, 222, 227–228, 280

Depression and Bipolar Support Alliance, 118

Dermatitis, 137–140
  contact, 137–138
  seborrheic, 115

Detoxification, 8, 71, 165

Devil's claw, 24, 29

DEXA scans, 241

DHA, 119–120, 125, 222, 223, 253, 254, 310

DHGLA, 179

Diabetes, 37, 62, 74, 113, 144, 196, 243
  type 1, 123
  type 2, 123–126, 261

Diaphragms, 113

Diarrhea, 70, 104, 106, 127–130, 168
   chronic, 128, 240
Diet, 3, 15, 18, 46, 48, 61, 63–64, 65, 67, 74,
      77, 79, 81, 84, 86–87, 91, 119, 121, 123,
      124, 131–132, 147, 153, 164, 193–193,
      198, 219, 226, 263
   Beaming with Health. *See* Diet, low-starch.
   bland, 230
   candida, 74–75, 116, 151, 161, 272
   gluten-free, 170
   iron-rich, 12, 13, 187
   low-fat, 212, 232, 245, 248
   low-iron, 187
   low-starch, 62, 244–247, 248
   high-fat, 125, 163
   Mediterranean, 119
   Pritikin, 36, 248
   raw, 63, 79, 84, 144
   vegetarian and vegan, 10, 27–28, 37, 46, 48,
      63, 71, 232, 258, 261, 263
Digestion, 12, 13, 18, 24, 150, 155, 211, 269
   babies', 153
Dinner, 246
Diverticulitis, 130–133
Diverticulosis, 130
DNA, 198
Dong quai, 12, 64, 79, 142, 199, 227, 258
Dopamine, 120
Douches, 75
Drinks, 269
   energy, 207
   soft, 173, 245
   sports, 183, 234
Drugs, recreational, 221
Dry mouth, 40
Dysbiosis, 137, 149, 157, 202
Dysmorphia, body, 13, 14, 16, 57

E. coli, 127
Ear candles, Hopi, 135–136
Ear infections, 133–136
Ears, 133–136
Eating, 18, 149, 212, 238, 251
   disorders, 13–16, 56–59
   emotional, 244, 248

   excessive, 56–59, 238, 244
Echinacea, 8, 29, 32, 41, 46, 48, 64, 68, 70, 75,
      82, 91, 94, 98, 99, 102, 114, 131, 132, 134,
      138, 155, 161, 166, 167, 176, 204, 216, 230,
      233, 272, 291
Eczema, 48, 137–140, 263
Effleurage, 289
EGCG (epigallocatechin gallate), 28, 65, 232
Ejaculations, 262
Elastin, 79
Elder, 41, 110, 272
Elecampane, 32
Electrical fields, 209
Electrolytes, 183
Elephants, 221
Emotional Intelligence (Goleman), 224
Emotions, 56, 58, 84, 145, 165, 227, 238, 257,
      259, 282, 295
Emphysema, 51
Endometriosis, 141–143
Endorphins, 120
Energy, 278, 284
Environment, 31
Enzymes, digestive, 151, 155, 158, 204, 213, 269
EPA, 23, 24, 28, 32, 119–120, 125, 142, 194,
      232, 247, 253, 254, 258, 310
Epictetus, 120
Epigenetics, 61
Epilobium, 262
Epi-pens, 154
Epithelium, 38
EPO. *See* Oils, evening primrose.
Epsom salts, 106, 132, 181, 209, 282
Equilibrium, 236
Erectile dysfunction (ED), 143–146
Esophagus, 109
Essential oils, 305–306
   atlas cedarwood, 114, 265
   basil, 121, 224
   bay, 44
   bergamot, 50, 121, 195, 228, 283, 195
   black pepper, 85, 108, 213, 216
   cajeput, 35, 52, 82, 100, 265, 273
   cardamom, 108, 151, 238
   carrot seed, 108, 174

chamomile, 21, 50, 55, 82, 96, 121, 132, 139, 210, 271
clary sage, 44, 117, 259, 283
coriander seed, 174
cypress, 9, 47, 80, 96, 162, 228, 289
eucalyptus, 30, 35, 111, 162, 273, 275, 291
everlasting, 52, 139, 271, 273
frankincense, 21, 121, 283
geranium, 55, 96, 162, 216, 259, 275, 289
ginger, 25, 44, 84, 195, 238
grapefruit, 50, 108, 174
jasmine, 145
jojoba, 121, 139
juniper, 30, 44, 80, 108, 174
kunzea, 85
lavender, 9, 50, 55, 75, 82, 96, 111, 121, 132, 139, 210, 216, 265, 271, 283
lavender spike, 25, 30
lemon, 85, 224, 289
lemon myrtle, 96
lemongrass, 47, 117, 162
mandarin, 151, 238
myrrh, 139, 162
neroli, 121, 195, 210, 259
palmarosa, 271
patchouli, 145
peppermint, 35, 82, 97, 213, 216, 224, 238, 275
pine, 195
ravensara, 52, 96, 100, 273
red myrtle, 289
rose, 145, 200
rose otto, 259
rosemary, 44, 117, 195, 216, 224
rosewood, 47
sandalwood, 9, 52, 100, 114, 210, 275
sage, 224
spearmint, 151, 235
sweet fennel, 25, 35, 228
sweet marjoram, 30, 85, 213
tea tree, 9, 75, 82, 96, 114, 117, 162, 265, 291
therapeutic properties, 293–293
thyme, 84, 111, 275
vetiver, 21, 210
Virginian cedar wood, 265

yarrow, 55, 271
ylang ylang, 21, 121, 141, 195
See also Carrier oils; Oils.
Estrogen, 63, 79, 141, 142, 197, 225, 226, 227, 240, 258, 261
Euphorbia, 110
Eustachian tubes, 135
Exercise, 3, 13, 16, 25, 26, 29, 31, 37, 66, 71, 72, 85, 92, 99, 107, 120, 123, 126, 142, 145, 147, 151, 167, 174, 184, 185, 190, 205, 208, 213, 216, 220, 227, 248, 255, 262, 282, 289
  aerobic, 19, 38, 79–80, 88, 194–195, 248, 259
  weight-bearing, 241, 248
Eyebright, 41, 102, 134, 178, 184, 272
Eyes, 102, 185, 278
  lens, 76
  pupils, 278
Eyestrain, 185
Eyewashes, 102

Facials, 8
False unicorn root, 199, 258
Familial hypercholesterolemia, 86
Fasting, 64, 97, 202, 204
Fatigue, 146–148, 215
Fats, 7, 15, 36, 43, 62–63
  artificial, 127
  saturated, 86, 232
  trans, 77, 86, 204
Fear, 47
Fecal leakage, 127
Feet, 47
Feldenkrais method, 25, 34
Fennel, 213
Fenugreek, 125
Fetal alcohol syndrome, 253
Feverfew, 64, 186
Fevers, 82, 229
Fiber, 7, 40, 63, 86, 87, 104, 105, 106, 131, 132, 164, 185, 189, 190, 203
  soluble, 107, 124, 132, 165, 237, 245, 258, 264, 288, 313
Fight-or-flight syndrome, 277, 278
Fish, 23, 28, 32, 86, 138, 141, 194, 198, 222, 232, 253, 254, 258, 263

Flatulence, 148–152
Flavonols, 308
Fletcher, Horace, 104, 149
Flossing, 41, 176
Flu, 97–101, 274
Fluid retention, 79
Fluids, drinking of, 7, 23, 32, 39, 40, 46, 77,
　　79, 81, 98, 104, 105–106, 110, 113, 116,
　　128, 131, 134, 138, 164, 166, 173, 178,
　　182, 183, 185, 189, 194, 215, 218, 222,
　　234, 236, 237, 255, 261, 263, 267, 272,
　　274, 281
Fluoride, 229, 230
Folate. *See* Vitamin B9.
Folic acid. *See* Vitamin B9.
Food hygiene, 234
Food poisoning, 127, 234–235
Foods, 153, 155, 198–199, 226, 266
　　acid-forming, 23, 28, 64, 173, 241, 316–318
　　alkaline-forming, 23, 28, 63–64, 316
　　bitter, 11–13, 150, 151, 269
　　calcium-rich, 40, 241
　　dairy, 40, 74, 98, 110, 178, 184, 242, 258,
　　　263, 272, 284
　　fermented, 65
　　high fat, 164, 237, 238
　　iodine-rich, 286
　　iron-rich, 12
　　prebiotic/probiotic, 40, 170–171, 203, 212
　　raw, 286
　　rotation of, 155
　　sodium-rich, 178, 193
　　sources, 307–315
　　starchy, 246
　　sweet, 18
Free radicals, 87, 198
Fried's rule, 4
Frostbite, 83
Fructose, 157, 212–213
　　malabsorption, 149, 150, 157–158, 212
Fruits, 64, 77, 91, 129, 157, 199, 245, 246, 253
Fucoidan, 65
Fumitory, 264
Fungal infections. *See* Infections, fungal.
Fungi, 160

Galactose, 156
Galen, 60
Gallbladder, 164, 165, 237
Gallstones, 163–165, 237–238
Gamma-linoleic acid (GLA), 232, 258–259
Garagiola, Joe, 42
Gargling, 274–275
Garlic, 32, 39, 38, 39, 49, 64, 65, 71, 75, 79, 84,
　　88, 98, 99, 102, 110, 113, 124, 131, 132,
　　134, 135, 161, 171, 176, 178, 184, 193, 194,
　　272, 291
Gas, 38
Gastritis, 238, 250
Gastroesophageal reflux disorder (GERD). *See*
　　Reflux.
Generall Historie of Plantes (Gerard), 223
Genes. *See* Heredity.
Genistein, 262
Gentian, 41, 150
Gerard, John, 223
Giardia, 127
Ginger, 24, 25, 29, 43, 58, 70, 79, 84, 98, 125,
　　129, 132, 142, 156, 164, 173, 174, 183, 213,
　　232, 235, 236, 237, 247, 255, 256, 267, 272
Ginger ale, 234
Gingivitis. *See* Gum disease.
Ginkgo biloba, 37, 38, 44, 54, 70, 77, 84, 125,
　　145, 176, 190, 199, 216, 223, 269, 289
Ginseng
　　American, 37, 38, 125
　　Korean, 64, 70, 71, 91, 92, 147, 199, 215,
　　　223, 281
　　panax, 68, 119, 145, 167, 227
　　Siberian, 32, 64, 68, 70, 71, 91, 92, 147, 167,
　　　215, 223, 247, 281
GLA. *See* Gamma-linoleic acid (GLA).
Glands
　　endocrine, 286
　　sebaceous, 6
Glandular fever, 166–168, 274
Globus hystericus, 274, 275
Glucosamine, 24
Glucose, 64, 77, 119, 123, 156, 182, 207, 219,
　　221, 222, 236, 238, 248, 280

Glue ear, 135

Glutamine, 58, 156, 171, 204, 223, 252, 262, 267

Glutathione, 65

Gluten, 104, 105, 127, 141, 168–172, 202, 203, 229, 230, 267

Gluten intolerance, 168–172, 196, 240, 263, 266, 286

Gluten sensitivity. *See* Gluten intolerance.

Glycemic index, 124, 245

Goat's rue, 125

Goiters, 284

Goitrogens, 286

Goldenrod, 41, 102, 134, 178, 184, 272

Goldenseal, 29, 32, 38, 41, 49, 64, 75, 91, 98, 102, 131, 132, 134, 138, 139, 150, 156, 161, 167, 178, 184, 230, 252, 267, 272

Goleman, Daniel, 224

Gotu kola, 79, 139, 189, 190, 215, 221, 223, 264, 269, 270, 281

Gout, 172–174

Grains, 168, 248

Grapeseed, 54, 176, 190, 269, 270, 289

Gravel root, 174

Grazing, 245

Green, James, 150

Grindelia, 32, 110

Guaiacum, 24

Guanine, 173

Guarana, 247

Gum, 41, 149, 175, 212, 230, 251

Gum disease, 39, 41, 42, 175–177

Gymnema, 125, 247, 258

Gynecological disorders, 197

Hair, 42–45
    analysis, 242
    follicles, 43, 48

Hair products, 115, 117

Halitosis. *See* Bad breath.

Hand creams, 139

Handwashing, 234

Hangovers, 238

Hashimoto's thyroiditis, 285

Hats, 84, 270

Hawthorn, 194

Hay fever, 134, 157, 177–180

Headaches, 181–186
    caffeine withdrawal (CWHs), 183–183
    constipation, 184–185
    dehydration, 182
    eyestrain, 185
    food chemical sensitivities, 182–183
    hangover, 183
    hormonal, 184
    hypertension, 184
    lack-of-sleep, 184
    low blood sugar, 182
    sinus, 184, 271
    stress and tension, 181–182
    "your neck is out," 183
    See also Migraines.

Heart attacks, 38, 86, 243

Heart beat, 224

Heart disease, 37, 87, 124, 225, 243, 281

Heartburn. *See* Reflux.

Heartsease, 139

He-Gu (acupuncture point), 181–182, 185, 235, 236, 237, 238

Helicobacter pylori, 39, 238, 250, 251, 266, 267

Hemochromatosis, 12, 187–188

Hemoglobin, 11, 33, 319

Hemorrhoids, 189–191, 255

Herbal bitters, 70, 106–107, 150, 151, 155, 164, 237, 269

Heredity, 17, 22, 27, 36, 44, 61, 83, 86, 116, 123, 137, 164, 169, 173, 177–178, 187, 189, 202, 218, 232, 243, 263, 269, 285, 288

Hernias, hiatus, 266

Herpes, 94–96

Herpes simplex virus type 1 (HSV-1), 94

Herpes simplex virus type-2 (HSV-2), 94, 95

Hesperidin, 288

Heterocyclic amines (HCAs), 62

High-sensitivity C-reactive protein (hsCRP), 87

Hippocrates, 203

Histamine, 31, 32, 158, 183

Homeopathy, 29

Honey, 24, 98, 178
    manuka, 70, 251

Honeycombs, 178

Hops, 18, 215, 207, 227, 262
Horehound
    black, 236
    white, 32, 110
Hormone replacement therapy (HRT), 76, 226
Hormones, 6, 7–8, 17, 44, 45, 61, 116, 118,
    141, 183, 185, 211, 222, 224, 227, 257
Hornbeam, 147, 167
Horny goat weed, 145
Horse chestnut, 54, 84, 189, 190, 269, 289
Horseradish, 41, 84, 98, 178, 184, 272
Hot flashes, 226, 227, 228
Hot toddies, 110, 274
Houses, damp, 160, 161
HRT. *See* Hormone replacement therapy (HRT).
Human growth hormone (HGH), 206, 207
Human papillomavirus (HPV), 290
Humidifiers, 34, 52, 111
Hunger, 245
Hydration. *See* Fluids, drinking of.
Hydrochloric acid, 10, 56, 58, 155, 250, 269
    low. *See* Hypochlorhydria.
Hydrogen breath test, 157, 212
Hyperglycemia, 123
Hypertension. *See* Blood pressure, high.
Hyperventilation, 19, 35
Hypnotherapy, 19, 30, 145, 209
Hypochlorhydria, 149, 150, 269
Hypoglycemia, 123
Hypotension. *See* Blood pressure, low.
Hypothyroidism, 244, 284–285

IBD. *See* Inflammatory bowel disease (IBD).
IBS. *See* Irritable bowel syndrome (IBS).
Immune system, 27, 32, 48, 61, 68, 70, 82, 153,
    155–156, 161, 166, 230, 233, 257, 280, 281
Immunoglobulin E (IgE), 152
Impotence. *See* Erectile dysfunction (ED).
Indole-3-carbinol, 199
Indoles, 65
Infections, 110, 211
    bronchial, 51
    colon, 130–133
    fungal, 160–163, 272
    respiratory, 31, 32, 51

throat, 40, 274–276
Infertility, 196–201
Inflammation, 60–61, 62, 65, 130, 131, 285
Inflammatory bowel disease (IBD), 201–205, 240
Influenza. *See* Flu.
Inner child, 16
Insomnia, 17, 18, 206–210, 227, 244
Insulin, 61, 123, 245
Insulin resistance, 123, 247
Intestines, 69, 73, 156, 168, 170–171, 201–205,
    211–214
Inversion tables, 25
Iodine, 43, 162, 247, 253, 254, 255, 284, 285,
    286, 311
Ipecac, 111
Ipecacuanha, 235, 237
Iridology torches, 278
Iron, 10, 11–12, 43, 44, 70, 105, 107, 118, 120,
    147, 171, 187–188, 204, 232, 254, 310
Irritable bowel syndrome (IBS), 56, 105, 141,
    157, 211–214
Isothiocyanates, 65
Isovaleric acid, 45
Itchiness, 81, 82, 137, 139

Jala neti, 179
Jet lag, 214–217
Jock itch, 160
Joint disease, degenerative. *See* Arthritis, osteo-.
Joints, 22–23, 26
Juices, 246
    carrot-cabbage, 204, 251
    cranberry, 113
    fruit, 166
    green, 63, 69
    pineapple, 51, 54, 110
    red, 63
    vegetable, 23, 28, 46, 102, 144, 147, 164,
        166, 167, 171, 173, 246, 281
Juicing, 63, 91
Juniper, 79, 174

Kava, 18, 46, 91, 106, 139, 185, 194, 207, 215,
    227, 233, 258, 281
Kegel exercises, 190

Kelp, 247

Keratin, 43

Kidney stones, 218–220

Kidneys, 112, 192, 219, 220

Kinesiology, 30, 209

Lactase, 128, 156, 169, 170

Lactobacillus plantarum, 107

Lactobacillus salivarius, 41

Lactoferrin, 156, 171

Lactose, 156

Lactose intolerance, 6, 7, 9, 39, 127, 128, 149, 156–157, 169, 170

L-alanine, 262

Laughter, 224

Lauric acid, 291

Lavender, 227

Lavender spike, 30

Laxatives, 56, 105, 106

Lazarev, N. V., 92

Lead, 90

Leaky gut, 73, 153, 263

Lecithin, 165

Ledum, 29

Leeks, 65

Legs, elevation of, 255, 289

Legumes, 84, 125, 150

Lemon balm, 18, 20, 44, 58, 95, 119, 132, 171, 194, 207, 213, 223, 281, 291

Lemonade, 234

Leptin, 247

L-glycine, 262

Libido, 227, 280

Licorice, 32, 44, 68, 91, 92, 95, 107, 108, 132, 167, 204, 223, 247, 252, 281, 287, 291

Life, control of, 14

Lifting, 189

Limbic system, 121

Linseeds, 105, 107, 132, 165, 190, 198, 203, 222

Lipoprotein(a) levels, 87

Lipoproteins, 87

Lithium, 285

Liver, 68, 71, 88, 125, 165, 167, 228, 237, 238, 258, 263

Liver (food), 11

Logic, 20

Losses, traumatic, 14, 17

L-tryptophan, 120

Lunch, 246

Lungs, 35, 109, 110, 111

Lupus erythematosus, 43

Lutein, 77, 185

Lycopene, 65, 77, 185, 199, 261

Lymphatic system, 79, 98, 166, 274

Lysine, 94, 95, 200

Maca, 145

Magnesium, 18, 34, 37, 46, 88, 91, 106, 110, 120, 125, 131, 142, 165, 181, 182, 183, 184, 185, 194, 199, 204, 208, 212, 219, 219, 241, 242, 254, 258, 281, 311

Magnolia, 18, 58, 194, 281

Maimonides, Moses, 31, 98

Malassezia furfur. See *Pityrosporum ovale.*

Malic acid, 162

Manganese, 29, 182, 241, 311

Margarines, 87, 125

Marijuana, 70–71, 196, 235

Marshmallow, 110, 204, 219, 252

Massages, 19, 34, 70, 79, 145, 181, 259, 289

    gum, 176

    scalp, 44, 181–182

Masters and Johnson, 143, 144

Mattresses, 34

Meadowstreet, 58, 129, 171, 252, 255

Meals, 18, 69, 84, 105, 119, 124, 147, 166, 182, 207, 215, 222, 235, 236, 237, 245, 246–247, 251, 256, 258, 267, 281

Meat, 11, 62, 86, 125, 141, 219, 251, 261, 263

Medications, 39, 43, 266

    antiacid, 10, 230

    antiemetic, 70, 235

    prescription, 5, 196, 222, 244

    sleep, 209

    topical, 304–305

Medicine

    evidence-based, 1

    herbal, 4, 8, 12, 18, 24, 32, 68, 110, 301–306

    natural, 3, 8, 63, 67, 99, 203

Traditional Chinese, 13, 142
Meditation, 47, 66, 71, 73, 93, 139, 147, 195,
    216, 221, 228, 248, 282
Melatonin, 120, 121, 208, 215, 216
Memory, 70, 221–225, 280
Men, 36, 42, 218, 254–255
    infertility and, 197, 199
Menopause, 113, 225, 225–229, 240
Menstruation, 10, 141, 184, 227, 229
Metabolic ash, 64, 316
Metabolic rate, 248
Metabolism, 284
Metals, heavy, 91, 93, 240, 241, 261
Metastatis, 60
Methionine, 24
Microbiome, 39, 137, 169, 203
Microflora, 39, 48, 58, 70, 73–75, 104–105,
    127, 129, 137, 148, 149, 169, 202, 203,
    211, 230, 264
Migraines, 185–186, 238
Mind, 18–19
Minerals, malabsorption of, 240
Miscarriages, 199, 236, 256
Mites
    dust, 34, 274, 275
    hair follicle, 269, 270
Molds, 34
Monoamine oxidase inhibitors (MAOIs), 119
Mononucleosis. *See* Glandular fever.
Morning sickness, 236, 256
Motion sickness, 236–237
Mouth taping, 322
Mouth ulcers. *See* Ulcers, mouth.
MS. *See* Multiple sclerosis (MS).
MSG, 158, 183
Mucopolysaccharides, 23, 28, 204, 251
Mucus, 31, 32, 38, 51, 98, 109, 110, 178, 179,
    238, 271
Muira puama, 145
Mullein, 32, 110
Multiple sclerosis (MS), 27, 231–233
Mumps, 196
Muscles, 107, 111, 243, 248, 280
    abdominal, 105, 107, 132
    neck and shoulders, 181

smooth, 37, 38, 105, 107, 142, 182, 213, 219,
    266, 275, 319
Mushrooms, 65
Music, 224
Myelin sheath, 231
Myringotomy, 135
Myrrh, 41, 167, 176

Nails, 10, 160, 161
Naps, 209
Nasal polyps, 271–272
Nasturtiums, 98
Nattokinase, 216
Nausea, 70, 234–239
Nervous system, 144, 227, 233, 276
    parasympathetic (PNS), 85, 107, 111, 194,
        209, 213, 224, 282, 320
    sympathetic (SNS), 276, 320
Neti pots, 40, 41, 179, 184, 272
Nettles, 8, 12, 44, 46, 49, 79, 84, 138, 174, 262
Neurotransmitters, 118
Niacin. *See* Vitamin B3.
Nightingale, Florence, 121
Nitrates, 182
Nitric oxide (NO), 37, 38, 273, 320
Nonspecific urethritis (NSU), 112
Notes on Nursing (Nightingale), 121
NSAIDs, 23, 250
Nuts, 65, 131
Nux vomica, 235

Oats, 82, 91, 95, 114, 119, 139, 147, 170, 194,
    281
Obesity. *See* Weight, high.
Objects, beautiful, 121
Oil infusions, 306
Oils, 106, 116, 135, 246
    apricot kernel, 116, 323
    arnica, 323
    avocado, 323
    borage, 324
    calendula, 162, 324
    carrot, 324
    castor, 190
    cedarwood, 44

chamomile, 20

clove, 161

coconut, 86, 161, 291

cod liver, 52, 99, 102, 110, 135, 264

eucalyptus, 100, 161

evening primrose, 8, 116, 138, 178–179, 184, 227, 232, 258, 264, 324

fish, 24, 28, 88, 116, 138, 173, 194, 204, 223, 232, 247, 254, 255

garlic, 135

grapeseed, 323

jojoba, 324

juniper, 174

krill, 88

lavender, 31, 44, 82, 116, 138, 139, 161, 181, 182, 264, 282

macadamia, 323

neem tree, 44

olive, 86, 116

peppermint, 213, 228

pine scotch, 47

rosehip, 324

rosemary, 116, 181

sandalwood, 116

sesame, 323

sunflower, 323

sweet almond, 116, 323

tea tree, 8, 34, 49, 75, 82, 116, 132, 138, 139, 161, 270, 275, 291

thyme, 44, 161

wheat germ, 324

See also Essential Oils.

Oligomeric proanthocyanidin complexes (OPCs), 28, 232, 289, 312

Olive leaf, 68, 98, 161, 167, 176, 194

Omega-3 fatty acids, 198, 203, 222, 253, 254, 263

Onions, 32, 65, 84, 102, 110, 113, 125, 134, 178, 272

syrup, 52, 110

Onychomycosis, 160

Orange (color), 145

Oranges, 22, 23, 28, 248

Oregano, 161

Oregon grape, 264

Orgasms, female, 200

Osteoarthritis (OA). *See* Arthritis, osteo- .

Osteopenia, 240, 241

Osteoporosis, 14, 225, 240–242

Ovaries, 225

Overweight. *See* Weight, high.

Ovulation, 197, 200

Oxalates, 218

Oxalic acid, 11

Oxygen, 11, 33, 198, 215, 319–320

Oxygen radical absorbance capacity (ORAC), 199

Oysters, 144

Paeonia, 142, 258

Panic attacks, 17

Parsley, 174

Passionflower, 18, 20, 44, 46, 58, 91, 106, 139, 182, 185, 194, 207, 215, 227, 233, 258, 281

Pau d'arco, 75

PCOS. *See* Polycystic ovarian syndrome (PCOS).

Pectin, 87, 165

Peony, 44, 199

Pepper, 110

Peppermint, 58, 129, 132, 164, 165, 171, 204, 213, 236, 237, 255, 266

Pepsin, 250

Peptic ulcers. *See* Ulcers, peptic.

Perimenopause, 225, 226, 227

Peristalsis, 105, 106, 212

Perniosis. *See* Chilblains.

Personalities, 295

Pets, 162

pH, 47, 58, 63–64, 74, 197, 257, 316

Phlebotomy. *See* Venesection.

Phytates, 11

Phytic acid, 11

Phytoestrogens, 65, 227, 241

Pilates, 34

Piles. *See* Hemorrhoids.

Pillows, 209

Pimples. *See* Acne.

Pine bark, 54, 190, 269, 289

Pineal gland, 120

Pineapples, 51, 54, 110

Pink eye. *See* Conjunctivitis.

Pityrosporum ovale, 115

Plants, 301–306
  drying, 302
  gathering, 301–302
Plaque, dental, 175
Plastic wrap, 304
PMDD. *See* Premenstrual dysphoric disorder (PMDD).
PMS. *See* Premenstrual syndrome (PMS).
Pneumonia, 51
Podophyllum, 129
Poke root, 49, 91, 167, 275
Pollen, 178
Pollution, 274
Polycosanol, 88
Polycyclic aromatic hydrocarbons (PAHs), 62
Polycystic ovarian syndrome (PCOS), 43, 44, 244, 247
Polyphenols, 175
Postnasal drip (PND), 39
Postpartum thyroiditis, 285
Postural drainage, 111
Posture, 31, 34, 183
  inverted, 44, 100, 116–117, 289
Potassium, 29, 46, 56, 193, 194
Poultices, 304–305
Prebiotics, 106, 170–171, 203, 212
Pregnancy, 4, 29, 43, 113, 164, 175, 189, 197, 199, 236, 253–256, 266, 288
Premenstrual dysphoric disorder (PMDD), 257
Premenstrual syndrome (PMS), 257–260
Prickly ash, 44, 84, 176
Pritikin, Nathan, 36, 248
Proanthocyanins, 269
Probiotics, 41, 58, 68, 69–70, 75, 106, 107, 113, 116, 128, 129, 138, 150, 151, 155, 156, 158, 161, 171, 203, 204, 212, 213, 234, 235, 251–252, 264, 267
Progesterone, 105, 255, 258
Propionic acid, 45
Propolis, 41, 99, 176, 179, 230, 275
Prostate, 112, 197, 261–262
Protein, 15, 68, 91, 119, 157, 198, 219, 222, 241, 245, 246, 281
  powders, 246
Prunes, 105, 189

Psoriasis, 263–265
Psychoneuroimmunology, 61
Psyllium, 41, 70, 87, 89, 107, 108, 124, 129, 132, 165, 185, 190, 204, 213, 245, 248, 255
Puberty, 46, 116
Pulsatilla, 142, 184, 236, 258
Purging, 56
Purines, 173, 218–219
Pygeum, 262

Qi gong, 92
Quasimodo (character), 240
Quercetin, 32, 35, 52, 54, 68, 77, 84, 87, 110, 173, 178, 183, 190, 255, 269, 312

Radiation, 285
Radiotherapy, 71–73
Raspberry leaf, 129, 142, 199, 255
Ratanhia, 176
Raynaud's syndrome, 83
Red (color), 84
Red clover, 46, 49, 138, 227, 264
Red yeast rice, 88
Reflexology, 289
Reflux, 39, 69, 109, 255, 266–268, 274
Rehmannia, 12, 29, 91, 167, 199, 227, 233, 247, 281, 287
Relationships, 35, 200
Remedies, natural, 3–5, 67, 99, 301–306
  children and, 4
  dosages, 3–4
  interactions with prescription medications, 5
  pregnancy and, 5
  reactions to, 7
Rescue Remedy. *See* Bach flowers, Rescue Remedy.
Resting, 25, 91–92, 97, 100, 166, 167
Resveratrol, 28, 54, 65, 84, 87, 176, 190, 232, 269, 270, 312
Rheumatoid arthritis (RA). *See* Arthritis, rheumatoid.
Rhodiola, 64, 91, 119, 147, 223, 227, 247, 281, 287
Rhubarb, 107
Rice, 128
Rice water, 128

Ringworm, 43, 160
Rome III criteria, 211
Rosacea, 268–271
Rosemary, 64, 221, 223
Ross River fever, 91
Royal jelly, 120, 147
Ruta, 54
Rutin, 54, 84, 189, 190, 255, 269, 288

Saccharomyces boulardii, 129
S-adenosylmethionine. *See* SAM-e (S-adenosyl-
    methionine).
Saffron, 110
Sage, 129, 176, 223, 227
Salads, 84, 129
Salicylates, 158
Salicylic acid, 291
Saliva, 40, 41, 175, 176
Salt, 32, 37, 38, 79, 178, 179, 184, 193, 219, 241,
    254, 258, 272, 284
    Dead Sea, 264
SAM-e (S-adenosylmethionine), 24, 120
Sanitary pads, 114
Santich, Rob, 4
Sarsaparilla, 8, 138, 264
Sauerkraut, 250
Saw palmetto, 8, 145, 199, 262
Scarves, 100
Schizandra, 64, 92, 223, 247, 281
Scurvy, 54, 175, 176
Seafood, 188, 253
Seasonal affective disorder (SAD), 120
Seawater, 8, 84, 116, 264
Seaweed, 65, 71
Sebum, 6, 8, 43
Selenium, 29, 64, 65, 77, 116, 198, 254, 262,
    264, 286, 312
Self-talk, negative, 120–121
Selye, Hans, 277
Semen, 261
Senna, 106
Sensitivities, dairy. *See* Lactose intolerance.
Sensitivities, food. *See* Allergies, food.
Sensitivities, gluten. *See* Gluten intolerance.
Sepia, 236

Septic loci, 27, 29
Serotonin, 15, 56, 58, 118, 120, 211, 280
Sexual intercourse, 113, 114, 200, 290
Sexual performance anxiety, 144, 145
Sexuality, 14
Shakespeare, William, 144, 221
Shampoos, 116, 264
Shatavari, 142, 199, 219, 227
Shaving, underarm, 47
Shepherd, Sue, 157, 212
Shift work, 206, 209
Shingles, 81, 94–96
Shoes, 25, 47, 84, 216
Shower curtains, 34
Showers, 34
Silicea, 255, 288
Silicon, 241
Silver, colloidal, 49, 162, 176, 270, 275
Silymarin, 199
Sinuses, 39, 178, 184
Sinusitis, 40, 179, 271–273
Sitting, 149, 189, 288
Skin, 6–7, 8, 46, 54, 71, 78–79, 116, 137, 139,
    161, 240, 263, 268–271
    dry, 264
    pH, 47
Skullcap, 20, 44, 106, 155, 182, 207
Sleep, 147, 185, 206–210, 222, 227, 244, 267
    cycles, 207, 208
Sleep apnea, 206
Sleeplessness. *See* Insomnia.
Slippery elm, 41, 58, 69, 129, 131, 132, 171, 190,
    204, 230, 251, 255, 267
Sloths, 22, 25
Smell, 224
S-methylmethionine, 204, 251
Smoking, 27, 37, 38, 40, 41, 44, 45, 61, 66, 77–78,
    80, 84, 111, 126, 144, 145, 175, 196, 200,
    202, 226, 240, 241, 250, 252, 255, 266, 267
Smoothies, 246, 251
Snacks, 247
Snoring, 206, 274
Soaps, 139, 264
Social media, 20
Sodium benzoate, 158

Sodium. *See* Salt.

Solanaceae family (plants), 23, 28

Sorbitol, 77, 212

Sore throat, 274–276

Soups, 31, 32, 98, 166

Soy, 65, 227, 228

Sperm, 196, 197, 199, 200, 253, 254, 256

Sphincters, 107

Sphygmometers, 192

Spina bifida, 253

Spirulina, 46, 147

Sportswear, 47

Sprouts, alfalfa, 44

St. John's wort, 15, 44, 46, 58, 82, 91, 96, 119, 139, 182, 194, 227, 228, 233, 258, 281, 291

St. Mary's thistle, 64, 68, 71, 88, 150, 164, 167, 183, 237, 264

Standing, 189, 255, 288

Statins, 88

Steam inhalation, 52, 111

Steiner, Rudolf, 62

Stomach, 250

Stomach acid. *See* Hydrochloric acid.

Strawberries, 173

Stress and stress management, 6, 27, 32, 34, 37, 38, 39, 43, 44, 61, 66, 72, 74, 86, 88, 90, 92, 94, 95, 104, 113, 116, 118, 126, 127, 129, 137, 139, 142, 145, 149, 151, 181, 194, 199, 200, 202, 204, 206, 211, 213, 221, 223, 226, 229, 230, 232, 233, 238, 241, 247, 248, 251, 252, 263, 264, 266, 267, 270, 274, 276–283, 285, 286–287

stages, 277–278

Strokes, 38, 86, 221, 243

Strontium, 241

Styes, 48, 49

Sugar, 6, 40, 48, 62, 68, 69, 86, 91, 94, 98, 102, 113, 116, 119, 124, 132, 134, 138, 147, 150, 156, 161, 166, 171, 175, 182, 202, 203, 222, 226, 230, 232, 235, 241, 245, 251, 258, 261, 263, 272, 274, 281, 291

Sulfur, 46

Sulphites, 158

Sunlight, 8, 62, 77, 95, 120, 216, 241, 264

Supplements, 3–5

weight loss, 238

Support groups, 58, 66, 171

Suppositories, 190

Surgery

cancer, 68

cataract, 76–77

Sweat, 45, 139

Sweat glands, 46

Sweeteners, artificial, 125, 127, 212, 245

Swimming, 25, 29, 135, 213, 216, 255, 270

Swimming suits, 161

Synovial membranes, 26

Tablets and capsules, 303–304

Tai chi, 29, 92

Tampons, 114, 142

Tape, 291

Taste buds, 150

Taurine, 200

Teas, 11, 40, 51, 98, 102, 222, 241, 302, 303

black, 32, 37, 38, 187, 199, 234, 275

chamomile, 131, 267

dandelion and dandelion root, 68, 164, 258

elder, 82

fenugreek, 184

ginger, 70, 131, 234, 235, 237, 267

green, 37, 38, 65, 175, 187, 199, 232, 247, 262, 270

herbal, 4, 8, 46, 48, 102, 110, 113, 202, 275

horsetail, 44

lemon balm, 131, 267

licorice, 267

lime flowers, 82

meadowsweet, 267

peppermint, 82, 131, 234, 235

senna, 107

thyme, 116

yarrow, 82

Teeth, 56, 58, 131, 175

Tempeh, 261

Temperature, atmospheric, changes in, 31

Terpenes, 305

Testicles, 197, 256

Testosterone, 44, 144, 145, 280

Theanine, 222

Theophylline, 32

Therapy, psychological, 15, 19, 58, 118, 120, 248–249, 270, 282

Thrombus, 38

Thrush, 74, 75, 160, 230, 257

Thuja, 64, 291

Thyme, 32, 75, 84, 110, 161, 176, 230, 724

Thyroid gland, 43, 118, 120, 170, 192, 247, 284–287

    hormones, 285

    testing, 285

Thyroid stimulating hormone (TSH), 285

Tinctures, 303

Tisanes, 303

Tissue salts

    Ant. tart., 111

    Calc. fluor., 190, 255, 267, 288

    Calc. sulph., 49

    Ferrum. phos., 82, 184

    Kali. mur., 82

    Kali. phos., 18, 20, 181

    Kali. sulph., 116

    Mag. phos, 18, 20, 34, 110, 181

    Nat. phos., 24, 174

    Nat. sulph., 259

    Silica, 24, 44, 46, 79, 174, 313

Toes, 160, 162, 172

Tofu, 261

Toilet paper, 190

Toilets, 107, 190

Tomatoes, 22, 23, 28, 65, 199, 261

Tongue scrapers, 41

Tonsillitis, 274

Toothbrushes, 176, 230, 275

Toothpastes, 176

Tophi, 172

Toxins, environmental, 62, 90, 91, 93, 200, 261, 285

Transit time, bowel, 6, 7, 39, 63, 70, 104, 149

Traumas, 17, 30

Treatise of Asthma, A (Maimonides), 31

Tribulus, 88, 119, 145, 199, 227

Trichophyton rubrum, 160

Tryptophan, 207

Tulsi, 91, 223, 281

Tumors, 60

Turmeric, 23, 24, 28, 29, 37, 38, 64, 65, 71, 75, 84, 142, 156, 164, 171, 173, 174, 183, 188, 199, 232, 237

Tyramine, 119, 183

Tyrosine, 247

Ulcers

    duodenal, 250

    gastric, 250

    mouth, 70, 229–231

    peptic, 238, 250–252

    triple therapy for, 250, 251, 267

Underpants, 114, 256

Urethra, 112, 113

Uric acid, 172, 173

Urinary tract infections (UTIs). *See* Cystitis.

Urination, 114, 261, 262

Urine, 114, 121

Uvaursi, 219

Vaccinations, 81

Vagina, 227

Vagus nerve, 150, 155

Valerian, 18, 33, 46, 91, 106, 182, 185, 194, 207, 213, 215, 227, 281

Valvular incompetence, 288

Varicocele, 197

Vasoactive amines, 182–183

Vegetables, 64, 77, 91, 157, 164, 198–199, 246, 253

    Brassicas (cruciferous), 65, 87, 142, 151, 286

Veins, 189, 197, 288

    varicose, 255, 288–290

Venesection, 187–188

Verbena, 119, 227

Vertebrae, 149, 151, 183

Vervain, 182, 194, 207, 233, 281

Vicks VapoRub, 100, 111, 272

Villi, 168, 169

Vinegar

    apple cider, 24, 49, 82, 95, 116, 151, 162, 174, 269

    white, 75, 135

Viruses, 61, 91, 97–101, 202
    Epstein-Barr, 91, 166, 232
    herpes, 91, 94–96, 200
    spread of, 100
    varicella-zoster, 81
Visualization, 66, 139
Vitamin A, 8, 33, 64, 82, 99, 102, 110, 114, 116, 139, 171, 198, 204, 252, 264, 267, 286, 287, 313
Vitamin B-complex, 44, 70, 91, 94, 119, 125, 145, 147, 173, 182, 183, 207, 230, 233, 247, 258, 262, 281, 287
Vitamin B3, 37, 88, 120, 314
Vitamin B5, 120, 147
Vitamin B6, 8, 79, 120, 142, 184, 213, 219, 224, 236, 258, 259, 307
Vitamin B9, 28, 29, 70, 173, 232, 253, 255, 264, 310
Vitamin B12, 54, 147, 232, 264, 314
Vitamin C, 3, 11, 13, 29, 32, 41, 49, 54, 64, 68, 70, 77, 82, 84, 87, 91, 95, 98, 99, 102, 110, 114, 125, 128, 135, 139, 161, 167, 173, 174, 175, 176, 178, 184, 185, 187, 188, 189, 190, 198, 199, 219–220, 230, 254, 269, 272, 275, 288, 291, 307
Vitamin D, 29, 33, 64, 99, 110, 125, 139, 232, 241, 254, 264, 314
Vitamin E, 29, 64, 77, 82, 84, 87, 95, 125, 142, 145, 162, 198, 200, 216, 227, 258, 315
Vitamin K, 54, 241, 315
Vitamins, multi- , 15, 24, 58, 142, 184, 198, 204, 254, 255, 258
Vitex agnus-castus, 44, 79, 142, 184, 185, 227, 258
Voice, overuse of, 274, 275
Vomiting, 234–239
    See also Bulimia.

Waist, measurement of, 243
Walking, 108, 244
Warts, 290–291
    common, 290
    genital, 290
    plantar, 290, 291
    subungual/perungual, 290

Water
    bottled, 129
    drinking of. *See* Fluids, drinking of.
Wax treatments, 24–25, 29
Weight
    high, 22, 25, 37, 38, 60, 86, 88, 124, 142, 144, 163, 165, 174, 184, 189, 195, 197, 243–249, 256, 266, 267, 288
    low, 83
    See also Anorexia nervosa; Body fat.
Wheat, 22, 23, 28, 155, 178
Wheatgrass, 46, 147
Wild yam, 142, 227
Willow bark, 24, 29, 174
Wine, 124, 199, 215, 216, 246, 253
Witch hazel, 82, 190, 289
Withania, 12, 18, 20, 64, 68, 70, 71, 91, 139, 145, 167, 199, 223, 227, 247, 281, 286, 287
Women, 90–91, 105, 112, 170, 226, 231, 244, 255–256, 257–260
    hormones and, 225–229, 257–260
    images of, 16
    infertility and, 197, 199
    red-haired, 141
    skin of, 79
World Health Organization, 128
Wormwood, 150

Xanthines, 32, 258
Xylitol, 175–176

Yeasts, 73, 150, 151, 161, 263
Yellow dock, 8, 12, 71, 107
Yoga, 19, 34, 92–93, 228, 262, 289
Yogurt, 57, 113, 129, 157, 245, 251

Zeaxanthin, 77, 185
Zinc, 8, 11, 12, 15, 28, 29, 41, 49, 64, 68, 70, 82, 87, 91, 94, 99, 110, 114, 116, 119, 125, 135, 139, 144, 145, 156, 161, 167, 171, 176, 182, 183, 188, 198, 199, 204, 230, 232, 241, 252, 254, 255, 258, 261, 262, 264, 267, 275, 286, 291, 315
Zizyphus, 18, 20, 46, 58, 91, 139, 194, 227, 232, 281

ABOUT THE AUTHOR

Mim Beim has been practicing natural medicine for nearly twenty-five years. She has written eight health and cookbooks, including *Grow Your Own Medicine,* published in 2011 by ABC Books. She currently writes a naturopathy column for *The Sunday Telegraph's* "Body+Soul," and for their website bodyandsoul.com.au. Over the years Mim has had regular columns with the *Sun Herald, Good Medicine,* and *Family Circle.* Mim currently lectures at the Australasian College of Natural Therapies in Sydney and is recent past head of naturopathy at the Australian Traditional Medicine Society. She also sees patients in her Bowral clinic in the Southern Highlands. In the 1990s Mim was the Triple J naturopath, and afterward gave advice on Tony Delroy's *Nightlife.* Mim starred in the *LifeForce* TV series on Foxtel. She has been a consultant to Liptons, Nokia, and Big Brother. In the last five years she has created a range of therapeutic (and delicious) herbal teas called Beaming with Health (www.beamingwithhealth .com.au/). Mim lives in Kangaroo Valley with her husband, two dogs, and two cats.